Domains	Definitions	Classes
Health Promotion	The awareness of well-being or normality of function and the strategies used to maintain control of and enhance that well-being or normality of function	**Health Awareness** Recognition of normal function and well-being **Health Management** Identifying, controlling, performing, and integrating activities to maintain health and well-being
Nutrition	The activities of taking in, assimilating, and using nutrients for the purposes of tissue maintenance, tissue repair, and the production of energy	**Ingestion** Taking food or nutrients into the body **Digestion** The physical and chemical activities that convert foodstuffs into substances suitable for absorption and assimilation **Absorption** The act of taking up nutrients through body tissues **Metabolism** The chemical and physical processes occurring in living organisms and cells for the development and use of protoplasm and the production of waste and energy, with the release of energy for all vital processes **Hydration** The taking in and absorption of fluids and electrolytes
Elimination and Exchange	Secretion and excretion of waste products from the body	**Urinary System** The process of secretion, reabsorption, and excretion of urine **Gastrointestinal System** Excretion and expulsion of the end products of digestion **Integumentary System** Process of secretion and excretion through the skin **Respiratory System** The process of exchange of gases and removal of the end products of metabolism
Activity/ Rest	The production, conservation, expenditure, or balance of energy resources	**Sleep/Rest** Slumber, repose, ease, relaxation, or inactivity **Activity/Exercise** Moving parts of the body (mobility), doing work, or performing actions often (but not always) against resistance **Energy Balance** A dynamic state of harmony between intake and expenditure of resources **Cardiovascular/Pulmonary Responses** Cardiopulmonary mechanisms that support activity and rest **Self-Care** Ability to perform activities to care for one's body and bodily functions
Perception/ Cognition	The human information processing system including attention, orientation, sensation, perception, cognition, and communication	**Attention** Mental readiness to notice or observe **Orientation** Awareness of time, place, and person **Sensation/Perception** Receiving information through the senses of touch, taste, smell, vision, hearing, and kinesthesia and the comprehension of sense data resulting in naming, associating, or pattern recognition **Cognition** Use of memory, learning, thinking, problem solving, abstraction, judgment, insight, intellectual capacity, calculation, and language **Communication** Sending and receiving verbal and nonverbal information
Self-Perception	Awareness about the self	**Self-Concept** The perception(s) about the total self **Self-Esteem** Assessment of one's own worth, capability, significance, and success **Body Image** A mental image of one's own body
Roles/ Relation-ships	The positive and negative connections or associations among persons or groups of persons and the means by which those connections are demonstrated	**Caregiving Roles** Socially expected behavior patterns by persons providing care who are not healthcare professionals **Family Relationships** Associations of people who are biologically related or related by choice **Role Performance** Quality of functioning in socially expected behavior patterns

Using NANDA International Taxonomy II (*continued*)

Domains	Definitions	Classes
Sexuality	Sexual identity, sexual function, and reproduction	***Sexual Identity*** The state of being a specific person in regard to sexuality, gender, or both ***Sexual Function*** The capacity or ability to participate in sexual activities ***Reproduction*** Any process by which human beings are produced
Coping/Stress Tolerance	Contending with life events and life processes	***Post-Trauma Responses*** Reactions occurring after physical or psychological trauma ***Coping Responses*** The process of managing environmental stress ***Neurobehavioral Stress*** Behavioral responses reflecting nerve and brain function
Life Principles	Principles underlying conduct, thought, and behavior about acts, customs, or institutions viewed as being true or having intrinsic worth	***Values*** The identification and ranking of preferred modes of conduct or end states ***Beliefs*** Opinions, expectations, or judgments about acts, customs, or institutions viewed as being true or having intrinsic worth ***Value/Belief/Action Congruence*** The correspondence or balance achieved between values, beliefs, and actions
Safety/ Protection	Freedom from danger, physical injury or immune system damage; preservation from loss; and protection of safety and security	***Infection*** Host responses after pathogenic invasion ***Physical Injury*** Bodily harm or hurt ***Violence*** The exertion of excessive force or power so as to cause injury or abuse ***Environmental Hazards*** Sources of danger in the surroundings ***Defensive Processes*** The processes by which the self protects itself from the nonself ***Thermoregulation*** The physiologic process of regulating heat and energy within the body for the purposes of protecting the organism
Comfort	Sense of mental, physical, or social well-being or ease	***Physical Comfort*** Sense of well-being or ease or freedom from pain ***Environmental Comfort*** Sense of well-being or ease in or with one's environment ***Social Comfort*** Sense of well-being or ease with one's social situations
Growth/ Development	Age-appropriate increases in physical dimensions, maturation of organ systems, or progression through the developmental milestones	***Growth*** Increases in physical dimensions or maturity of organ systems ***Development*** Progression or regression through a sequence of recognized milestones in life

Source: Adapted from NANDA International (2009). *NANDA International nursing diagnoses: Definitions and classification 2009–2011.* Oxford: Wiley-Blackwell, pp. 370–380.

FIFTH EDITION

Nursing Process & Critical Thinking

Judith M. Wilkinson, PhD, ARNP

Pearson

Boston   Columbus   Indianapolis   New York   San Francisco   Upper Saddle River   Amsterdam
Cape Town   Dubai   London   Madrid   Milan   Munich   Paris   Montreal   Toronto
Delhi   Mexico City   Sao Paulo   Sydney   Hong Kong   Seoul   Singapore   Taipei   Tokyo

Library of Congress Cataloging-in-Publication Data
Wilkinson, Judith M. (date)
    Nursing process and critical thinking /
Judith M. Wilkinson, PhD, ARNP. — Fifth edition.
        p. ; cm.
    Includes bibliographical references and index.
    ISBN-13: 978-0-13-218162-4 (alk. paper)
    ISBN-10: 0-13-218162-2 (alk. paper)
    1. Nursing.   2. Critical thinking.   I. Title.
    [DNLM 1. Nursing Process.   2. Decision Making.
    3. Patient Care Planning. WY 100]
    RT41.W57 2012
    610.73—dc22
                                    2010053331

Publisher: Julie Levin Alexander
Executive Assistant: Regina Bruno
Senior Acquisitions Editor: Kelly Trakalo
Development Editor: Lauren Sweeney
Managing Production Editor: Patrick Walsh
Production Liaison: Yagnesh Jani
Manufacturing Manager: Ilene Sanford
Design Director: Maria Gulielmo-Walsh
Director of Marketing: David Gesell
Marketing Specialist: Michael Sirinides
Marketing Assistant: Crystal Gonzalez
Digital Media Product Manager: Travis-Moses Westphal
Media Product Manager: Rachel Collett/Leslie Brado
Composition: PreMediaGlobal, Inc.
Printer/Binder: Edwards Brothers
Cover Design: Jayne Conte
Cover Image: © Huntstock

Pearson® is a registered trademark of Pearson plc

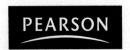

www.pearsonhighered.com

10 9 8 7 6 5 4 3 2 1
ISBN: 0-13-218162-2
ISBN-13: 978-0-13-218162-4

Contents

1

Overview of Nursing Process

2
Critical Thinking 29

3

Assessment   65

4
Diagnostic Reasoning   117

5
Diagnostic Language   157

6
Planning: Overview and Outcomes   197

7
Planning: Interventions   237

8
Implementation 267

9
Evaluation

10
Creating a Care of Plan
339

Preface

Students find this text easy, even enjoyable to use. Nevertheless, it is a serious text, with in-depth treatment of concepts. Because nurses need conceptual understanding of nursing process as well as the practical ability to plan and implement nursing care, this text balances conceptual and practical aspects. For example, Chapter 4 describes a diagnostic process, and Chapter 5 explains how to write diagnostic statements; Chapters 6 and 10 contain detailed explanations of how to create working care plans for real patients, while Chapters 6 and 7 discuss concepts related to choosing outcomes and interventions. There are also several new features in this edition:

- Updated NANDA terminology to latest guidelines
- New addition of Student Resources website. Website contains additional content, critical thinking questions and answers, and NCLEX questions and answers.
- New Take-Away Points that are incorporated throughout the book and summarize key points
- New What Do You Know—questions that are throughout the text to help students stop and think about what they have read and learned.
- New Think & Reflect—this feature gives students questions to reflect on and discuss in class

Content

The nursing process provides a basic framework within which nurses apply the unique combination of knowledge, skills, and caring that constitute the art and science of nursing. The purpose of this book is to promote professional practice through effective use of the nursing process. To that end, the text integrates the following topics into the discussion of each nursing process step:

- **Collaborative Practice and Delegation.** The text acknowledges the changing face of nursing and healthcare by emphasizing collaborative practice and expanding discussion of work delegation by nurses. Case management and critical pathways are treated extensively, as well.
- **Critical Thinking.** Critical thinking is important for nurses—perhaps in different degrees and for different uses, but at all levels of practice. The nursing process provides an excellent vehicle for encouraging critical thinking. Chapter 2 presents concepts of critical thinking as it relates to nursing, and subsequent chapters integrate critical thinking into assessment, diagnosis, planning, implementation, and evaluation. In addition, the "Nursing Process Practice" exercises are designed to foster

critical thinking while learning nursing process. Each chapter includes a special "Critical Thinking Practice" exercise, designed to teach a specific critical-thinking skill. These are excellent for class discussion or small-group projects. The "Case Study" at the end of each chapter provides opportunity for students to use *both* critical thinking and the nursing process to practice clinical decision making safely in simulated situations.

- **Standardized Nursing Language.**   Standardized vocabulary for problems, outcomes, and interventions is introduced and integrated throughout each chapter to help students prepare to use computerized information systems. The text includes discussions and illustrations of NANDA International, NIC, NOC, the Omaha System, and the Clinical Care Classification system for home health.

- **Culture and Spirituality.**   To reflect our multicultural society and promote holistic care, cultural and spiritual dimensions of each step of the nursing process are explored. For example, Chapter 3, "Assessment," includes tools for both cultural and spiritual assessment.

- **Ethical and Legal Issues.**   To increase awareness of ethical issues embedded in the practice of nursing, each chapter includes ethical and/or legal principles and considerations pertinent to that particular nursing process phase (e.g., maintaining confidentiality of client data in the assessment phase).

- **Home, Family, and Community Care.**   Examples and discussions are greatly expanded in this edition, reflecting the expanding role of nursing in homes and other community settings.

- **Nursing Frameworks/Theories.**   Nursing models are integrated into the explanation of each nursing process phase in order to encourage theory-based practice. For example, assessment tools and nursing diagnoses are categorized according to different frameworks. In order to maintain flexibility, no one model was chosen. Instead, several nursing frameworks are summarized and used. For some courses, teachers may choose not to use the nursing theories; for others, a particular framework could be chosen and emphasized.

- **Professional Standards of Care.**   Nurses are more than just the means to organizational ends. Even in a bottom-line, outcomes-driven environment, nurses are accountable for the quality of the care they give: for what they know and what they do. To this end, the ANA Standards of Practice are linked to each phase of the nursing process. These standards enable nurses to evaluate their own behaviors—not merely the patient outcomes they help produce.

- **Wellness Concepts.**   Wellness language and examples are interspersed throughout the text in order to promote awareness of health promotion as a vital part of nursing practice. Most chapters include a section in which wellness concepts are related to the chapter material; the end-of-chapter exercises also include wellness examples.

Teaching/Learning Features

I have used these chapters as learning units to teach nursing process to students of various levels, as well as in continuing education for practicing nurses. Student response has been overwhelmingly positive.

- **Interactive Format.**   Neither nursing process nor critical thinking can be mastered by memorizing facts and principles. Students need to practice applying the concepts; they need to "work problems," just as they do in a math class. This text provides many practice problems. The exercises are not just "recall and fill in the blanks." They are application exercises, designed to promote high-level thinking skills. In addition to the "What Do You Know?" and "Think & Reflect!" questions interspersed within each chapter, "Take-away points" are also integrated to help students summarize and recall what they have just read.

- **Learning Aids.**   Each chapter begins with Learning Outcomes and a figure that serves as a visual guide to chapter content. Each chapter ends with a summary of chapter content.

- **Case Studies.**   In addition to the features "What Do You Know?" and "Think & Reflect!" each chapter also contains a case study ("Critical Thinking and Clinical Reasoning: A Case Study") to help students apply critical thinking and nursing process to real-life situations, using the concepts and principles they have learned in the chapter. These cases focus on critical thinking and nursing process. They are *not* intended to teach in-depth content about medical conditions and pathophysiology. Even beginning students can use the case studies.

- **Student Resources.**   Students have access to interactive exercises entitles "What Do You Know About [insert chapter title]" and "Critical Thinking Practice." The "What Do You Know" questions assist with recall and comprehension of chapter content, and allow students to use critical thinking within the framework of the nursing process. The "Critical Thinking Practice" teaches a different specific critical thinking skill (e.g., making inferences) in each chapter. Approximately 15 NCLEX-style questions are also included—again, to help students recall and apply chapter content and practice taking NCLEX-style tests.

- **Detailed Answer Keys.**   For questions in the book and on the Student Resources site, the answer keys provide the rationale for both correct and incorrect answers and frequently demonstrate the thinking process used to arrive at the answers. This detailed feedback provides for truly interactive learning, as well as the kind of student-instructor dialogue that is so important for learning nursing process. Students are easily frustrated by the many ambiguities and seeming contradictions that arise when applying abstract nursing process concepts to concrete specific situations. The answer key discussions are vital for easing this frustration and modeling the thinking inherent in the process. Because answers can vary widely, the answer keys for critical thinking questions and case studies provide suggested, not comprehensive, responses.

- **Versatility.**   This text is suitable for nursing students as an introduction to nursing process, or for use in the continuing education of professionals who may need refresher information and practice. It is effective for students who have had nursing process early in the curriculum and who later have difficulty applying it in a clinical course—simply assign a chapter and exercises to remediate the difficulty. The text is organized to accommodate the instructor's professional judgment—that is, it can be used in whole or in part, and for students of different levels, depending on what the instructor chooses to assign or emphasize. For example, for instructors who believe the concept of "possible problems" is too difficult for beginning students, that portion of Chapter 4 could be omitted without damaging the continuity of the material. Some teachers may choose to present Chapter 5 before Chapter 4. Some use Chapter 10 as a sort of road map, presenting it after Chapter 2; others prefer to use it at the end of the course, after all the phases of the nursing process have been taught. All approaches are workable.

- **Independent Study.**   This text can be used for independent study and for distance learning, but it is in no way limited to that approach. It can be used as a text to supplement lectures, either in a separate course or when the nursing process is integrated in the curriculum.

- **Care Plans—or not.**   This text makes clear that nursing process and a written plan of care are *not* one and the same. For teachers who question the exclusive use of written care plans as a teaching strategy, this text will be helpful. I have found that the time I previously allotted to lecture can be used to discuss student questions about nursing process and patient care. Even more exciting, I assign fewer traditional care plans, and I need to make fewer comments on the plans they do write. I also spend less time in remedial conferences helping students with nursing process. If you use care maps instead of columnar care plans, students still need to learn the nursing process. The *process* is the same, regardless of whether they record the plan in columns or as a care map. To assist with care mapping, the text provides a section on care mapping in Chapter 10.

- **Terminology.**   I use both *client* and *patient* in this book. Either can be appropriate, depending on the context. *Client* implies that nurses have independent functions, are increasingly accountable to individuals rather than institutions, and are not setting-bound; it also stresses that people are increasingly active in managing their own healthcare. However, most nursing still does occur in hospitals, and with ill people who are in a dependent state. Furthermore, most nurses are paid by an employing health agency rather than directly by a client. In these situations, the term *patient* seems more accurate.

   I use a similar approach for denoting gender. I acknowledge and welcome the presence of men in nursing and, further, realize that patients are both men and women. However, terms like *s/he* and *she/he* are artificial and awkward to read, so I do not use them. Both nurses and patients are arbitrarily assigned gender and referred to either as *he* or *she*.

   In this text I often speak to the reader directly as "you" instead of "the nurse" or "the student." For one thing, this suits my informal nature. But more importantly, I hope this will empower and engage the reader personally, promoting active involvement with the text.

Reviewers

I am grateful to the following for their comments and suggestions provided in their review of this manuscript:

Rose Marie Caballero, MSN, RN, CCM
Assistant Professor
Del Mar College – West Campus
Corpus Christi, TX

Laura B. Hammond, BSN, MN, RN
Nursing Instructor
Seattle Central Community College
Seattle, WA

Kathleen Hopkins, MA, RN
Nursing Faculty
Rockland Community College
Suffern, NY

Faith L. Johnson, BA, BSN, MA, RN, CNE
Nursing Faculty
Ridgewater College
Wilmar, MN

GN Niere, RN, BSN, MSN
Faculty Member
College of Central Florida
Ocala, FL

Eric J. Williams, RN, BSN, MSN, DNP
Professor of Nursing
Santa Monica College
Los Angeles, CA

Students: Getting the Most from Your Reading

The following suggestions should help you make best use of this text. Because people learn in different ways, you should adapt them to fit your particular learning style.

1. **Read the chapter objectives first**. These give you a blueprint of the chapter and direct your reading.
2. **Key terms** are in bold print in the chapter text. Be sure you can recognize and define these terms.
3. **Read the chapter content.**
   A. Pay attention to headings and subheadings. Because they give you a concept label for the paragraphs that follow them, they can focus your thinking and help you to remember what you have read.
   B. Also pay attention to the Take-Away Points. They summarize key points for you. You can also use them later to help you review the material.
   C. Make notes in the margins. Writing reinforces your learning.
   D. As you read, stop and answer the questions for What Do You Know? and Think & Reflect! Doing so will help you remember what you have read. Be sure you understand the rationale provided in the answer keys, and refer to the chapter text as you need to.
4. **Work through the case study at the end of each chapter.** The case studies provide practice in applying critical thinking and nursing process together. They are a safe way for you to practice making clinical judgments before you actually need to do so in a clinical setting.
5. **Take advantage of the materials in the online Student Resources.** In order to learn the nursing process, you must apply it, not simply memorize what you read about it. As a nurse, you will be applying the nursing process, not simply recalling facts about it, so begin learning to do that now. Work the exercises before you look at the answer keys. Write your answers, make notes, and discuss these with your instructor and/or your classmates to be sure you are on the right track. Discuss your thinking processes—*how* you arrived at your answers. The "suggested responses" to critical thinking exercises focus on correct use of the *thinking skill*, not on the *correct answer*. Critical thinking skills can be acquired best through discussion with others, either individually or in class.
6. **You will find four types of learning materials on the Student Resources site:**
   - *Figures, tables, and boxes relating to chapter content*—These are not in all chapters
   - *What Do You Know About [Chapter Title]*—A set of recall and application exercises to help you learn and remember the chapter content

- *Critical Thinking Practice*—A set of exercises, each teaching you a specific critical thinking skill (such as making inferences)
- *NCLEX®-Style review questions*—Ten to 20 questions to provide practice in taking NCLEX®-type questions and to help you review chapter content

If you have difficulty with any of the exercises, reread the chapter and try again. If you are still having trouble, ask your instructor to suggest additional exercises, audiovisual materials, or further readings.

Overview of Nursing Process

Introduction

Because nursing process texts (and teachers) talk about *concepts*, *ideas*, and *processes*, students sometimes wonder what all this has to do with taking care of patients—with the "real world," as you may hear nurses refer to it. In this book, you will learn that the **nursing process** is a special way of thinking that nurses use. It is also what nurses *do* when giving patient care. In other words, the nursing process is a thinking-doing *approach* that nurses use in their work. Keeping this general idea in mind will help you as you work through the more detailed explanation developed in this chapter. The six phases (processes) of the nursing process are shown in Figure 1–1.

What Is Nursing?

A broad understanding of nursing will help you to understand the nursing process and how it fits into the way you think and practice as a nurse. **Nursing** has the following unique combination of characteristics. It is:

- A blend of art and science
- Applied within the context of interpersonal relationships
- Done for the purpose of promoting wellness, preventing illness, and restoring health
- Used when caring for individuals, families, and communities

The Art of Nursing

Think about the difference between a painting you might make and one you would find hanging in an art gallery. Now apply that to nursing. It should be assumed that you

LEARNING OUTCOMES

After completing this chapter, you should be able to do the following:

- Define *human responses* in the context of nursing.
- Compare and contrast the concerns of nursing and medicine.
- Define *nursing process* in terms of purpose, characteristics, and organization.
- Name and describe the six phases of the nursing process.
- Describe qualities a nurse needs to use the nursing process successfully.
- Explain the importance of the nursing process to patients and nurses.
- Discuss the use of the nursing process in wellness and health promotion.

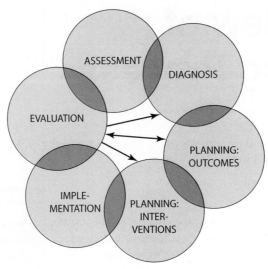

FIGURE 1–1

The interconnected phases of the nursing process

will have the theoretical knowledge and technical skills to provide safe nursing care. However, *nursing art* goes beyond this. It involves sensitivity, creativity, empathy, and the ability to adapt care—either to meet a patient's unique needs or in the face of uncertainty (Finfgeld-Connett, 2008), and it includes the ability to:

1. Develop meaningful connections with clients
2. Grasp the meaning in client encounters.
3. Perform nursing activities skillfully.
4. Use rational thinking to choose appropriate courses of action.
5. Conduct one's nursing practice ethically (Johnson, 1994).

> **Take-away point:** Art is not so much what you know or what you do but more about your *approach* to what you do.

Defining Nursing

Florence Nightingale (1859/1969, p. 133), the first nurse theorist, said that what nurses do "is to put the patient in the best condition for nature to act upon him." This fits with the holistic idea that people have innate abilities for growth and self-healing and that the nurse's role is to nurture and support these abilities. The American Nurses Association (ANA), the professional organization for U.S. nurses, defines nursing this way:

> Nursing is the protection, promotion, and optimization of health and abilities, prevention of illness and injury, alleviation of suffering through the diagnosis and treatment of human response, and advocacy in the care of individuals, families, communities, and populations (ANA, 2004, p. 7).

The ANA *Social Policy Statement* describes six essential features of contemporary nursing practice (2003). Nurses:

1. Do not focus only on problems—they consider a range of human experiences, including health, disease, and illness within the environment.
2. Integrate patients' subjective experience with objective data.
3. Use critical thinking to apply scientific knowledge to diagnosis and treatment processes.
4. Provide a caring relationship that facilitates health and healing.
5. Advance professional nursing knowledge through scholarly inquiry.
6. Influence social and public policy to promote social justice.

Take-away point: Nursing is not limited to problem solving. It also includes patient perspective, critical thinking, caring relationships, lifelong learning, and promotion of social justice.

Nursing Theory

Nursing **theory** offers a way of looking at the discipline in clear, explicit terms that can be communicated to others. Theories help to explain the unique place of nursing in the interdisciplinary team. They are based on the theorist's values and assumptions about health, patients, nursing, and the environment. Each theory describes those concepts and explains how they are related. Think of a theory as a lens through which to view nursing and patients: the color and shape of the lens affect what you see. That is why there are so many definitions of nursing and why your theory of nursing affects your use of the nursing process. To see how several nurse theorists define nursing, see Resources: Table 1–1 at Pearson Nursing Student Resources.

Although definitions and theories vary, most agree that even though nurses care for patients with health problems, nursing is not limited to disease processes and that nursing concerns are different from medical concerns. Overall, nursing theories (models) describe nursing as:

- An art and a science with its own evolving, scientific body of knowledge
- Holistic, or concerned with the client's physical, psychosocial, cultural, and spiritual needs
- Involving caring
- Occurring in a variety of settings
- Concerned with health promotion, disease prevention, and care during illness

Take-away point: Nursing is a unique blend of art and science (knowledge and problem-solving processes) within person-to-person relationships. Its purpose is to promote wellness; prevent illness; and restore health in individuals, families, and communities.

Nurses Treat Human Responses

Nurses view patients holistically, so they are concerned with **human responses**— *reactions* to an event or stressor such as disease or injury. Nurses diagnose, treat, and prevent patient responses to diseases rather than the disease itself. For example, if a patient has diabetes, the nurse would be concerned about the patient's lack of knowledge about diet and possible loss of self-esteem; the primary care provider would prescribe insulin to treat high blood sugar. Reactions (responses) may be biological, psychological, social, and spiritual.

EXAMPLE: Consider the following possible patient responses to a heart attack:

Physical response:	Pain
Psychological response:	Fear
Sociological response:	Returning to work before she is well
Spiritual response:	Praying

An infinite variety of possible human responses occurs at all levels: cells, organs, systems, interpersonal, cultural, and so on. The stressors that cause health problems are often diseases or microorganisms, but they can also be:

- Environmental—e.g., too much exposure to the sun produces a sunburn.
- Interpersonal—e.g., adapting to parenthood causes stress after a baby is born.
- Spiritual—e.g., guilt about falling away from one's religion may lead to depression.

Interdisciplinary Practice

Increasingly, healthcare is delivered by multidisciplinary teams. This is also referred to as **collaborative practice** and **interdisciplinary practice**. This means that nurses, physicians, and other professionals work together to plan and provide patient care (Box 1–1). This does not mean that nurses must become invisible; each discipline retains its identity even as they collaborate.

Although some functions may be shared, nursing is different from medicine. Physicians focus on diagnosis and treatment of disease; nurses focus on giving care during the cure. This is sometimes referred to as *curing versus caring*. Caring in this sense refers to the activities that nurses perform in *taking care of* patients, not the subjective feeling of *caring about* patients. That feeling may, of course, be involved, but it does not

---

BOX 1–1

COLLABORATIVE (MULTIDISCIPLINARY) PRACTICE

Collaboration is a collegial working relationship with another healthcare provider in the provision of (to supply) patient care. Collaborative practice requires (may include) the discussion of patient diagnosis and cooperation in the management and delivery of care (ANA, 1992).

Collaboration among health care professionals involves recognition of the expertise of others within and outside one's profession and referral to those providers when appropriate. Such collaboration also involves some shared functions and a common focus on the same overall mission (ANA, 2003).

TABLE 1-1   Comparison of Nursing and Medicine

Medical Focus	Nursing Focus
1. Diagnose and treat disease. 2. Cure disease. 3. Focus on pathophysiology and biological, physical effects. 4. Teach patients about the treatments for their disease or injury.	1. Diagnose, treat, and prevent human responses. 2. Care for the patient. 3. Take a holistic approach—consider the effects on the whole person (biological, psychosocial, cultural, spiritual). 4. Teach clients self-care strategies to increase independence in daily activities. 5. Promote wellness activities.

necessarily differentiate nursing from medicine. Table 1–1 summarizes the differences between nursing and medicine. If you would like to learn some strategies for improving relationships among health professionals, see Resources: Box 1–1 at Pearson Nursing Student Resources.

> **Take-away point:** In actual practice, all health team members contribute to implement a plan of care.

Nursing in Wellness and Illness

Nursing is concerned with the whole person, ill or well. Nurses support ill people and help them to (a) solve or reduce their health problems and (b) adapt to and accept problems that cannot be treated. They help those who are terminally ill to achieve a peaceful death. For well people, nurses aim to prevent illness and promote wellness. This may involve a variety of activities, such as role modeling a healthy lifestyle; being an advocate for community environmental changes; or teaching self-care strategies, decision making, and problem solving.

> **EXAMPLE:** Cara Wolinski is a nurse in a factory. She promotes health by organizing and supervising a daily exercise class for employees. Cara also provides nutrition counseling for those who request it.

1-1 WHAT DO YOU KNOW?

1. What is meant by describing nursing as an art?
2. True or false? The ANA says that critical thinking is an essential feature of contemporary nursing practice.
3. What are human responses?
4. How is nursing different from medicine?

See answer to #1-1 What Do You Know? in Appendix A.

nursing.pearsonhighered.com

Why Is Nursing Process Important?

There are many reasons for learning and using nursing process. Because the client is the focus of nursing, the most important reasons are the ways the nursing process benefits clients. However, nursing process is good for nurses and the nursing profession as well. The nursing process:

- **Promotes collaboration.** When all team members value a systematic, organized approach, communication improves. Each person feels satisfaction from delivering effective, individualized care, and the work atmosphere becomes more positive.
- **Is cost efficient.** By improving communication, the nursing process prevents errors and expedites diagnosis, treatment, and prevention of patient problems. This means shorter hospital stays and lower costs for healthcare agencies.
- **Helps people understand what nurses do.** Because nursing is complex, it is sometimes difficult for nurses to define their role to others. To be valued by employers and patients, nurses must show that they contribute to better outcomes and decreased costs. A record of nursing assessments and interventions can be used to show how nurses prevent complications and hasten recovery.
- **Is required by professional standards of practice.** Successful use of the nursing process will help you to meet the professional standards of practice, to which nurses are held accountable (e.g., Box 1–2).
- **Increases client participation in care and promotes client autonomy.** Self-care is very important in our cost-driven healthcare environment. Clients are often discharged from the hospital while still in need of care and treatment. Involving clients in each step of the nursing process helps them to realize the importance of their contributions, learn more about their bodies, improve their health decisions, and regain their independence more quickly.
- **Promotes individualized care.** Human responses (e.g., to a disease) are infinitely variable. With a care plan to point out specific, unique needs, nurses can avoid the tendency to categorize and give standardized care based solely on a patient's medical diagnosis.

  EXAMPLE: The standardized care plan for a patient with a hysterectomy includes monitoring for complications and teaching for self-care. Because Carol Wu's care plan also states that she has a hearing problem, the nurses are careful to position themselves so that Ms. Wu can read their lips and understand the discharge teaching.

  Notice that the interventions for Ms. Wu's hearing deficit are not related to her surgical diagnosis (hysterectomy). Because nurses focus on the person instead of her surgical diagnosis, Ms. Wu's needs are successfully met.

- **Promotes efficiency.** Duplication wastes time and can be tiring and irritating for patients. A systematic approach helps you organize and prioritize care and prevents omissions and duplications.
- **Helps you develop good thinking habits** so you will be able to think critically in class and in providing patient care.

  EXAMPLE: Melissa Carpenter has just given birth and is on a unit that uses a checklist for teaching needs as a part of the plan of care. When the evening nurse

BOX 1–2

AMERICAN NURSES ASSOCIATION STANDARDS OF PRACTICE

1. **Assessment**
The registered nurse collects comprehensive data pertinent to the patient's health or the situation.

2. **Diagnosis**
The registered nurse analyzes the assessment data to determine the diagnoses or issues.

3. **Outcomes Identification**
The registered nurse identifies expected outcomes for a plan individualized to the patient or the situation.

4. **Planning**
The registered nurse develops a plan that prescribes strategies and alternatives to attain expected outcomes.

5. **Implementation**
The registered nurse implements identified plan.

   5A. **Coordination of Care**
The registered nurse coordinates care delivery.

   5B. **Health Teaching and Health Promotion**
The registered nurse employs strategies to promote health and a safe environment.

   5C. **Consultation**
The advanced practice registered nurse and the nursing role specialist provide consultation to influence the identified plan, enhance the abilities of others, and effect change.

   5D. **Prescriptive Authority**
The advanced practice registered nurse uses prescriptive authority, procedures, referrals, treatments, and therapies in accordance with state and federal laws and regulations.

6. **Evaluation**
The registered nurse evaluates progress toward attainment of outcomes.

Note: This material is from the draft for public comment (ANA, 2010, in press); its wording may be somewhat changed in the final published version (August 2010). For that version of the ANA standards, visit http://www.nursingworld.org.

Source: Reprinted with permission from American Nurses Association (2010, in press). In *Nursing: Scope and standards of practice* (2nd ed.). (Public Comment draft, January). Silver Spring, MD. Available at http://nursebooks.org.

---

arrives, she sees that the day nurse has checked off "episiotomy care," so she does not reteach that information. Instead, she spends her time helping Ms. Carpenter learn to bathe her baby.

■ **Fosters continuity and coordination of care.** A written care plan ensures that all caregivers are informed of patient needs. Hospitals are staffed 24 hours a day, so a patient usually receives care from two or three registered nurses each day. Each nurse may be competent, but if they do not function in a coordinated manner, patients may doubt their competence and lose confidence that their needs will be met.

EXAMPLE: A new mother is having difficulty breastfeeding her baby. The day nurse has told her she should wake the baby and try to feed him every two hours. The evening nurse tells her to feed the baby on demand because he will wake up when he is hungry. The mother is becoming confused and discouraged. She says to her partner, "Maybe we should bottle feed the baby; this is really too hard to do."

- **Increases job satisfaction.** Many of the rewards in nursing come from realizing that you have helped someone. As you begin to see how the nursing process increases your ability to help, you will take satisfaction in a job well done. Good care plans also save you time, energy, and frustration, thereby increasing your ability to find creative solutions to client problems. Creativity helps prevent the burnout that can result from a repetitive "cookbook" approach to your daily work.

Take-away point: Nursing process helps you think like a nurse and benefits both clients and nurses.

1-1 THINK & REFLECT!

- Are all registered nurses professional nurses?
- Are all professional nurses registered nurses?
- The term "professional nurse" is used often. Who are the "nonprofessional" nurses, and what do they do?

See suggested responses to #1-1 Think & Reflect! in Appendix A.

What Is Nursing Process?

The nursing process is a special way of thinking and acting. It is a systematic, creative approach used to identify, prevent, and treat actual or potential health problems; identify patient strengths; and promote wellness. The nursing process can be more completely explained by describing its relationship to nursing and caring, as well as its background, purpose, characteristics, and six-step organization.

Take-away point: The nursing process provides the framework in which nurses use their knowledge and skills to express human caring.

History of Nursing Process

The following is a time line of the development of the nursing process:

- 1955: Hall first described nursing as a *process*.
- 1959 to 1963: Johnson (1959), Orlando (1961), and Wiedenbach (1963) were among those who first used the term *nursing process*. They described the process of nursing as a series of steps.
- 1970s: The process evolved from a three-step to a five- or six-step process (e.g., Vitale, Schultz, & Nugent, 1974). This text uses a six-step process to reflect both the current outcomes-driven healthcare environment and the organization of the ANA standards of practice (2004).
- 1973: The ANA developed standards for evaluating the quality of care that nurses deliver. Publication of the ANA standards encouraged most states to revise their

nurse practice acts to include assessment, diagnosis, planning, implementation, and evaluation as legitimate features of the nursing role.

■ 1987: The Canadian Nurses Association published standards for practice that were also organized around the nursing process.

■ The present: Since the publication of the ANA standards, virtually all nurses have accepted the nursing process as the basis of their practice. The most recent ANA standards of practice (2004) are shown in Box 1–2. Currently, Canadian standards are developed by provincial and territorial associations. These, too, usually include the nursing process and critical thinking in their standards for practice. To see some examples of Canadian Nurses Association standards of nursing practice, see Resources: Box 1–2 at Pearson Nursing Student Resources.

The nursing process is now taught in nearly every school of nursing. The National Council Licensure Examination for registered nurses (NCLEX, or "state board exams") integrates the phases of the nursing process into its questions. National accrediting bodies (e.g., The Joint Commission and the National League for Nursing) include aspects of the nursing process in their criteria for evaluating hospitals, schools of nursing, and other healthcare agencies.

Relationship to Nursing and Caring

You may have noticed that the definitions of *nursing* and *nursing process* are similar. They are certainly interrelated, but nursing is more than just nursing process. On one hand, a nurse may have an organized, systematic, deliberate approach that is, nevertheless, mechanical and lacking in warmth and caring. On the other hand, a nurse can feel deeply for a patient, want to help, and yet not have the necessary problem-solving skills to do so. Although the nursing process is systematic and logical, its use does not diminish the caring aspect of nursing. As you master the nursing process, it will become second nature to you and actually facilitate your caring.

Nurses view caring in various ways—for example, as comforting, involvement, kindness, nurturing, tenderness, and concern. Here is what some nurse theorists have to say:

■ Care is the essence of nursing and there can be no cure without caring (Leininger, 1978).

■ Carative factors are nursing interventions that are related to human care (Box 1–3) (Watson, 1988, p. 75).

■ Caring "sets up the conditions of trust that enable the [patient] to accept the help offered and to feel cared for" (Benner & Wrubel, 1989, pp. 1–4).

Purpose and Characteristics

The purpose of the nursing process is to provide a framework within which nurses can identify clients' health status and assist them in meeting their health needs. The nursing process is a deliberate but flexible guide for planning, implementing, and evaluating effective, individualized nursing care. Often (but not always) the vehicle for this is a written nursing or multidisciplinary care plan.

Take-away point: The nursing process is more than just a written plan of care!

nursing.pearsonhighered.com

BOX 1–3

WATSON'S CARATIVE FACTORS: INTERVENTIONS RELATED TO HUMAN CARE

1. *Forming a humanistic-altruistic system of values.* This involves obtaining satisfaction through giving and extending the sense of self.
2. *Instilling faith and hope* through development of an effective nurse-client relationship.
3. *Cultivating sensitivity to one's self and others.* This includes the ability to recognize and express one's own feelings.
4. *Developing a helping-trust (human care) relationship.* This involves effective communication, empathy, and nonpossessive warmth.
5. *Expressing positive and negative feelings* (e.g., feelings of sorrow, love, and pain) and accepting expression of those feelings from patients.
6. *Using a creative problem-solving caring process.* This links caring to the nursing process.
7. *Promoting transpersonal teaching and learning.* This factor differentiates caring from curing and shifts responsibility for wellness to the client.
8. *Providing a supportive, protective, or corrective environment.* This includes assessing the internal and external environment and the client's ability to cope with mental, physical, sociocultural, and spiritual changes and making changes in the environment as needed.
9. *Helping with the gratification of human needs.* This includes recognizing and attending to the physical, emotional, social, and spiritual needs of the client.
10. *Being sensitive to existential-phenomenologic-spiritual forces.* This means that you are alert to the mind-body-soul data of the immediate situation, allowing you to better understand the client's experience.

Source: Adapted from Watson, J. (1988). *Nursing: Human science and human care. A theory of nursing.* National League for Nursing Publication No. 15-2236. New York: National League for Nursing.

The following paragraphs describe characteristics of the nursing process and expand on its definition. The nursing process is:

- **Dynamic and cyclic.** Nurses evaluate changing patient responses to nursing interventions so they can make necessary revisions in the plan of care. Previously completed phases (e.g., assessment) are constantly reexamined for accuracy and appropriateness. Because the phases, or steps, are interrelated, there is no absolute beginning or end to the process.
- **Client centered.** In the nurse–client relationship, the client's needs always take precedence. Clients are encouraged to exercise control over their health and to make decisions about their care to the extent they are able.
- **Holistic.** Nurses see each patient as a unique individual, and they consider the whole person—body, mind, spirit, and culture.

- **Planned and outcome-directed.** Interventions are carefully chosen and based on principles and research rather than tradition (e.g., "We've always done it that way"). Nursing interventions are chosen for the purpose of achieving desired patient outcomes.
- **Evidence based.** The nursing process requires nurses to make judgments and choose interventions based on the best available evidence.
- **Flexible.** Nursing process provides an organized approach to care but it is not carried out in rigid, stepwise fashion. You give care according to a plan but realize that the plan will change continually.

   EXAMPLE: According to the plan of care, Mr. Akers was to be up in a chair for 15 minutes. However, as soon as he was out of bed, he became pale and dizzy, so his nurse helped him back to bed instead of continuing toward the chair.

- **Universally applicable.** Nursing process can be used with clients of all ages, with any medical diagnosis, and at any point on the wellness–illness continuum. It is useful in any setting (e.g., schools, hospitals, clinics, home health, industries) and across specialties (e.g., hospice nursing, maternity nursing, surgical nursing). It is used to provide care for individuals, families, groups, and communities.
- **Health status oriented.** This means that plans of care are organized according to statements about the patient's health status. These are usually problem statements; however, they may also be statements describing healthy conditions or patient strengths. Of course, the nursing process cannot prevent or eliminate every patient problem (e.g., chronic health problems, such as the pain and immobility associated with arthritis). When problems cannot be eliminated, the nurse provides available relief, supports the patient's strengths in coping with the problems, and helps the patient to understand and find meaning in his situation.
- **A cognitive (thinking) process.** Nursing process requires you to use intellectual skills in solving problems and making decisions. Nurses use critical thinking to apply nursing knowledge systematically and logically to client data, enabling them to determine its meaning and plan appropriate care. This characteristic is discussed further in Chapter 2.

1-2 WHAT DO YOU KNOW?

1. Nursing was first described as a process in:
    a. The 1940s.
    b. The 1950s.
    c. The 1960s.
    d. The 1970s.
2. True or false? Using a systematic, logical process such as the nursing process interferes with the nurse's ability to focus on caring.

See answer to #1-2 What Do You Know? in Appendix A.

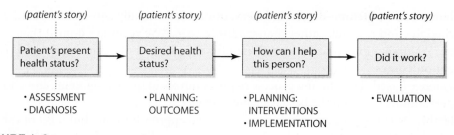

FIGURE 1–2
Overview of the nursing process

What Are the Phases of Nursing Process?

Explained very simply, the nurse using the nursing process listens to the patient's story in order to answer the following questions:

- What is the person's present health status?
- What is the person's desired health status?
- How can I help this person?
- Did it work?

Figure 1–2 shows how these questions fit with the six phases of the nursing process.

Some authors organize the nursing process into five phases: assessment, diagnosis, planning, implementation, and evaluation. A few authors still combine assessment and diagnosis into a single "assessment" phase; their phases are assessment, planning, intervention, and evaluation. This text divides the nursing process into six phases (or steps) because it is easier to learn in smaller "chunks." This helps you to learn the planning processes gradually and in more detail. Don't be too concerned about such inconsistencies. All such divisions are artificial anyway because of the dynamic nature of the nursing process (see later sections on "Phases are Sequential," "Phases," and "Phases Overlap"). The following is an overview of the six nursing process phases. Table 1–2 summarizes them.

TABLE 1–2 Phases of the Nursing Process

Phase	Activities
Assessment	Collect and organize data.
Diagnosis	Identify present health status (problems and strengths).
Planning: **O**utcomes	Choose desired patient outcomes.
Planning: **I**nterventions	Choose nursing interventions.
Implementation	Carry out the plan of action.
Evaluation	Determine if the plan was effective.

Assessment—Getting the Facts

In this phase, you will collect, organize, validate, and record data about the patient's current health status. You will obtain data by examining patients, talking to them and their families, and reading charts and records. You do not draw conclusions about the data in this phase.

EXAMPLE: After Maura Greenberg's baby was born, the home health nurse performed a comprehensive assessment. She recorded on the nursing history Ms. Greenberg's statements that she is often constipated, snacks frequently, does not drink much, and does not take laxatives.

Diagnosis—What Is the Patient's Present Health Status? What Is Contributing to It?

In this phase, you will (a) sort, cluster, and analyze the data to identify the patient's present health status (actual and potential health problems and strengths), (b) write a precise statement describing the patient's health status and the factors contributing to it, (c) prioritize the diagnoses, and (d) decide which diagnoses will respond to nursing care and which must be referred to another healthcare professional.

EXAMPLE: The nurse wrote the following diagnosis on Ms. Greenberg's care plan: "Constipation related to insufficient intake of fiber and fluids."

NANDA International has developed a set of standardized labels for nurses to use in writing nursing diagnoses (NANDA International, 2009). This list is found on the inside front cover of this text. It is discussed further in Chapter 6.

Planning: Outcomes—What Is the Desired Patient Health Status?

In this phase, you will work with the client to choose the desired outcomes. That is, you will decide exactly how you want the client's status to change and within what period of time. The outcomes chosen in this phase are the criteria you will use in the evaluation phase.

EXAMPLE: The nurse wrote the following outcomes on Ms. Greenberg's care plan:
- Will have soft, formed bowel movement at least every other day by May 15.
- Will be able to name at least six high-fiber foods before next visit on May 15.

There is also a standardized vocabulary for describing patient outcomes thought to be sensitive to nursing interventions—the *Nursing Outcomes Classification (NOC)* (Moorhead, Johnson, Maas, & Swanson, 2008). Chapter 7 discusses in more detail how nurses can use the NOC in planning and evaluating care.

Planning: Interventions—How Can You Help Achieve the Desired Outcomes?

In this phase, you will choose interventions for promoting wellness or preventing, correcting, or relieving health problems. You will plan specific interventions for the outcomes associated with each nursing diagnosis. The end product of the planning phases may be a written plan of care. However, in some cases, planning is simply the mental process of choosing what to do. You will often act without a written plan but never without a plan.

EXAMPLE: The nurse wrote the following nursing orders on Ms. Greenberg's care plan:

1. Give the pamphlet "Fiber in Your Diet" to Ms. G.
2. Help Ms. G. make a meal plan using high-fiber foods.
3. Explain the relationship of fiber and fluids to bowel elimination.
4. Reassess bowel elimination status in one week (5/15).

There is also a standardized classification of nursing interventions, called the Nursing *Interventions Classification (NIC)* (Bulechek, Butcher, & Dochterman, 2008). Chapters 8 and 10 describe more fully how nurses use this vocabulary to plan care and record nursing work.

 ### Implementation—Doing, Delegating, and Documenting

In this phase, you will communicate the plan of care to other members of the healthcare team and carry out the interventions indicated on the plan or delegate them to others. The final activity in this phase is to record the care given and the client's responses.

EXAMPLE: The nurse took the pamphlet to Ms. Greenberg and talked with her about the importance of fiber and fluids and preventing constipation in the postpartum period. She recorded these interventions in the nursing progress notes.

Evaluation—Did It Work?

In this phase, after implementing the plan, you will compare the patient's health status with the desired outcomes identified in the planning outcomes phase. You will determine which interventions were or were not helpful in achieving desired outcomes and revise the care plan as needed. The nursing process is cyclic: You will keep reexamining all the phases (assessment, diagnosis, outcomes, interventions, and implementation) to determine what is effective and what should be changed.

EXAMPLE: On the nurse's May 15 return visit, Ms. Greenberg was able to identify high-fiber foods but reported that she had not had a bowel movement since May 12. The nurse advised her to drink more fluids, including some prune juice, and to call her primary care provider if she did not have a bowel movement within the next 24 hours.

Take-away point: The phases of the nursing process are assessment, diagnosis, planning outcomes, planning interventions, implementation, and evaluation.

Phases Are Sequential and Systematic

Nursing process phases are organized and systematic. They are also sequential in that each step depends on the activities of preceding steps. For example:

1. **Assessment → Diagnosis.** You must have accurate data (assessment phase) to make the correct diagnosis (diagnosis phase).
2. **Diagnosis → Planning outcomes.** Desired outcomes are developed directly from your diagnoses. In the preceding example of Ms. Greenberg, the diagnosis was "Constipation . . ." and an expected outcome was that she would have a "soft, formed bowel movement . . ."
3. **Planning outcomes → Planning interventions.** The desired outcomes direct your choice of interventions. You choose interventions that you expect will produce the outcomes.
4. **Planning outcomes and interventions → Implementation.** The plan of care guides the activities you perform during implementation.
5. **Implementation → Evaluation.** You identified the client's present health status in the diagnosis phase. You must carry out the plan (implementation) in order to produce a change in health status that you can evaluate.

However, "sequential" does not mean that the phases always occur in the ADP_OP_IIE order. That is, you will not always complete one step before proceeding to the next. For example, nurses do not always gather complete data about a patient before taking action. In an emergency, for instance, you would quickly think of an action (planning interventions) and implement it immediately (implementation) before doing formal data collection or writing a plan of care. Of course, you would have had to make *some* observations (assessment) to realize that action was needed, but you would have only limited data, and you probably would not have consciously formulated a problem statement. After acting, you would evaluate whether the emergency was over and then return to a more thorough and systematic collection and analysis of data. The following is another example of nonsequential phases:

> **EXAMPLE:** A teacher has brought Carlene to the school nurse's office. Carlene is crying and saying, "My stomach hurts so much!" (data). She seems very anxious, so before attempting a complete assessment, the nurse first acts (implementation) to calm Carlene. After evaluating that Carlene is calm enough to answer questions (evaluation), the nurse proceeds with the interview and physical examination (assessment).

Phases Overlap

This text describes the phases of the nursing process separately to help you learn them. However, in practice, they overlap a great deal. For example, even though the first encounter with a client usually begins with some form of data collection, assessment actually continues at each patient contact. While you are bathing a patient (implementation), you may at the same time observe the skin over his bony prominences (assessment). If you observe some redness (assessment), you may conclude that the patient has *Impaired Skin Integrity* (diagnosis).

The evaluation phase overlaps with all phases of the nursing process because you will constantly examine what you have done in previous phases. After performing interventions and determining their effect on client health status, you will examine the:

- *Assessment phase* to see if your data are complete and accurate.
- *Diagnosis phase* to see if the diagnoses are accurate and if any need to be added to or removed from the list.
- *Planning outcomes phase* to check whether the outcomes were appropriate or realistic.
- *Planning interventions phase* to see whether the most effective interventions were chosen.
- *Implementation phase* to determine whether the plan was actually carried out properly and whether activities were delegated appropriately.

Take-away point: Nursing process phases are usually sequential; but they are overlapping and do not always occur in ADP_OP_IIE order.

Relationship of Nursing Process and the Problem-Solving Process

Problem solving is the process of identifying a problem and then planning and taking steps to resolve it. Said another way, it is the process used when you recognize a difference between what is occurring and what should be occurring. Because the nursing process also considers wellness and strengths, it is not limited to problems. However, it is similar to other formal problem-solving methods.

The scientific method is a systematic, logical approach to problem solving based on data and hypothesis testing. The first step is to identify the problem. The next step is to define it carefully. The problem statement serves as a guide for setting criteria by which to evaluate possible solutions. Scientists then collect data relating specifically to the problem and generate solutions (formulate hypotheses). After considering the consequences of each, the preferred solution is put it into effect, and the results are evaluated (hypothesis testing).

EXAMPLE: Suppose you are on your way to an important job interview when your car breaks down. Your analysis of the situation is that your most important and immediate need is to get a job, not to repair the car. You have specified the exact nature of your problem: possible loss of a job opportunity caused by being late to the interview. You have the following data: (a) it is too far to walk and (b) no one is at home to come get you. You make a quick plan. Your goal is to get there on time. You decide to walk to the nearest telephone and call a taxi for yourself and a tow truck for the car (hypothesis). The outcome of your plan is a fabulous job and a new car—you evaluate that the plan was successful.

When using the nursing process, the problem is not usually so obvious. The nurse often begins with comprehensive data collection and uses the data to identify problems

TABLE 1–3　Comparison of Formal Problem Solving, the Research Process, and the Nursing Process

Research Process	Formal Problem Solving	Nursing Process
State a research question or problem.	Recognize that a problem exists.	Assessment: Perform comprehensive assessment (collect data).
Identify the purpose of or rationale for the study.		
Review related literature.	Gather information about the problem.	
Formulate hypothesis and define variables.	Define the exact nature of the problem.	Diagnosis: Formulate the nursing diagnoses.
Select method to test hypotheses.	Develop solutions and decide on a plan of action.	Planning: ■ Choose patient outcomes. ■ Generate and choose nursing interventions and activities.
Collect the data.	Implement the plan of action.	Implementation: Carry out the nursing interventions.
Analyze the data; interpret the results.	Monitor the situation over time (collect data about the effects of the plan).	
Evaluate the hypothesis.	Evaluate the plan or solution to ensure initial and continued effectiveness.	Evaluation: Collect data about patient responses to interventions; judge whether outcomes were achieved.

or health risks. In the scientific method, the problem is identified before extensive data are collected, and the only information gathered is that which pertains to the problem. Table 1–3 provides further comparisons.

Intuition is a problem-solving approach that relies on use of one's "inner sense." Expert nurses describe instances in which they "just had a feeling" that something was wrong even though they could not say what prompted the feeling. Although it is neither systematic nor data based, intuition is gaining credibility as a legitimate aspect of expert clinical judgment that is acquired through knowledge and experience. For example, a nurse might develop expertise in cardiovascular nursing through continuous experience with patients' responses to cardiovascular problems. The knowledge base of expert nurses enables them to recognize patient cues and patterns and begin to make correct decisions. They are able to judge quickly which evidence is most important and act upon that limited evidence. Thus, intuition describes a leap in (or a condensing of) the critical thinking element of considering evidence.

The danger in using intuition is that sometimes the nurse's inner sense is true, but sometimes it is not. Critical thinkers realize how easy it is to confuse intuitions and prejudices. They follow their "inner sense that something is so" but only with a healthy sense of intellectual humility. Intuition is not a reliable problem-solving method for novice nurses or students because they lack the knowledge and clinical experience on which to base their judgments. Used by a novice, intuition may be little more than guessing. As a beginning practitioner, you should be cautious about flashes of intuition and discuss them with more experienced colleagues before acting on them.

> **Take-away point:** As a novice, you should not rely on intuition. Discuss with an experienced nurse before acting on intuition.

In the **trial-and-error** method, you would try a number of solutions until you found one that worked. However, without considering alternatives systematically, you cannot know why one solution worked and another did not. This method is not recommended for nurses because it is inefficient and because the patient might be harmed if a solution is not appropriate.

1-3 WHAT DO YOU KNOW?

Define "intuition."

See answer to #1-3 What Do You Know? in Appendix A.

1-2 THINK & REFLECT!

Why do you think the scientific method of problem solving would not work well in planning care for a patient?

See suggested responses to #1-2 Think & Reflect! in Appendix A.

What Qualities Does a Nurse Need?

The nursing process is only as good as the nurse who uses it. The following qualities and attitudes contribute to successful use of the nursing process. You can improve all of these qualities through awareness, effort, and practice.

> **Take-away point:** As a nurse, you will need a combination of thinking, interpersonal, and psychomotor skills, including creativity, cultural sensitivity, and the ability to work with technology.

Cognitive (Intellectual) Skills

The nursing process is a guide to systematic thinking in nursing practice. Intellectual skills used in the nursing process are problem solving (discussed in the preceding section), decision making, and critical thinking.

- **Decision making** is the process of choosing the best action to take—the action most likely to produce the desired outcome. It involves deliberation, judgment, and choice.

Decision making is important in the problem-solving process, but not all decisions involve problem solving (e.g., you decided what to wear today).

- **Critical thinking** is careful, goal-oriented, purposeful thinking that involves many mental skills, such as determining which data are relevant, evaluating the credibility of sources, and making inferences. It is essential to good problem solving and decision making.

Creativity and Curiosity

Creativity and curiosity are essential to the nursing process and critical thinking. You need vision and insight to find new and better ways of doing things. Always ask yourself, "Why are we doing this?" and "Why are we doing it this way?" Excellent nurses understand the rationale for every nursing activity. If they cannot find a reason for the activity or cannot show that it is having the desired effect, they work to have it discontinued.

EXAMPLE: A hospital's procedures specify the use of draw sheets. Mauricio works on a unit where most of the patients are ambulatory. One day as he is changing bed linens, he wonders, "What good is this draw sheet? We never use it for anything, and we use fitted bottom sheets." He talks to the unit manager, who changes the unit procedures, saving both money and nursing time.

Interpersonal Skills

Interpersonal skills are the activities used in person-to-person communication. They include:

- Oral and written communication
- Knowledge of human behavior and social systems
- Nonverbal behaviors such as body posture and movement, facial expression, and touch.

Success in developing a trusting relationship with patients depends on your ability to communicate—to listen and to convey compassion, interest, and information. Successful outcomes depend on successful nurse-patient relationships.

EXAMPLE: Elsa Banayos is the primary nurse for a group of patients. When she notices that the patient care assistant is not using correct body mechanics to help Mr. Davis out of bed, she draws on her interpersonal skills. She must intervene to ensure the safety of both Mr. Davis and the assistant but without embarrassing the assistant or undermining the patient's confidence in her.

Communication skills are important, but *what* you communicate is just as important. You can promote good relationships by having a positive attitude and sense of humor; being open, honest, patient, and frank; by demonstrating humility, accountability, and reliability; admitting when you are wrong; and giving credit to others who deserve it.

Cultural Competence

Cultural competence means that the nurse works within the client's cultural belief system to resolve health problems. This requires the nurse to be aware of similarities and differences among cultural groups and to be culturally sensitive. Although cultural competence can be called an interpersonal skill, it also involves knowledge and attitudes.

Psychomotor Skills

Nurses use **psychomotor skills**, especially in the implementation phase of the nursing process when giving hands-on care. Good psychomotor skills help to gain client trust and achieve desired client outcomes.

> **EXAMPLE:** Turning a patient smoothly minimizes pain and helps establish trust and rapport. If you are clumsy with the turning, the patient may think you are not competent and will be less likely to trust you in other situations. He may hesitate to ask you for information or help, and you may be unable to obtain important assessment data from him.

Technological Skills

Nurses work with high-technology equipment, such as heart monitors and ventilators, much of which contains programmable computer chips.

> **EXAMPLE:** In the past, nurses regulated intravenous infusions by counting drops and visualizing markings on the container. Now they must perform several steps to program a computerized pump to deliver the correct fluid rate and measure the amount infused.

Many nurses use computers for planning and documenting patient care. Some carry hand-held computers, which they use to record assessments, retrieve laboratory results, and document interventions. In addition, nurses are making on-unit use of the Internet to find information they need to choose the best nursing interventions.

1-4 WHAT DO YOU KNOW?

Give six examples of psychomotor skills a nurse might use.

See answer to #1-4 What Do You Know? in Appendix A.

1-3 THINK & REFLECT!

1. Describe an incident in which you observed a nurse demonstrating cultural competence. What did the nurse do and say? (Or describe a nurse who was not culturally competent.)

> **2.** Describe an incident in which you demonstrated either curiosity or creativity in patient care. If you have not yet given patient care, describe a different situation in which you showed those qualities.
>
> **See suggested responses to #1-3 Think & Reflect! in Appendix A.**

Nursing Process and Wellness

Consider the characteristics of the nursing process as it is applied in the following case study of a well client.

CASE STUDY

A 40-year-old corporate executive has come to the company nurse for her required annual physical examination.

Assessment   The nurse takes a complete health history, which reveals no past medical problems, except that the client's father died of a heart attack at age 62 years. The client's laboratory results and chest radiographs are normal. The nurse performs a complete physical examination, with normal findings, including a blood pressure of 120/74 mm Hg and a pulse of 84 beats/min. The client is 10 lb overweight. The nurse asks about the client's health habits and lifestyle and discovers that she works long hours and often takes work home; her only exercise is an occasional golf game. She eats a balanced diet, sleeps about 7 hours a day, and smokes a half-pack of cigarettes per day.

Diagnosis   If nursing were concerned only with illness, the nurse would analyze the data, diagnose that no problem exists, and conclude that no interventions are needed. However, the nurse takes a holistic perspective and understands the importance of disease prevention and health promotion. The nurse diagnoses that the client has unmet health-promotion and disease-prevention needs.

Planning: Outcomes   Using client input, the nurse develops broad outcomes: The client will (a) become aware of ways in which her lifestyle can either increase or decrease her risk of disease and (b) experience improved health status, as evidenced by smoking cessation, beginning an exercise program, and maintaining her current weight. The nurse does not include a goal for the client to reduce her work hours because the client insists that she needs to work long hours, enjoys it, and has no interest in changing that behavior.

Planning: Interventions   Based on the desired outcomes, the nurse chooses nursing interventions and writes the care plan. The nurse plans to (a) talk with the client about the effect of smoking on coronary circulation and about the relationship of exercise and diet to weight control and a healthy heart and (b) give the client pamphlets about basic nutrition, smoking cessation, and aerobic exercises.

Implementation   Before the client leaves, the nurse encourages her to attend the company-sponsored smoking cessation clinic. The nurse does not refer her to a dietitian because she seems adequately informed and motivated to avoid gaining weight.

Evaluation The client and the nurse included in the plan that the client will return in one month to be weighed and to evaluate her efforts to stop smoking and begin exercising. If desired outcomes are being achieved, the nurse plans to assess the client's stress level and coping mechanisms at the one-month follow-up to be sure that she is still showing no effects from her strenuous work schedule. At that time, they may modify her plan of care.

From the case study, you should see that nursing process is not limited to use with clients who are ill. Nurses frequently work with well clients, focusing on health promotion, health protection, and disease prevention. **Health promotion** activities (e.g., daily exercise) are directed toward achieving a higher level of wellness; they are not aimed at avoiding any particular disease. In health promotion, the client is seen as having more control and expertise, and the nurse serves as a facilitator. **Health protection** focuses on activities that decrease environmental threats to health (e.g., air pollution). **Disease prevention** involves actions that help to prevent specific health problems or diseases (e.g., immunizations, prenatal care).

Although most of the national health budget is spent on care and treatment of illnesses, health-promotion initiatives are receiving attention from government agencies. The U.S. Public Health Service, in *Healthy People 2020* (2010a), outlines a national strategy for improving the health of the nation during this decade. The report acknowledges that health promotion and disease prevention provide the best opportunities for preserving our healthcare resources. It outlines four broad goals:

1. Eliminate preventable disease, disability, injury, and premature death.
2. Achieve health equity and eliminate health disparities.
3. Create social and physical environments that promote good health for all.
4. Promote healthy development and healthy behaviors at every stage of life.

Nursing Process and Community Health

Consider the characteristics of the nursing process as it is applied in the following case study of a well client.

CASE STUDY

Parish nurse Patti Munoz wishes to identify the parish community's health needs and priorities so that she can provide an effective health education program.

Assessment Patti develops a survey and distributes it to church members. She collects data about their wellness behaviors and beliefs in four categories: physical, emotional/relational, spiritual, and health system relationships/knowledge base.

Diagnosis From the data, Patti identifies several groups of parishioners who are at risk. One such group consists of adults younger than age 50 without regular blood pressure (BP) screening.

Planning: Outcomes For this group, Patti develops a desired outcome based on national public health standards: "Increase to at least 95 percent the proportion of adults who have had their blood pressure measured within the preceding 2 years and can state whether their blood pressure was normal or high" (U.S. Department of Health and Human Services, 2010b).

Planning: Interventions To achieve this outcome, Patti plans an annual health fair. One of the activities to be included is BP screening. She also plans to place related literature in the church library and write an article about heart disease prevention for the monthly newsletter.

Implementation Patti places literature in the library, writes the article, and holds the health fair as planned. At the health fair, nursing students from the local college conduct the BP screening.

Evaluation A year later, after implementing her plan, Patti again surveys the congregation regarding their health beliefs and behaviors. She discovers the desired outcome regarding BP screening has been met and decides to continue with the same interventions, except for the newsletter article, which she will not use this year.

Case created from Miskelly, S. (1995). A parish nursing model: Applying the community health nursing process in a church community. *Journal of Community Health Nursing, 12*(1): 1–14.

From the case study, you can see that nursing process is not limited to caring for individual patients. Community health nurses use nursing process to focus on the health needs of groups of persons (e.g., communities and systems). Parish nurses, for example, holistically address the physical, emotional, and spiritual needs of members of a church congregation (community). They provide teaching, counseling, health screening, and advocacy. Hands-on care, although provided, is not their main focus.

1-5 WHAT DO YOU KNOW?

1. In the wellness case study, the nurse provided teaching to help the client stop smoking. What kind of intervention was this?
   a. Health promotion
   b. Health protection
   c. Disease prevention
2. In the parish nursing case study, the nurse conducted blood pressure screenings to identify those who might have an elevated blood pressure. What kind of intervention was this?
   a. Health promotion
   b. Health protection
   c. Disease prevention

See answer to #1-5 What Do You Know? in Appendix A.

Ethical and Cultural Considerations

Professional standards of practice require nurses to apply the nursing process in an ethical and culturally sensitive manner. For example, nurses are ethically responsible for evaluating the quality of the care they give and for maintaining the knowledge they need to give good care. The ANA *Code of Ethics for Nurses* (2001), found in Appendix B, and Standard 12 of the *Standards of Professional Performance* (ANA, 2010, in press) specifically require that nurses' decisions be made in an ethical manner (Box 1–4).

BOX 1–4

AMERICAN NURSES ASSOCIATION PROFESSIONAL PERFORMANCE STANDARD 7—ETHICS

The registered nurse integrates ethical provisions in all areas of practice.

Competencies

The registered nurse:
1. Uses the *Code of Ethics for Nurses with Interpretive Statements* (ANA, 2001) to guide practice.
2. Delivers care in a manner that preserves and protects patient autonomy, dignity and rights, values, and beliefs.
3. Respects the centrality of the patient/family as core members of any health care team.
4. Upholds and advocates for patient confidentiality within legal and regulatory parameters.
5. Serves as a patient advocate assisting patients in developing skills for self-advocacy and informed decision-making.
6. Maintains a therapeutic and professional patient-nurse relationship with appropriate professional role boundaries.
7. Demonstrates a commitment to practicing self-care, managing stress, and connecting with self and others.
8. Contributes to resolving ethical issues of patients, colleagues, community groups, systems, and other stakeholders.
9. Takes appropriate action regarding instances of illegal, unethical, or inappropriate behavior that can endanger or jeopardize the best interests of the patient or situation.
10. Cooperates in an interprofessional team to make ethical decisions regarding the application of technologies and the acquisition and sharing of data.
11. Demonstrates professional comportment (openness, honesty, integrity, and authenticity).
12. Speaks up when appropriate to question health care practice when necessary for safety and quality improvement.

Note: There are additional standards for advanced practice registered nurses and nurses in a nursing role specialty. This material is from the draft for public comment (ANA, 2010, in press); its wording may be somewhat changed in the final published version (August 2010). For that version of the ANA standards, visit http://www.nursingworld.org.

Source: American Nurses Association (2010, in press). *Nursing: Scope and standards of practice* (2nd ed.). (Public Comment draft, January). Silver Spring, MD. Available at http://nursebooks.org

BOX 1–5

AMERICAN NURSES ASSOCIATION STANDARDS OF PROFESSIONAL PERFORMANCE

Standard 7	**Ethics.** The registered nurse integrates ethical provisions in all areas of practice.
Standard 8	**Education.** The registered nurse attains knowledge and competency that reflects current nursing practice.
Standard 9	**Evidence-Based Practice and Research.** The registered nurse integrates research findings into practice.
Standard 10	**Quality of Practice.** The registered nurse systematically enhances the quality and effectiveness of nursing practice.
Standard 11	**Communication.** The registered nurse uses a wide variety of communication skills and formats in all areas of practice.
Standard 12	**Leadership.** The registered nurse provides leadership in the professional practice setting and the profession.
Standard 13	**Collegiality.** The registered nurse interacts with and contributes to the professional development of peers and colleagues.
Standard 14	**Collaboration.** The registered nurse collaborates with patient, family, and others in the conduct of nursing practice.
Standard 15	**Professional Practice Evaluation.** The registered nurse evaluates one's own nursing practice in relation to professional practice standards and guidelines, relevant statutes, rules, and regulations.
Standard 16	**Resource Utilization.** The registered nurse considers factors related to safety, effectiveness, cost, and impact on practice in the planning and delivery of nursing services.
Standard 17	**Environmental Health.** The registered nurse integrates the principles of environmental health for nursing in all areas of practice.

Note: This material is from the draft for public comment (ANA, 2010, in press); its wording may be somewhat changed in the final published version (August 2010). For that version of the ANA standards, visit http://www.nursingworld.org.

Source: Reprinted with permission from American Nurses Association (2010, in press). In *Nursing: Scope and standards of practice* (2nd ed.). (Public Comment draft, January). Silver Spring, MD. Available at http:/nursebooks.org.

The other ANA professional performance standards (Box 1–5) indirectly imply the ethical nature of nursing. Many institutions have an ethics committee for addressing ethical issues in patient care. It is important for nurses to participate in such committee work.

In addition, there are cultural variations in the ways caring is expressed and received. Nurses should try to understand how clients of different cultures view care and then work toward providing culture-specific care (Leininger, 1978).

SUMMARY

Nursing process:

- Is a systematic approach to delivering holistic care to well and ill clients.
- Identifies the client's present health status (problems and strengths) and focuses on desired outcomes.
- Is used to provide care for individuals, families, and communities.
- Is not limited to treatment of illnesses but is used in health promotion, health protection, and disease prevention.
- Benefits clients, nurses, and the nursing profession.
- Is organized in six interrelated phases: assessment, diagnosis, planning outcomes, planning interventions, implementation, and evaluation.
- Is patient-centered, flexible, dynamic, and cyclic.
- Requires special nursing knowledge and skills to be used successfully.
- Must be used with cultural sensitivity and in an ethical manner in order to meet standards of professional practice.

CRITICAL THINKING AND CLINICAL REASONING: A CASE STUDY

Alma Boiko has been in an intermediate care facility since having a stroke that left her unable to care for herself. When she developed pneumonia, she was transferred to a hospital. Juan Apodaca, RN, *settles her comfortably in bed* and briefly *interviews her* about her symptoms. He *obtains a temperature* of 101°F, pulse of 120 beats/min, respirations of 32 breaths/min, and blood pressure of 100/68 mm Hg. Juan *examines Ms. Boiko's chart* to obtain a history of her illness and a record of her nursing care. He *administers oxygen by nasal cannula*, as ordered by the physician. When *performing the physical examination*, Juan notices a reddened area over Ms. Boiko's coccyx.

Because Ms. Boiko is unable to move about in bed, Juan *writes a diagnosis of* "*Risk for Impaired Skin Integrity* over coccyx related to constant pressure to bony prominences caused by inability to move about in bed." From the list on the computer, he *chooses an outcome* that the skin on Ms. Boiko's coccyx will remain intact and that the redness will be gone within 2 days. He *writes nursing orders for skin care*; a schedule for turning Ms. Boiko every 2 hours; and orders for frequent, continued observation of her skin.

Two days later, while *bathing Ms. Boiko*, Juan *observes that her coccygeal area is still red*, a small area of skin is peeling off, and there is some serous drainage. Juan *concludes that the outcome has not been achieved*. He is sure his data were adequate, and he changes his nursing diagnosis to "*Impaired Skin Integrity* over coccyx. . . ." The other staff members assured Juan that they had carried out the 2-hour turning schedule except for 6 hours at night when they left Ms. Boiko to sleep undisturbed. Even though turning every 2 hours while awake was a standard of care on the unit and had been adequate for other clients,

Juan concludes that it was not often enough for Ms. Boiko. He *changes the order on the plan of care* to read: "Turn every 2 hours around the clock."

1. Label the italicized activities A, D, P_O, P_P, I, or E, according to the phase of the nursing process represented by the activity.
2. List all the client data (human responses).
3. Circle the activities that show the dynamic or cyclic nature of the nursing process.
4. List all the nursing orders that Juan wrote. Note that some are summarized here instead of being fully written out in nursing-order format.
5. Where in the case study do you see the most obvious example of overlapping nursing process phases?
6. How did the nurse demonstrate creativity?
7. Which characteristic(s) of the nursing process was/were demonstrated when Juan ordered a turning schedule that was more frequent than the unit routines?

See suggested responses to Critical Thinking and Clinical Reasoning: A Case Study, in Appendix A.

Pearson **Nursing Student Resources**

Find additional review materials at **www.nursing.pearsonhighered.com**
Prepare for success with additional NCLEX®-style practice questions, interactive assignments and activities, Web links, animations and videos, and more!

Critical Thinking

2

Why Do Nurses Need to Think Critically?

"... How do you choose between a butterfly or an IV intracath? [You] have to consider why you want that line in. And just learning the insertion alone is difficult. You take into consideration ... whether it's a short-term, keep-open IV with limited medications, then the butterfly IV is more comfortable and presents less of a threat of phlebitis. Doctors vary in their preferences as well, and you have to take that into consideration. And of course, the condition of the patient and his veins makes a great deal of difference. For example, with older patients special skill is required. They look as if they are going to be so easy to get in because the veins look large, but they are so fragile. If you do not use a very, very slight tourniquet, the ... vein will just pop open" (Benner, 1984, pp. 124–125).

That exemplar, presented by an expert nurse, illustrates that nursing is both thinking and doing. Learning to be a nurse requires more than just memorizing facts. Nurses use stored-up facts along with new information to make decisions, generate new ideas, and solve problems (Figure 2–2). In order to transfer nursing knowledge into nursing practice, they must use critical thinking—a purposeful mental activity in which ideas are produced and evaluated and judgments are made.

Take-away point: "Most professional practice situations are characterized by complexity, instability, uncertainty, uniqueness, and the presence of value conflicts" (Schön [1983] as cited in Gaberson & Oermann, 1999, p. 4).

After completing this chapter, you should be able to do the following:

- Give a definition of *critical thinking*.
- Explain why critical thinking is important for nurses.
- Compare and contrast five types of nursing knowledge.
- Describe some important critical thinking skills and attitudes.
- Use intellectual standards to evaluate your own thinking.
- Discuss the relationship between critical thinking and nursing process.
- List guidelines to aid in developing critical thinking.

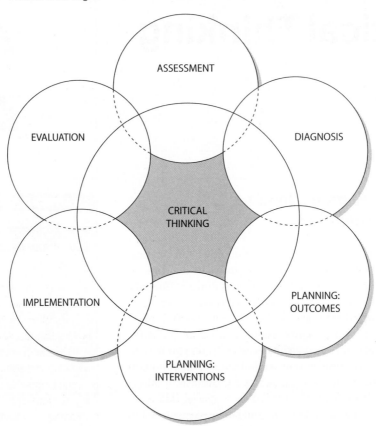

FIGURE 2–1
Critical thinking and nursing process

Nursing Is an Applied Discipline

Nurses apply a basic core of knowledge to each new client situation. In an academic discipline (e.g., mathematics), problems are well structured, and the right answer can usually be found by applying the right theory or formula. In an applied discipline (e.g., nursing), problems are messy and confusing. There may be insufficient or conflicting data, an unknown cause, and no single "correct" or "best" answer or solution. To manage such problems, you must know how to identify knowledge and data gaps, find and use new information, and initiate and manage change. All of these skills require critical thinking.

Nursing Draws on Knowledge from Other Fields

Some professionals, such as chemists and mathematicians, concentrate almost completely on the single body of knowledge that makes up their field. This is not so for nurses. Because nursing deals holistically with a wide range of human responses, nurses use information and insights from other subject areas, such as physiology and

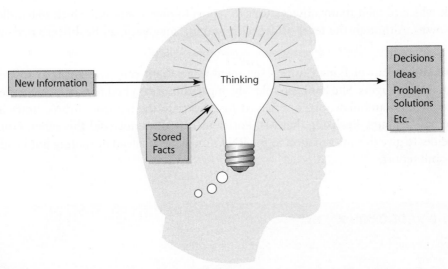

FIGURE 2–2
Critical thinking

psychology, in order to understand the meaning of patient data and to plan effective interventions. This, too, requires critical thinking.

Nurses Deal with Change in Stressful Environments

Nurses work in fast-paced, rapidly changing, and often hectic situations. Therefore, routine behaviors and "the usual procedure" may not be adequate for the situation at hand. For example, knowing the routine for giving 9 o'clock medications may not help a nurse to deal with a patient who is frightened of injections or one who does not wish to take a medication. Treatments, medications, and technology change constantly, and a patient's condition may change from minute to minute. When anticipating or reacting to changes, nurses must base their decisions on knowledge and rational thinking in order to respond appropriately under stress.

> **EXAMPLE:** Dwayne has been admitted to the hospital after an automobile accident. After being moved from the emergency department to the orthopedic unit, he becomes lethargic and sleepy, and his speech is slurred. The primary care provider tells the nurse that tests do not indicate a significant head injury. When the nurse makes her initial full assessment, she reads in the history that the patient is a diabetic. She finds his blood sugar is only 60 mg/dL. She obtains medical orders for insulin, and the patient improves dramatically.

Nurses Make Frequent, Varied, and Important Decisions

Nurses make many decisions during a workday. These are not trivial decisions; they often involve a client's well-being or even survival. Nurses use critical thinking to collect and interpret information and to make sound judgments and good decisions (e.g., to decide which of their many observations to report to physicians and which to handle on their own). Although the level of decision making may vary, all healthcare personnel need to use critical thinking.

EXAMPLE: Part of Edna Chin's assignment as a patient care assistant is to answer patients' call lights. She has been told which patients are on bed rest and which ones need help to ambulate. She has helped Ms. Porter to the bathroom three times in the past 3 hours. Realizing that Ms. Porter usually does not void this often, Edna decides to give this information to the RN immediately instead of waiting until end-of-shift report.

?

2-1 WHAT DO YOU KNOW?

Discuss four reasons why nurses need to think critically.

See answer to #2-1 What Do You Know? in Appendix A.

What Is Critical Thinking?

By now you may be wondering, What is critical thinking? Am I doing it? How can I tell when others are (or I am) doing it? Box 2–1 contains questions to help you evaluate and develop your thinking.

BOX 2–1

ARE YOU A CRITICAL THINKER?

Do you:
- Explore the thinking and assumptions that underlie your emotions and feelings?
- Base your judgments on facts and reasoning, not personal feelings, self-interest, or guesswork?
- Suspend judgment until you have all the necessary data?
- Support your views with evidence (e.g., principles and research)?
- Evaluate the credibility of sources you use to justify your beliefs?
- Differentiate among facts, opinions, and inferences?
- Distinguish relevant from irrelevant data and important from trivial data?
- Ask for clarification when you don't understand?
- Use knowledge from one subject, discipline, or experience to shed light on other situations?
- Turn mistakes into learning opportunities by determining what went wrong and by thinking of ways to avoid that mistake in the future?
- Fight the tendency to believe that you should have all the answers?

Some Definitions of Critical Thinking

Critical thinking is both an attitude and a reasoning process involving several intellectual skills. It is "the art of thinking about your thinking while you're thinking so as to] *what?!* make your thinking more clear, precise, accurate, relevant, consistent, and fair" (Paul, 1988, pp. 2–3). Critical thinking is disciplined, self-directed, rational thinking that supports what we know and makes clear what we don't know. Some other definitions of critical thinking are found in Box 2–2.

BOX 2-2

SOME DEFINITIONS OF CRITICAL THINKING

Critical thinking is:

". . . reflective reasonable thinking that is focused on deciding what to believe or do" (Ennis, 1962).

". . . a rational response to questions that cannot be answered definitively and for which all the relevant information may not be available . . . an investigation whose purpose is to explore a situation, phenomenon, question, or problem to arrive at a hypothesis or conclusion about it that integrates all available information and that can therefore be convincingly justified" (Kurfiss, 1988, p. 2).

". . . the skill and propensity to engage in an activity with reflective skepticism" (McPeck, 1981).

". . . skillful, responsible thinking that facilitates good judgment because it (1) relies on criteria, (2) is self-correcting, and (3) is sensitive to context" (Lipman, 1988).

". . . the intellectually disciplined process actively and skillfully conceptualizing, applying, analyzing, synthesizing, and/or evaluating information gathered from, or generated by, observation, experience, reflection, reasoning, or communication, as a guide to belief and action . . ." (Scriven & Paul, 1987).

". . . that mode of thinking – about any subject, content, or problem – in which the thinker improves the quality of his or her thinking by skillfully taking charge of the structures inherent in thinking and imposing intellectual standards upon them" (Paul & Elder, 2001).

". . . involv[es] the ability to explore a problem, question, or situation; integrate all the available information about it; arrive at a solution or hypothesis; and justify one's position" (Warnick & Inch, 1994, p. 11).

". . . thinking that attempts to arrive at a judgment only after honestly evaluating alternatives with respect to available evidence and arguments" (Hatcher & Spencer, 2000).

". . . an attitude of inquiry involving the use of facts, principles, theories, abstractions, deductions, interpretations, and analysis of arguments" (paraphrased from Mathews & Gaul, 1979).

". . . both a philosophical orientation toward thinking and a cognitive process characterized by reasoned judgment and reflective thinking. Critical thinking is predicated on an intellectual disposition toward challenging accepted visions of truth and an openness to identifying new possibilities and explanations" (Jones & Brown, 1993, p. 72).

Characteristics of Critical Thinking

As you might expect of such a complex process, there is no single, simple definition that explains critical thinking. However, it has some characteristics that will help you to know when it is taking place.

- **Critical thinking is rational and reasonable.** This means that the thinking is based on reasons rather than prejudice, preferences, self-interest, or fears. Suppose you decide to vote for the Republican candidate in an election because your family has always voted for Republicans. That decision is based on preference, prejudice, and, possibly, self-interest. By contrast, suppose you took time to reflect on what the candidate said about the issues in the election and based your choice on that. In that case, even though you might still vote for the Republican, you would be thinking rationally, using facts and observations to draw your conclusions.

- **Critical thinking involves conceptualization.** Conceptualization is the intellectual process of forming a concept. A **concept** is a mental image of reality. It is formed by generalizing an abstract idea from particular instances, and it exists as a symbol (e.g., a word or picture) in the mind. Concepts are ideas about events, objects, and properties, as well as the relationships among them.

  EXAMPLE: By experiencing headaches and minor injuries (e.g., falling down when you were a child), by observing others in pain, and perhaps by reading about pain, you have an abstract idea of pain. "Pain" is not just *this* headache; it applies to many different situations.

  Nurses use concepts about **properties** (the way things are) and **processes** (the way things happen). A property concept, for example, might be about the patient's *anxiety* or whether there is infection in the patient's incision. A process concept might be about *how morphine works in the central nervous system.*

- **Critical thinking requires reflection. Reflection** means to ponder, contemplate, or deliberate something. It takes time and cannot be done during an emergency. Reflective thinking integrates past experiences into the present and explores potential alternatives. In reflection, one considers an array of possibilities and reflects on the merits of each. When reflecting, one draws "if . . . then" conclusions (e.g., *if* you finish reading this chapter now, *then* you will have time to go to a movie later).

- **Critical thinking involves both cognitive (thinking) skills and attitudes (feelings).** To think critically, you must have thinking skills as well as the motivation and desire to use them. Critical thinking skills and attitudes are discussed fully in a later section.

- **Critical thinking involves creative thinking. Creative thinking** means breaking out of established patterns of thinking and approaching situations from new directions. It results in innovative ideas and products. Nurses use creative thinking when they encounter a new client situation or one in which traditional interventions are not effective.

BOX 2–3

CHARACTERISTICS OF CREATIVE THINKERS

- Able to generate ideas rapidly
- Flexible and spontaneous (i.e., able to discard one viewpoint for another or change directions in thinking rapidly and easily)
- Able to provide original solutions to problems
- Prefer complex thought processes to simple and easily understood ones
- Demonstrate independence and self-confidence even when under pressure
- Exhibit distinct individualism

EXAMPLE: Ned, a pediatric nurse, makes a home visit to 8-year-old Emily, who has been breathing shallowly after abdominal surgery. The surgeon has prescribed incentive spirometry breathing treatments, but Emily is frightened by the equipment, and she tires quickly during the treatments. Ned offers Emily a bottle of soap bubbles and a blowing wand, and she is delighted. Ned knows that the respiratory effort in blowing bubbles will promote alveolar expansion and suggests that Emily blow bubbles between incentive spirometry treatments.

Creative thinking creates original ideas by establishing relationships among thoughts and concepts. It involves the ability to break up and transfer a concept to new settings or uses. In the preceding example, Ned transferred a familiar play activity to a new use: breathing treatment. Refer to Box 2–3 for characteristics of creative thinkers.

- **Critical thinking requires knowledge.** Critical thinking does not occur in a vacuum. You will use it to apply a basic core of knowledge to each client situation. Your fund of knowledge affects your ability to use cognitive, interpersonal, and technical skills effectively. For example, if you did not know that normal body temperature is 98.6°F (37°C), you could not make good decisions about a client whose temperature is 102°F (38.9°C). The following section explains what is meant by *nursing knowledge*.

2-2 WHAT DO YOU KNOW?

List six characteristics of critical thinking.

See answer to #2-2 What Do You Know? in Appendix A.

Types of Nursing Knowledge

Five "ways of knowing" make up the basic core of nursing knowledge: nursing science, nursing art, nursing ethics, personal knowledge (Carper, 1978; Chinn & Kramer, 1991), and practice wisdom.

TABLE 2–1 Examples of Nursing Scientific Knowledge

Subject Matter	Purpose	Example
Helping relationships, including verbal and non-verbal communication	To communicate with patients, families, and other health team members	Conveying caring and support to a patient during insertion of a urinary catheter
Effect of sociocultural and developmental factors on client behavior	To choose effective interventions and understand client behaviors	Understanding how a client's religious beliefs influence his cooperation with the treatment plan
Change theory and motivational theory	For effective team functioning	Supervising team members who are performing delegated tasks
Facts and information needed to perform technical and technologic skills	Hands-on, task-oriented skills, often involving direct contact with the client (Done well, they promote patient confidence and successful nursing actions.)	Operating a slide projector when teaching a class about sexually transmitted diseases Keeping bed linens taut and wrinkle free to prevent Impaired Skin Integrity

Nursing Science

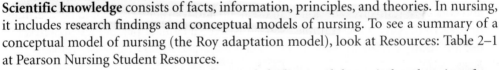

Scientific knowledge consists of facts, information, principles, and theories. In nursing, it includes research findings and conceptual models of nursing. To see a summary of a conceptual model of nursing (the Roy adaptation model), look at Resources: Table 2–1 at Pearson Nursing Student Resources.

Scientific knowledge also consists of research findings and theoretical explanations from other disciplines (e.g., physiology, psychology). Such knowledge is used to describe, explain, and predict. Table 2–1 provides examples of some subjects that make up nursing science.

There is a strong movement in nursing—in all health care—to use evidence-based interventions and treatments. **Evidence-based practice (EBP)** is an approach that uses firm scientific data rather than anecdote, tradition, intuition, or folklore in making decisions about medical and nursing practice. In nursing, it includes blending clinical judgment and expertise with the best available research evidence and patient characteristics and preferences. The goal of EBP is to identify the most effective and cost-efficient treatments for a particular disease, condition, or problem.

Nursing Art

The art of nursing is the way in which nurses apply their knowledge. Nurses express caring through their art; therefore, their art must include attitudes, beliefs, and values. Scientific knowledge is acquired by scientific investigation; in contrast, art includes feelings gained by subjective experience. Scientific knowledge can be verified or explained to others, but nursing art is more difficult to describe. Sensitivity and empathy (the ability to imagine what another person is feeling) are important to this artistic knowing, and they enable the nurse to be aware of a client's perspective and be attentive to verbal and nonverbal cues to his psychological state. This enhanced awareness makes available to the nurse a wider range of interventions.

Nursing Ethics

Ethical knowledge refers to knowledge of professional standards of conduct. It is concerned with matters of obligation, or what ought to be done, and it consists of information about basic moral principles and processes for determining right and wrong actions. Nurses are accountable to clients and to each other for the ethical performance of their work. A **professional code of ethics** is a formal set of written statements reflecting the goals and values of the profession. Formal codes define professional expectations and provide a framework for making ethical decisions. Appendix B, the American Nurses Association's *Code of Ethics for Nurses* (2001), is an example of a formal code of ethics for nurses.

The informal ethics of a profession are based on **conventional moral principles**—unwritten values that are widely held in a profession, expressed in practice, and enforced by rewards and sanctions (e.g., the approval or disapproval of fellow professionals). The following conventional moral principles of nursing are rooted in nurses' more general views of morality, their experiences, and the history of the profession. Nurses should:

- be competent.
- have patient good as their primary concern.
- be loyal to each other.
- not use their position to exploit patients (Jameton, 1984, p. 73).

2-1 THINK & REFLECT!

For each of the conventional moral principles above, write an example to illustrate how a nurse might demonstrate the principle. Compare your answers with those of a peer.

See suggested responses to #2-1 Think & Reflect! in Appendix A.

Personal Knowledge

Personal knowledge is about knowing and actualizing one's self. It involves knowing self in relation to another human being and interacting on a person-to-person rather than a role-to-role basis. This kind of knowledge enables nurses to approach patients as people rather than objects and to establish therapeutic relationships. Highly developed self-awareness and self-knowledge, along with a good self-concept, enable you to be more attuned to your patients. The "Critical Thinking Practice" in Chapter 1 of Pearson Nursing Student Resources is an example of developing self-knowledge.

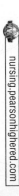

Practice Wisdom

Practice wisdom is acquired from intuition, tradition, authority, trial and error, and clinical experience (Ziegler et al., 1986). It provides the basis for much of the nursing care that is given. As nursing develops a broader, research-based body of knowledge, nurses will come to depend less on practice wisdom. Meanwhile, you should refine and use your critical thinking skills to evaluate interventions that are based on practice wisdom and continue to seek new scientific and ethical knowledge as it becomes available.

Take-away point: The five types of nursing knowledge are nursing science, nursing art, nursing ethics, personal knowledge, and practice wisdom.

Critical Thinking Attitudes

Take-away point: Attitudes and character profoundly influence the ways in which people use their thinking skills

---

Without a critical attitude, it is easy to use thinking skills to justify prejudice, narrow-mindedness, and intellectual arrogance. Richard Paul, an expert in the area of critical thinking, identifies several interdependent traits of mind (attitudes) essential to high-level critical thinking (Paul, 1990). Progress with one attitude invariably leads to progress in others. For example, as you begin to fairly examine ideas or viewpoints toward which you have strong negative emotions (intellectual courage), you will become more aware of the limits of your knowledge (intellectual humility).

Independent Thinking

Critical thinkers think for themselves. They do not passively accept the beliefs of others or simply go along with the crowd. People acquire many beliefs as children because they are rewarded for them or because they do not question, not because they have rational reasons for believing. As they mature and learn, critical thinkers examine and analyze their beliefs, holding those they can rationally support and rejecting those they cannot.

Independent thinking does not mean ignoring what others think and doing whatever you please. It means that critical thinkers consider a wide range of ideas, learn from them, and then make their own judgments about them. Because they will not accept or reject a belief they do not understand, critical thinkers are not easily manipulated. Nurses must be willing to challenge orders and rituals that have no rational support.

EXAMPLE: Nurses traditionally wore white, starched caps in order to prevent hair and hair-borne contaminants from getting on patients and equipment. However, those head coverings evolved into small caps perched on the top of the head. Eventually, most nurses and institutions gave up the caps when they realized they no longer served the original purpose.

Intellectual Humility

Intellectual humility means being aware of the limits of your knowledge and realizing that the mind can be self-deceptive. Critical thinkers are not afraid to admit that they don't know. Admitting lack of knowledge or skill can enable you to grow professionally.

> **EXAMPLE:** A nurse has just begun working on a dialysis unit. He feels insecure and unsure about how to proceed. He requests a meeting with the nurse manager to discuss his strengths and areas of inexperience and to develop a plan for gaining the needed knowledge and skills. Admitting insecurity and requesting help enables the nurse to get support and learn unit policies and procedures rapidly.

Intellectual humility also means rethinking conclusions in light of new knowledge. In the 1960s, for example, physicians and nurses believed that a client recovering from a myocardial infarction (heart attack) should stay on complete bed rest for 2 or 3 days, which meant using a bedpan for elimination. Research later demonstrated that bed rest was not necessary and that using a bedpan was actually more stressful than using a bedside commode. You should assume that you will continue to learn something new or that new evidence may be discovered that will change currently accepted knowledge.

Intellectual Courage

An attitude of intellectual courage means being willing to consider and examine fairly your own beliefs and the views of others, especially those to which you may have strongly negative reactions. This type of courage comes from recognizing that beliefs are sometimes false or misleading and that ideas considered dangerous or absurd are sometimes rationally justified. Inevitably, after carefully examining such ideas, you will come to see some truth in those you considered wrong and some questionable elements in the ideas you so strongly believed to be true. You need courage to be true to your thinking in such cases, especially if social penalties for nonconformity are severe.

> **EXAMPLE:** Evelyn is a nurse in a community where there is prejudice toward homosexuality and acquired immune deficiency syndrome (AIDS). Her friends believe that the homosexual lifestyle is wrong and that AIDS is a punishment. In caring for clients with AIDS, Evelyn learns to view them as individuals rather than labeling and condemning them. Because some of her friends have difficulty accepting her view, Evelyn risks losing them. She needs courage to stand up for what she knows to be right.

New ideas may cause discomfort, and old beliefs can provide a sense of security. Therefore, a lack of courage can cause people to become resistant to change. Nurses need intellectual courage to deal with the constant changes in their practice environments.

Intellectual Empathy

Intellectual empathy is the ability to imagine yourself in the place of others so you can understand them and their actions and beliefs. It is easy to misinterpret the words or actions of a person from a different cultural, religious, or socioeconomic background, and it requires imagination to understand the feelings of a person experiencing a situation that you have not experienced yourself.

> **EXAMPLE:** Ginny Yamamura has cancer. Her husband does not wish her to know her diagnosis. Dave Glen, their nurse, believes that the patient has a right to know, and his first reaction is irritation toward Mr. Yamamura. However, as he begins to reflect on what to do, Dave thinks, "I wonder why Mr. Yamamura has made that decision. What is their relationship like? What are his views about marriage, caring, and the right to know? What was his reasoning?"

Intellectual empathy also requires the ability to reconstruct the viewpoints and reasoning of others and to reason from their viewpoints. People frequently make the mistake of believing that the way they see things is the way things really are.

Intellectual Integrity

Intellectual integrity means being consistent in the thinking standards you apply (e.g., clarity, accuracy, completeness)—holding yourself to the same rigorous standards of proof to which you hold others. By nature, people are inconsistent. For example, if people are not thinking critically, they tend to overrate their own ideas and the ideas of those who like them and judge more harshly the ideas of those who dislike them. Knowing this, critical thinkers will question their own reasoning as quickly and thoroughly as they will challenge the reasoning of others. Critical thinkers honestly admit inconsistencies and error in their own thoughts and actions.

Intellectual Perseverance

Intellectual perseverance is a sense of the need to struggle with confusion and unsettled questions over an extended period of time to achieve understanding and insight. For nurses, this means looking for the most effective solutions to patient problems and not settling for the easy, obvious, or routine. Perseverance enables you to sort out issues despite difficulties even when others are opposed to your search. Important questions tend to be complex, confusing, and frustrating; therefore, they may require a great deal of thought and research. Critical thinkers resist the temptation to find a quick, easy answer.

Intellectual Curiosity

Intellectual curiosity is an attitude of inquiry. It means having a mind filled with questions: Why do we believe this? What causes that? How does that work? Does it have to be this way? Could something else work? What would happen if we did it another way? Who says this is so? Critical thinkers examine statements to see if they are true or valid rather than blindly accepting them. In response to a claim such as, "Fords are better than Chevrolets," a critical thinker might ask: (a) What do you mean by "better than"? Better in what ways? and (b) What information do you have to show that this is so? Questioners tend to challenge the status quo and remove the comfort of habit, so some people see them as dangerous. But far more dangerous are people or disciplines who are in a "thinking rut," not even realizing that their old beliefs and practices need to be reexamined (e.g., "This is how we do it here" or "Everyone knows this is the best way").

Faith in Reason

Faith in reason implies that people can and should learn to think logically for themselves despite the natural tendencies of the mind to do otherwise. Critical thinkers believe that well-reasoned thinking leads to trustworthy conclusions. Therefore, they have confidence in the reasoning process and use logic to examine emotion-laden arguments. Critical thinkers develop skill in both **inductive reasoning** (forming generalizations from a set of facts or observations) and **deductive reasoning** (starting with a generalization and moving to specific facts or conclusions that it suggests). The confident thinker is not afraid of disagreement and, indeed, is concerned when all agree too quickly. Reasoning is discussed in more detail later in this chapter.

Fair-mindedness

Fair-mindedness involves making impartial judgments. It means treating all viewpoints alike without favoring your own feelings or vested interests or those of your friends, community, or nation. Fair-minded thinkers understand that their personal biases or social pressures and customs could unduly affect their thinking. They actively examine their own biases and bring them to awareness each time they think or make a decision.

> **EXAMPLE:** A nurse spends a great deal of time trying to teach a diabetic client about his diet. The nurse is mystified when the client seems uninterested and fails to follow her advice. The nurse's egocentric tendency to assume that all clients are motivated and interested in preventive care (just because the nurse is) results in inaccurate assessment of the client's desire to learn. Both the nurse's and the client's time are wasted.

Interest in Exploring Thoughts and Feelings

Although we distinguish between thought and feeling in an effort to understand them, in reality they are inseparable. The critical thinker knows that emotions can influence thinking and that all thought creates some level of feeling. The feelings you have in response to a situation would be different if you had a different understanding of the situation.

> **EXAMPLE:** Todd's nursing instructor assigned him to care for a patient who required very little physical care. Todd was eager to use some of his newly learned psychomotor skills, so he was disappointed and angry. His instructor explained that this was an opportunity for Todd to concentrate on communicating with the patient and to focus on identifying and meeting the client's needs rather than his own need to practice skills. As Todd's understanding (thoughts) of the situation

BOX 2–4

DEALING WITH NEGATIVE EMOTIONS

To deal with strong, negative emotion, try these suggestions:

- Limit action for a while to avoid making hasty conclusions and impulsive decisions.
- Discuss negative feelings with a trusted peer or friend.
- Work off some of the energy generated by the emotion (e.g., by walking or exercising).
- Reflect on the situation and determine whether your emotional response was appropriate. After the strong emotion has moderated, you can then objectively move toward needed conclusions or make required decisions.

changed, so did his feelings. He was still disappointed that he would not have a chance to give an injection, but he was no longer angry.

Nurses need to identify, examine, and control or modify feelings that interfere with good thinking. Box 2–4 provides some suggestions for dealing with negative emotions.

2-3 WHAT DO YOU KNOW?

List and define at least five critical thinking attitudes.

See answer to #2-3 What Do You Know? in Appendix A.

2-2 THINK & REFLECT!

1. Which of the critical thinking attitudes do you believe to be your greatest strength? Explain your reasoning.
2. Which of the critical thinking attitudes do you most need to improve? Why do you think this?

See suggested responses to #2-2 Think & Reflect! in Appendix A.

Critical Thinking Skills

Cognition is the act of knowing. **Thinking** is an active, organized, purposeful mental process that links ideas together by making logical connections among perceptions, beliefs, knowledge, judgments, and feelings. **Cognitive critical thinking skills** are the intellectual activities used in complex thinking processes such as critical analysis, problem solving, and decision making. For example, when solving problems (*complex process*), nurses make inferences, differentiate facts from opinions, and evaluate the credibility of information sources (*cognitive critical thinking skills*). This text addresses only those

BOX 2-5

COGNITIVE CRITICAL THINKING SKILLS

Using Language

Using language precisely
Using critical thinking vocabulary

Perceiving

Avoiding selective perception
Recognizing differences in perception

Believing and Knowing

Distinguishing facts from interpretations
Supporting facts, opinions, beliefs, and preferences

Clarifying

Questioning to clarify meaning of words and phrases
Questioning to clarify issues, beliefs, and points of view

Comparing

Noting similarities and differences
Classifying
Comparing and contrasting ideals and actual practice
Transferring insights to new contexts

Judging and Evaluating

Providing evidence to support judgments
Developing evaluation criteria

Reasoning

Recognizing assumptions
Distinguishing between relevant and irrelevant data
Evaluating sources of information
Generating and evaluating solutions
Exploring implications, consequences, advantages, and disadvantages

skills most important for nurses. Refer to Box 2–5 for a list of cognitive skills covered in this section.

Although we study them separately, critical thinking skills are not used one at a time. They overlap, in that using one skill may require the use of others. For example, when *making an inference*, one would need to use the skills of *identifying relevant data* and *classifying (clustering) data*.

Using Language

You use language to understand your thinking and to communicate your thoughts. Improving your use of language also improves your ability to think and make sense of things. Critical thinkers avoid general, vague, and nonspecific descriptions such as the following, given at a change-of-shift report:

> Mr. Li had a *good* night.
>
> Susan is taking fluids and *tolerating them well.*
>
> Ms. Froelich ambulated *with no difficulty.*

Because of the vague wording, one nurse might think Mr. Li's "good night" means that he slept well. Another might think it meant he had very little pain. The nurse should have said, "Mr. Li slept from 10:00 P.M. until 6:00 A.M. and reports that he feels rested."

You should also avoid clichés (e.g., "haste makes waste"), slogans (e.g., "healthcare is a right"), jargon, and euphemisms. **Jargon** consists of expressions and technical terms that are understood by a particular group (e.g., nurses) but not by the general public; for example, "I'm giving you some *IV meds* because of your *elevated WBC*" or "I'm going to take your *vital signs.*" A **euphemism** is a supposedly more pleasant and less objectionable term that is substituted for a more direct or blunt expression. Euphemisms can be dangerous when they are used to create misperceptions. For example, an obese woman who describes herself as "pleasingly plump" may avoid dealing with the weight problem that is contributing to her diabetes and hypertension.

Take-away point: Avoid using clichés, euphemisms, and jargon.

Take-away point: Make your language more precise by asking: Who? What? When? How? Where? Why?

2-3 THINK & REFLECT!

What do you think about the following definitions? Are they too broad, too narrow, or just right? Explain your answer.
1. A nurse is a professional.
2. A nurse is a professional woman who works in a hospital.

See suggested responses to #2-3 Think & Reflect! in Appendix A.

Perceiving

Perception is the process of using the senses (sight, hearing, smell, touch, and taste) to experience the world. Perception brings sensations into your awareness; it involves three distinct activities:

1. *Selecting* certain sensations to pay attention to
2. *Organizing* these sensations into a design or pattern
3. *Interpreting* what the design or pattern means to you

Avoiding Selective Perception

You cannot possibly attend to all the stimuli that constantly bombard you. Your mind perceives selectively—that is, you unconsciously choose what you will notice and what you will not. Selective perception may cause you to focus on things that support your own ideas and tune out information that does not.

EXAMPLE: Elena believes that fat people are lazy. When an obese nurse on her unit sits to chart, Elena focuses on the fact that the nurse is sitting and thinks, "She is so lazy." Elena fails to notice the many times this nurse has offered to help her with her patients or that the nurse often tidies the medication and supply areas. Elena perceives only evidence that supports her prejudice.

Avoid selective perception by looking for details you haven't noticed before to balance your perceptions. When you notice that you are focusing on negative details, make a conscious effort to look for positive ones and vice versa.

Recognizing Differences in Perceptions

Different points of view are often a result of different perceptions rather than just different lines of reasoning. In the following example, two people have attended a meeting where one nurse consistently spoke in a quiet tone of voice.

Perception A: "What an unassertive woman. She must lack self-esteem."

Perception B: "How reassuring and confident she seems."

Take-away point: Critical thinkers do not assume that what they perceive is what is actually taking place nor that what they heard is what others heard. When you notice that your perception differs from the perception of others, you should examine the way they (and you) have been selecting, organizing, and interpreting sensory information.

2-4 THINK & REFLECT!

Recall an instance when you and a classmate heard a teacher's instructions differently (e.g., perhaps the teacher said to wear lab coats to orientation, but you thought you were supposed to wear your full uniform). Whose perception was inaccurate, and why?

See suggested responses to #2-4 Think & Reflect! in Appendix A.

Believing and Knowing

Beliefs are interpretations, evaluations, conclusions, and predictions about the world that we take to be true. Realizing that beliefs are subject to error, critical thinkers reflect on their beliefs and revise them in light of new information and experiences.

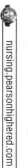

> ### BOX 2–6
>
> #### DISTINGUISHING FACTS FROM INTERPRETATION
>
> To distinguish facts from interpretations, ask the following questions:
> - Is this something that I can observe directly, or would I have to interpret what I see to arrive at this conclusion?
> - Could this be verified in principle? What would I need to do to verify it (e.g., dissect a cadaver, weigh a patient)?
> - Does this description stick to facts, or does it include reasoning and rationale?
> - Is this how *anyone* would describe the situation?

Distinguishing Facts from Interpretations

Take-away point: Statements about beliefs, issues, conclusions, and claims are not statements of fact. They are interpretations.

Facts are statements you can verify through observation and investigation (e.g., the nurse is wearing white shoes). You can check their accuracy. Statements that can be verified in principle are also considered facts. For example, it is a fact that arteries are less distensible than veins. Even though you cannot check it out at the moment, you could verify that statement if you dissected a cadaver. See Box 2–6 for help in distinguishing facts from interpretations.

Inferences are conclusions that are based on factual information but go beyond that information to make statements about something not presently known. If you want to practice making valid inferences, see Critical Thinking Practice: Believing and Knowing, in Chapter 3, at Pearson Nursing Student Resources.

Judgments are evaluations of information that reflect values or other criteria. **Opinions** are beliefs or judgments that may fit the facts or be in error. Consider the following example:

EXAMPLE: Ms. Albert comes to the clinic, where the nurse weighs her. The scale indicates 250 lb.

1. *Fact:* Ms. Albert weighs 250 lb.
2. *Inference:* Ms. Albert consumes more calories than she needs.
3. *Judgment:* Ms. Albert is greedy or has poor self-control.
4. *Opinion:* If someone really wants to lose weight, they can do it.

Statement 1 can be verified by the scale. Statement 2 would also be a fact if the nurse had actually observed Ms. Albert's eating patterns or counted her calories. But in this case, the nurse made an inference based on the fact of Ms. Albert's weight, together with the knowledge that excess calorie intake is the usual cause of obesity. Statement 3 is a judgment reflecting the nurse's value of self-control. For this nurse, that is a negative value judgment. However, not all judgments are negative (e.g., "What a pretty baby!"). Statement 4, an opinion, cannot be observed or "proven." It may or may not be in error.

TABLE 2–2   Supporting Facts and Opinions

Guideline	Example
■ If you state a fact that is not common knowledge or that cannot be easily verified, state where you got your information.	*Common knowledge, no source needed:* "For the average person, an intramuscular injection should be given at a 90-degree angle." *Source of information should be given:* "The average RN is over 40 years old."
■ If you state an opinion or view with which others might disagree, include answers to questions they might ask.	"Critical thinking is important for nurses *because they work in rapidly changing environments.*"
■ If you are not sure whether a statement is a fact or an opinion, treat it and state it as an opinion.	"*In my opinion,* the ventrogluteal site is the safest one for intramuscular injections." (If you can cite references or research, you could treat this statement as a fact.)

Supporting Facts, Opinions, Beliefs, and Preferences

Recall that facts are statements that can be verified through investigation. Some statements may be made in the form of facts but are actually incorrect. For example, if someone says, "Florence Nightingale wrote *Notes on Nursing* in 1959," it sounds as though she is stating a fact. However, Nightingale died in 1856, so that statement is actually an erroneous belief, not a fact.

Take-away point: You should be able to provide support for your facts, beliefs, and opinions when others challenge them (Table 2–2).

A personal preference is merely a statement of something one likes or dislikes (e.g., "I like strawberry ice cream better than chocolate"). You do not need to provide support for your preferences; however, when you express them in the form of opinions (e.g., "Strawberry ice cream is better than chocolate"), you should expect others to challenge them.

Clarifying

Critical thinkers ask questions to clarify and understand complex concepts, ideas, and situations. This helps to keep them from drawing superficial, inaccurate conclusions.

Questioning to Clarify or Analyze the Meaning of Words and Phrases

If you understand a word or concept being used, you should be able to give clear, obvious, concrete examples of it. For example, if someone says, "Students are special people," you could not agree or disagree with them until you clearly understand what they meant by "students" and "special." Concrete examples of "students" might include a child in kindergarten, a nursing student, or a couple taking square-dancing lessons. Concrete examples of "special" might include someone who is different from the group, someone

BOX 2–7

QUESTIONS FOR CLARIFYING

Questions to Clarify the Meaning of Words and Phrases

- What is a clear, concrete example of the concept X?
- Why is this an X?
- What would be an example of X's opposite? Or of something clearly not X?
- Why is this not an X? How is this case different from the clear-cut examples?
- What are some situations in which X would apply?

Questions to Clarify Statements and Conclusions

- Do I understand this issue?
- Did I state it fairly?
- How can we know whether this statement is true or false? What evidence do we need?
- Is there a clearer or more accurate way to word this statement?
- Would others accept this as a fair and accurate statement of the issue?
- What would count as evidence against this statement?
- How did you form that idea (or acquire that belief)? Have you always thought that? If not, why did you change your belief?
- Why do you believe this? What are some reasons that people believe this?
- Are there any exceptions to this view? What would someone say who disagrees with you? How would someone from a different culture see it?
- What are the consequences of this idea? What would have to be done to put this idea into action?
- What are the implications of this idea? If you believe that, wouldn't you also have to believe. . .?

you love, or someone with a disability. See Box 2–7 for questions to help you clarify words and phrases.

Questioning to Clarify Issues, Beliefs, and Points of View

In discussions with others, critical thinkers question and probe to gain deeper understanding. They ask questions not to embarrass others but to learn more about what they think and to evaluate their statements for themselves. See Box 2–7 for questions to help you clarify statements about issues, beliefs, and points of view.

Comparing

To **compare** is to examine similarities and differences among things in the same general category. For example, a nurse might compare and contrast the ways in which clients of different cultures express grief. Although each client might be from a different culture, they are all from the same general category: *people*. Making careful, systematic comparisons improves the quality of your decisions. Comparing also involves classifying things, comparing the ideal with the actual, and transferring your insights to new contexts. If you would like to practice the skill of comparing, see Critical Thinking Practice: Clarifying, Comparing, and Contrasting, in Chapter 5, at Pearson Nursing Student Resources.

Noting Similarities and Differences

Critical thinkers make careful, thorough observations and note significant similarities and differences, realizing that things that seem alike on the surface may be different in important ways.

> **EXAMPLE:** A nurse is caring for two middle-aged male clients with the same medical diagnosis: myocardial infarction (heart attack). Although these clients are similar in age and diagnosis, they are responding very differently to their disease. Mr. Jonassen is experiencing nausea, brought about by severe pain. Mr. Nguyen has no nausea and only mild pain. His main response is anxiety about being away from his business. The nurse recognizes that despite their similarities, they have very different needs.

Classifying

Classifying, or categorizing, is the process of grouping things on the basis of their similarities or common properties. For the most part, you classify things automatically and continuously as you organize and make sense of your experience. For example, the concept "thermometer" represents a type of object that nurses use to measure temperature. In order to determine whether an object is a thermometer, we focus on similarities: (a) it has a scale marked in increments, (b) it has numbers on it that represent degrees of temperature, and (c) it registers temperature changes. So you would classify a variety of instruments as thermometers (e.g., a glass thermometer, an electronic thermometer, a skin probe with a digital readout, a large thermometer that measures room temperature). Classifying also allows you to see how things are different—for example, to see how thermometers are different from other objects with numbers and incremental scales, such as sphygmomanometers or scales for weighing things. Chapter 4 points out some important ways in which nurses classify patient data (e.g., according to nursing theories). The "Critical Thinking Practice" in Chapter 6 of Pearson Nursing Student Resources provides practice in classifying.

Comparing and Contrasting Ideals and Actual Practice

It is important to recognize the gaps between facts and ideals. The more realistic your ideals, the more likely you are to achieve them. Unrealistic ideals, by contrast, may lead to frustration. For example, the statement, "Nurses give holistic care" has appeared so often in the nursing literature that many take it to be a fact. Yet some nurses find that their patient caseload is too heavy for them to attend to anything more than basic physiological and safety needs.

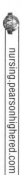

2-5 THINK & REFLECT!

Think about the nurses you have observed and about your own nursing experiences.
- What, exactly, is meant by "holistic" care?
- Do nurses always, or even usually, give holistic care?
- Is holistic care really a statement of what nurses are trying to achieve?
- What problems do nurses have in achieving this ideal?
- Is it realistic to try to achieve this ideal?

See suggested responses to #2-5 Think & Reflect! in Appendix A.

Transferring Insights to New Contexts

By making analogies between situations, critical thinkers are able to transfer insights and information from one situation to another. An **analogy** is a special kind of comparison that points out ways in which things from different categories are similar to each other. For example, people say, "Time is money." Time and money are from completely different categories, but the analogy brings out their similarities. That is, we have only a limited amount of each, both are important, we can save or spend them both, and so on.

Critical thinkers do not compartmentalize their knowledge. They use their understanding of one subject to gain insight into other subjects. For example, to gain understanding about the present status of nurses, you could use insights from the history of nursing, the historical status of women, the sociology of oppressed groups, and the social effects of technology on the labor market and healthcare. Nurses need to connect insights from many subjects (e.g., psychology, sociology, interpersonal communications, physiology, pharmacology, nutrition) in the care of each patient.

Take-away point: As you learn a new principle, you can enrich your understanding of it by applying it to new situations. Think, "What other situation is different but still like this one in some important ways? How would this principle work in that situation?"

Judging and Evaluating

Recall that facts are statements that can be verified and that judgments are evaluations of facts and information that reflect certain criteria, such as our values. Whereas facts and inferences describe what is happening, judgments express your evaluation of what is happening (see "Believing and Knowing" above). **Opinions** are longstanding beliefs that are formed by making judgments over time. In comparison, a judgment can be made more or less "on the spot" and can be a one-time thing.

Providing Evidence to Support Judgments

Disagreements with others are often a result of differences in judgment rather than differences in perceptions, definition of terms, or lack of clarity. Not all judgments are equally good. Their credibility depends on the criteria used to make them and the evidence given to support the criteria. When your judgment differs from someone else's, the following is an intelligent approach to use:

1. Make explicit the criteria, standards, or values used as the basis for the judgments.
2. Try to establish the reasons that justify these criteria.

For example, a nursing instructor's judgment, "That was a good injection" is based on the criteria that: (a) sterile technique is used, (b) the needle is inserted quickly at a 90-degree angle, (c) the student aspirates before injecting the medication, and so forth. These criteria are justified because they can be found in current nursing literature; they are also backed by the germ theory of disease and knowledge of anatomy.

Developing Evaluation Criteria

Evaluation, like judgment, is the process of determining the value or worth of something. Unlike judgment, evaluation requires that you first identify the criteria or standards to be used and then decide to what extent the thing you are examining meets those standards. Evaluation criteria should be: (a) made explicit, (b) stated clearly, and (c) applied consistently. Consider the following example:

Judgment: I really like that music.

Evaluation: I like this music because it has a beautiful melody and meaningful lyrics. The rhythm keeps the song moving along at an interesting pace.

Although the evaluation criteria are not explicit (the example does not say, "These are the criteria being used"), the evaluation statements imply that they included considerations of melody, lyrics, rhythm, and the ability of the music to capture one's attention. Undoubtedly, your instructors have openly stated the criteria they use to evaluate your clinical performance. Nurses develop evaluation criteria in the form of patient outcomes, or goals, that they intend to achieve with their nursing interventions. Chapter 6 discusses outcome (evaluation criteria) development in detail. Chapter 9 discusses evaluation as it is used in the nursing process.

Reasoning

Reasoning is logical thinking that links thoughts together in meaningful ways. Reasoning is used in scientific inquiry, in examining controversial issues, and in problem solving (e.g., in the nursing process). When reasons are given to provide support for a conclusion or position, it is called **argument**. Although they sometimes sound the same, arguments are different from explanations. The goal of an argument is to show *that* something is true; the goal of an **explanation** is to show *why* something is true.

EXAMPLE:

Argument: Penicillin is the drug of choice for many infections because of its low cost and low toxicity and its effectiveness against many gram-positive bacteria.

Explanation: Penicillin is effective against a variety of gram-positive bacteria because it interferes with cell wall formation, making the bacterium susceptible to destruction by osmotic processes and autolysis.

Nurses use both inductive and deductive reasoning. **Inductive reasoning** begins with specific details and facts and uses them to arrive at conclusions and generalizations.

EXAMPLE: If you observe in a large number of cases that ice melts when it is warmed to 32°F (0°C), you will reason that all ice melts at 32°F (0°C).

EXAMPLE: A patient complains of soreness at an intravenous (IV) site. The nurse observes that the site is cool, pale, and swollen and that the IV is not running. Having observed similar symptoms in many patients, the nurse reasons that the IV is infiltrated.

In good inductive arguments, the conclusion *probably* follows from the reasons, but one can never be absolutely certain that it will. Inductive arguments can be strong or weak, depending on the number of observations made and on the quality of the reasons given. Think about the difference in the certainty of the conclusions in the two preceding examples. When scientific induction leads to conclusions that are almost invariably true (e.g., ice melts at 32°F), those conclusions can then be used as the major premises for deductive reasoning.

Deductive reasoning begins with a major theory, generalization, fact, or major premise that generates specific details and predictions. Reasoning is from the universal to the particular—that what is true of a class of things is true of each member of that class.

EXAMPLE:

Fact (major premise): All ice melts at 32°F (0°C).

Fact (minor premise): It is warmer than 32°F (0°C) in this room.

Conclusion (correct): The ice in the patient's water pitcher will melt.

In deductive reasoning, if the facts in the premises are true, then the conclusion must be true. However, we sometimes assume that generalizations (major premises) are true when they might not be. The following is an example of wrongly assuming the truth of a major premise (the first statement).

EXAMPLE:

Fact (major premise): All infections cause fever.

Fact (minor premise): Mr. Annas's temperature is 102°F (a fever).

Conclusion (incorrect): Mr. Annas has an infection.

The major premise is incorrect in the preceding example because not all infections produce fever, although most do. In addition, factors other than infection can produce fever (e.g., dehydration, heat prostration). A reasoning error can also be made if the *minor premise* (the second statement in the example) is incorrect. If Mr. Annas had a hot drink before his temperature was taken or if the thermometer was calibrated incorrectly, the reading of 102°F (38.9°C) would not reflect his true body temperature, and the conclusion that he has an infection would again be in error.

Recognizing Assumptions

An **assumption** is an idea or concept that you take for granted (e.g., people once assumed the world was flat). Assumptions can be true or false. In the preceding example, you would incorrectly conclude that Mr. Annas has an infection if you incorrectly assumed that all infections cause fever. Of course, some assumptions are necessary for efficient performance of daily activities. For example, when you cross the street in a pedestrian crosswalk, you assume the cars will stop for you. When you take a patient's blood pressure, you assume the apparatus works properly. When you give medications, you assume the capsule marked "aspirin" is actually aspirin. These are all reasonable assumptions.

Nurses must recognize and examine their assumptions about patients and patient data. It is easy to recognize the assumptions hidden in some statements. "Have you stopped beating your wife?" assumes, first, that the person had a wife, and second, that he has beaten his wife. A more subtle assumption is hidden in this statement about a client: "If he wanted to get well, he would keep his clinic appointments." This statement assumes (a) that the client has transportation, (b) that he is capable of remembering the appointment, (c) that the client has had no emergency that prevented him from keeping his appointment, and (d) that keeping his appointments will actually help him to get well.

2-6 THINK & REFLECT!

1. What are some assumptions nurses commonly make about patients (e.g., patients are obligated to follow doctors' orders and to tell the truth when questioned about their symptoms)?
2. What are some assumptions you have about nurses (e.g., that they know what is best for patients; that they always chart accurate data)?

Compare your assumptions with those of another student. How are they alike or different? Are they well-founded assumptions or are they in error?

See suggested responses to #2-6 Think & Reflect! in Appendix A.

Distinguishing Between Relevant and Irrelevant Data

When making clinical judgments, nurses sift through a great deal of data. But even data that are confirmed and verified (i.e., *facts,* as defined earlier in this chapter), are useful only if they are relevant. Critical thinkers focus on relevant facts—that is, they stick to the point. **Relevant** statements or data are those that pertain to the issue at hand. Relevant data are facts that are important or significant. **Irrelevant** factors have nothing to do with the issue (problem, argument, and so forth), or they might be related but unimportant. The "Critical Thinking Practice" at the end of Chapter 7 will help you to differentiate between relevant and irrelevant data.

Evaluating Sources of Information

Critical thinkers thoughtfully examine others' statements before accepting them, and they provide credible information to support their own positions. When the source of information is something other than direct observation, they evaluate the credibility of the source. Box Box 2–8 provides questions to use when evaluating the credibility of sources. However, even when a credible expert provides information, it is often wise to seek the opinion of at least a second expert. Give more weight to information sources that:

- Have a good track record.
- Are in a position to know.
- Have a reputation for honesty.
- Have a reputation for consistency.
- Do not have a vested interest in the issue at hand.

Generating and Evaluating Solutions

When presented with a problem, critical thinkers do not cast about wildly for solutions nor do they accept the first solution that comes to mind. Instead, they take time to formulate problems carefully, ensuring that their problem statements are clear, accurate, and fair. They also identify and examine the causes of the problem. As you will see in Chapter 4, nurses do these things when they make nursing diagnoses.

Because problems usually do not come with ready-made solutions, nurses need creative thinking, including flexibility and imagination, to generate and evaluate possible solutions (e.g., nursing actions). For nurses, problem solving often means identifying or choosing the best nursing interventions. Chapter 7, "Planning: Interventions," addresses that in more detail. The following questions may be useful:

- Do I have all the relevant information?
- What solutions have previously been used for this problem? For similar problems?

BOX 2-8

QUESTIONS FOR EVALUATING CREDIBILITY OF INFORMATION SOURCES

- Is this person in a position to know?
- Could the source have directly seen or heard or did he have to reason his conclusion?
- Was the source able to make accurate observations?
- What is the person's interest in the issue? Does the person have anything to gain?
- What is the person's purpose for providing the information?
- What knowledge or experience would a person need to be an expert in this area? Does this person have those credentials?
- Has this source been reliable in the past?
- Who paid for the work that went into gathering the information?

- What makes some solutions better than others? What criteria should I use in deciding which solution is best?
- What solutions will solve the problem? What solutions will address the *cause* of the problem?
- Is this solution realistic?

Exploring Implications, Consequences, Advantages, and Disadvantages

It is certainly important to evaluate data and facts. However, when making decisions about problem solutions, policies, or actions (e.g., nursing interventions), you must consider other factors as well. It is especially important to consider implications and consequences. For example, if you believe in a policy of capital punishment, the *implication* is that you believe killing is acceptable, at least in some situations. If the belief in capital punishment is actually translated into law, then one *consequence* is that some people will be killed, albeit legally. To **imply** something is to express it indirectly, suggesting it without stating it. To accept a statement is to accept its implications or the logical connection between one statement and another (i.e., if X is true, then it follows that Y must be true). Words such as *therefore, so,* and *then* point to the logical connection between two statements and may be a clue that an implication is present. For example, "*If* Madeline is a registered nurse, *then* she uses the nursing process."

Consequences are different from implications in that they are more action oriented. A **consequence** is the effect or result that is caused by something (i.e., if one acts on X, then Y will occur). For example, "*If* a nurse gives morphine, *then* the client will experience pain relief" or "The nurse administered morphine; *therefore,* the client experienced pain relief." Refer to Box 2–9 for questions to help you explore possible consequences of nursing interventions. Chapter 7, "Planning: Interventions," further discusses choosing nursing interventions.

BOX 2-9

QUESTIONS FOR EXPLORING CONSEQUENCES

- What effect will this action probably have? (e.g., What therapeutic effect will this medication have? What undesirable side effects?)
- Are there other possible actions? What would their effects be?
- Has this worked in the past? What happened?
- What are the advantages and disadvantages of this action?
- If this action is implemented, who will be affected, and what will those effects be?
- Does the action (or problem solution) take into account everyone's best interests?

Complex Intellectual Activities

This chapter has presented individual critical thinking attitudes and skills one at a time to help you understand them. However, they overlap a great deal, and they are not used individually or in isolation. The cognitive skills are actually used in different combinations as a part of more complex intellectual processes. For example, when nurses are solving problems (a complex activity), they use the individual skills of making inferences, differentiating facts from opinions, and evaluating the credibility of information sources.

The complex thinking processes overlap, just as the individual skills do (e.g., recall from Chapter 1 that nursing process is related to problem solving and critical thinking), and even the experts do not always agree on how to define them. This section discusses the following terms and their relationship to critical thinking: critical analysis, problem solving, nursing process, clinical reasoning, decision making, clinical judgment, and reflective reasoning. Box 2–10 provides a summary of definitions of these terms. Recall

---

BOX 2–10

COMPLEX INTELLECTUAL PROCESSES

Critical thinking	Goal-oriented, purposeful thinking that involves many mental attitudes and skills, such as determining which data are relevant and making inferences. Critical thinking is essential when a problem is ill defined and does not have a single "best" solution.
Problem solving	The mental activity of identifying a problem (unsatisfactory state) and finding a reasonable solution to it. This requires decision making; it may or may not require the use of critical thinking.
Nursing process	A systematic, creative approach to thinking and doing that nurses use to obtain, categorize, and analyze patient data and to plan actions to meet patient needs. This type of problem-solving process requires the use of decision making, clinical judgment, and a variety of critical thinking skills.
Decision making	The process of choosing the best action to take—the action most likely to produce the desired outcome. It involves deliberation, judgment, and choice. Decisions must be made whenever there are mutually exclusive choices but not necessarily problems.
Clinical reasoning	Reasoning is logical thinking that links thoughts together in meaningful ways. Clinical reasoning is reflective, concurrent, and creative thinking about patients and patient care—the kind of reasoning used in the nursing process.
Reflection or reflective judgment	A kind of critical thinking that considers a broad array of possibilities and reflects on the merits of each in a given situation. Reflection is essential when a problem is complex and has no simple, "correct" solution.
Clinical judgment	Judgment is the use of values or other criteria to evaluate or draw conclusions about information. Clinical judgments are conclusions and opinions about patients' health, drawn from patient data. They may or may not be made using critical thinking.
Analysis or critical analysis	Analysis is a critical thinking skill. It is the process of breaking material down into component parts and identifying the relationships among them. Critical analysis is the questioning applied to a situation or idea to determine essential information and ideas and discard superfluous information and ideas. Critical thinking more than just analysis.

that critical thinking is careful, reflective, goal-oriented, purposeful thinking that involves a variety of mental attitudes and cognitive skills. It may be helpful to think of critical thinking as a broad umbrella for the complex thinking processes, all of which tend to be purposeful and deliberate.

Problem solving is the mental activity of identifying a problem (unsatisfactory state) and then planning and finding a reasonable solution to it. There are various methods of problem solving, including the *nursing process,* trial and error, and the scientific method. Depending on the nature of the problem, problem solving may or may not require the use of *critical thinking.* Many problems are well structured and have only a few reasonable answers, possibly only one. Such problems (e.g., simple math problems such as 2 + 2 = ?) do not require critical thinking. Problem solving requires the use of *decision making.*

Nursing process is a systematic, creative approach to thinking and doing that nurses use to obtain, categorize, and analyze patient data and to plan actions to meet a patient's needs. It is a type of *problem-solving* process requiring the use of *decision making, clinical judgment,* and a variety of *critical thinking skills.* It provides the framework for the type of critical thinking that nurses do.

Decision making is the process of choosing the best action to take—the action most likely to produce the desired outcome. It involves deliberation, judgment, and choice. Decision making is important in the *problem-solving* process and in all phases of the *nursing process,* but not all decisions involve problem solving. For example, nurses make value decisions (e.g., to keep client information confidential) and time management decisions (e.g., taking clean linens to the client's room at the same time as the medication in order to save steps). Decisions must be made whenever there are mutually exclusive choices. For example, when faced with several patients' needs at one time, the nurse decides which patient to assist first. *Critical thinking* improves decision making by providing a "broader menu of options with which to analyze problems and make decisions" (Adams, 1999, p. 111).

Clinical reasoning is reflective, concurrent, and creative thinking about patients and patient care—the kind of reasoning used in the *nursing process.* Recall that *reasoning* is logical thinking that links thoughts together in meaningful ways. Reasoning is used in scientific inquiry, in examining controversial issues, and in *problem solving,* as well as in clinical reasoning.

Reflection, or **reflective judgment,** is usually used to describe a kind of reasoning that considers a broad array of possibilities and reflects on the merits of each in a given situation. It is a type of *critical thinking* and is used by some experts to describe critical thinking (i.e., they would say that critical thinking *is* reflective reasoning). Reflection is useful in *decision making* and *problem solving,* and it is essential when the problem is complex and has no simple, "correct" solution. Nurses use reflective judgment when dealing with moral conflict and ethical problems, for example.

Clinical judgments are conclusions and opinions about patients' health, drawn from patient data. Clinical judgment is similar to *decision making* in that nurses make judgments (as well as decisions) about the meaning of patient data and about nursing actions that should be taken on the patient's behalf. Clinical judgments are made as a part of the *nursing process.*

Judging itself is a *critical thinking skill*, and other thinking skills are essential for making sound judgments. However, good clinical judgments can be made without using critical thinking skills. For example, a patient might complain of a dry mouth, and the nurse might respond correctly by offering a sip of water—without thinking critically. Using *critical thinking*, the nurse would assess the oral cavity, evaluate skin turgor and temperature, evaluate input and output, review the patient's medications and treatments, and so forth. This assessment would have a goal of identifying the source of the problem (dry mouth) and planning an intervention on that basis—an intervention that could include a sip of water. *Critical thinking skills* are used to expand and "flesh out" the nursing process (Adams, 1999, p. 112).

Analysis is the cognitive process of breaking material down into component parts and identifying the relationships among them (e.g., nurses use analysis to examine and interpret each piece of patient data to identify deviations from normal). **Critical analysis** is used to determine which information or ideas are essential in a situation. Analysis is used in *problem solving, decision making,* and *clinical judgment.* Although analysis is a critical thinking skill, *critical thinking* goes beyond analysis to focus on what to believe or what actions to take.

2-7 THINK & REFLECT!

1. Write a paragraph describing a problem you have solved recently. Identify the problem-solving method you used.
2. Describe a decision you made in the clinical setting that was *not* made for the purpose of solving a problem.

See suggested responses to #2-7 Think & Reflect! in Appendix A.

Standards of Reasoning

Recall that critical thinking is, in part, "thinking about your thinking" (*metacognition*). You should apply a basic set of intellectual standards whenever you are checking the quality of your thinking. That is, you should check your thinking for clarity, accuracy, precision, relevance, depth, breadth, and logic. Table 2–3 explains these intellectual standards. Subsequent chapters will show you how to apply these standards in each phase of the nursing process.

Critical Thinking and Nursing Process

Take-away point: Critical thinking and the nursing process are interdependent, but not identical.

Nurses function effectively some part of every day without thinking critically. Many decisions are based on habit, with little thinking involved (e.g., selecting what clothes to wear, choosing which route to take to work, and deciding what to eat for lunch).

TABLE 2-3   Standards of Reasoning

Standard	Evaluative Questions	Examples
Clarity—A statement must be clear in order to know whether it is accurate, relevant, and so on.	▪ Could you give an example? ▪ Can you express that point another way?	*Unclear:* After a clinic visit, the nurse instructs a parent to call the primary care provider if the child's fever recurs. *Clearer:* The nurse instructs the parent how often to check the temperature and tells her the acceptable range for a child's temperature (e.g., "Call if the temperature is more than 101°F [38.3°C]").
Accuracy—A statement can be clear but not accurate.	▪ Is that really true? ▪ How could you check it?	Most people weigh more than 300 lb (136 kg). (*Clearly stated but inaccurate*)
Precision—A statement can be clear and accurate but not precise.	▪ Could you give more details? ▪ Can you be more exact?	If Jack weighs 350 lb., the statement, "Jack is overweight" is clear and accurate. A *precise* statement would say, "Jack is 200 lb (91 kg) overweight."
Relevance—A statement can be clear, accurate, and precise but not relevant to the issue.	▪ How does that relate to the problem? ▪ How does that help us understand the issue?	Students sometimes think that the amount of effort they put into a course should determine their grade. However, effort does not always measure the quality of a student's learning. When that is so, effort is not relevant to the grade.
Depth—A statement can be clear, accurate, precise, and relevant—but superficial.	▪ How does the statement address the complexities of the situation? ▪ Are you taking into account the problems that statement creates? ▪ Does the statement deal with the most important factors?	The statement "Just say no," which is used to discourage youthful drug use, is clear, accurate, precise, and relevant. Still, it is superficial because it does not deal with the complexities of the issue.
Breadth—A line of reasoning can meet all the other standards, but be one-sided.	▪ Do we need to consider another point of view? ▪ Is there another way to look at this?	An argument from either a liberal or a conservative would get deeply into an issue such as the death penalty or abortion, but it would probably be narrow, presenting only one side of the question—either for or against.
Logic—Reasoning brings various thoughts together in some kind of order. When the thoughts make sense in combination, thinking is logical.	▪ Does this really make sense? ▪ Does the conclusion follow from what was just said (or from the data)? ▪ How can both these "facts" be true?	Someone who states both, "Killing is wrong" and "We should have capital punishment" is being illogical.

Source: Adapted from Paul, R. (1996). Universal intellectual standards. In *Critical thinking workshop handbook.* Dillon Beach, CA: Foundation for Critical Thinking. See http://www.criticalthinking.org.

Psychomotor skills, such as operating a familiar cardiac monitor, involve minimal thinking. But critical thinking is essential to the nursing process. According to the American Nurses Association, the nursing process provides the framework for critical thinking in nursing (2004). Nurses use critical thinking at each stage of the process. In the following discussion, critical thinking skills are shown in italics.

Assessment When assessing, nurses use an *attitude of inquiry* as they *use facts, principles, theories, abstractions, deductions, and interpretations* to gather *patient data and validate* what the patient says with what they observe. They must *make reliable observations* and *distinguish relevant from irrelevant data and important from unimportant data.* They also *organize* and *categorize* the relevant, important data in some useful manner, perhaps according to a theory-based nursing framework. In addition, *they identify missing information and fill in the gaps.*

> **EXAMPLE:** In assessing Mr. Wiley's skin, the nurse notes that it is dry, thin, and inelastic. This is relevant information the nurse uses to diagnose Risk for Impaired Skin Integrity. The nurse also notices a 4-inch contracted scar on Mr. Wiley's lower abdomen. It is obviously an old scar and is now irrelevant to the nursing diagnosis. The nurse also notices that Mr. Wiley, age 50 years, is balding. This information is relevant because it pertains to the topic of skin. However, it is a normal finding and not important in making the nursing diagnosis.

Diagnosis In the diagnosis phase, nurses analyze the data they have categorized to look for patterns and relationships among the cues and draw conclusions about them. Critical thinkers are careful to suspend judgment when they do not have enough data. This is what nurses do when they write a "possible" rather than an "actual" nursing diagnosis. In the following example, there are not enough data to be sure the inference is correct. The nurse should *question the patient to validate the observations.* Even after making a valid diagnosis, a critical thinker *remains open to all possibilities.*

> **EXAMPLE:** The nurse observes that a patient is grimacing and moving about restlessly in bed. The nurse's knowledge and previous experience suggest that these symptoms mean the client is in pain. This is only an *inference* and, until verified, is neither a fact nor a nursing diagnosis.

Planning: Outcomes In this phase, nurses *use reasonable, reflective thinking that is focused on deciding what to believe or do.* They *use knowledge* and reasoning skills (e.g., *forming valid generalizations and explanations*) to *predict patient responses* and *develop evaluative criteria (i.e., patient outcomes).* They use the outcomes developed in this stage as criteria for evaluating the client's progress and the success of the nursing actions.

Planning: Interventions Nurses make predictions and form valid generalizations and explanations when they plan and implement creative interventions. They make interdisciplinary connections when they use their knowledge of subjects such as physiology, psychology, and sociology to choose appropriate nursing actions and provide rationales for them. Finally, nurses hypothesize that certain nursing interventions will relieve the patient's problem or help achieve the stated health goals.

Implementation This is when nurses apply knowledge and principles from nursing and related courses to each specific patient-care situation. The ability to apply, not simply memorize, principles is a mark of critical thinking.

> **EXAMPLE:** A nursing student has learned the principles "heat is lost through evaporation" and "the normal newborn is at risk for cold stress." Although the student has never bathed a newborn and has not memorized the exact steps for doing so, she prevents cold stress by uncovering only the parts she is bathing and by drying the infant well.

Carrying out the nursing orders in the implementation phase can be compared to *hypothesis testing* in the scientific method. The nursing orders must be translated into action (or tested) in order to decide whether they were successful.

Evaluation When evaluating, nurses utilize *criterion-based evaluation* when they use new observations to determine whether patient goals have been met. They *analyze* outcomes to determine which nursing interventions (*hypotheses*) worked and which did not.

> **EXAMPLE:** When bathing a newborn, a student realizes she must evaluate the results of her actions; that is, she must determine whether she has kept the infant warm enough. The obvious criterion to use is that the infant's body temperature should be at least 98°F (36.7°C). Although no rule states that she should take the baby's temperature after a bath, she does so in order to evaluate whether she has achieved the goal of avoiding cold stress.

Critical Thinking and Nursing Ethics

Nurses often deal with ethical questions in their work. Even beginning students encounter ethical situations in their interactions with staff, patients, faculty, and peers. Because students may feel overwhelmed and uncomfortable in their new role, it is sometimes hard for them to recognize and define the ethical issues involved. The following are some examples (Ludwick & Sedlak, 1998):

- *Interactions with staff.* Students perceive nurses (and other health professionals) as experts, so it is particularly difficult when they observe nurses performing skills incorrectly, giving inappropriate care, or not paying attention when the student reports pertinent assessment findings.
- *Interactions with patients.* Students wonder, "What if I say the wrong thing? Or make a mistake?" Because of their inexperience, they may feel guilty if they do not perform perfectly 100 percent of the time. Pressure to be perfect may even tempt students to hide mistakes or falsify information.
- *Interactions with faculty.* Students rely on faculty as role models and as authority figures for handling clinical situations. Ethical questions arise when faculty ask them to do things they are afraid or unprepared to do, when a faculty member fails to use standard technique for a procedure, or when the student believes the teacher does not stand up to the staff regarding students' rights.

- *Interactions with peers.* Common questions include what to do when observing other students violating patient confidentiality (e.g., discussing patients at lunch), giving care incorrectly or incompletely (e.g., failure to change linens), relying on others for information about their assigned medications, falsifying patient information, or stealing supplies. Students usually do not want to "tattle," and there are questions about when and with whom to discuss such situations.

If you encounter such situations, critical thinking can help you to (a) think analytically and reflectively about what to do, (b) understand the basis for your decisions and the beliefs on which they are based, (c) identify your values and assumptions, and (d) examine your thinking processes for errors in reasoning.

Developing Critical Thinking

Critical thinking does not just "come naturally." By nature, people tend to believe what is easy to believe, what those around them believe, and what they are rewarded for believing. People develop and use critical thinking more or less effectively along a continuum. Some people make better evaluations than others; some believe information from nearly any source; and still others seldom believe anything without carefully evaluating the source. The following are some guidelines to enhance critical thinking (Berman, Snyder, Kozier, & Erb, 2008):

- *Perform a self-assessment.* Determine which critical thinking attitudes you already have and which need to be cultivated. Reflect on situations where you made decisions that you later regretted and analyze the thinking processes or attitudes that you used. This could also be done with a trusted colleague or as a group.
- *Tolerate dissonance and ambiguity.* For example, to develop fair-mindedness, you could practice being open to other viewpoints by deliberately seeking out information that is in opposition to your views. As another example, you could practice suspending judgment (or tolerating ambiguity). If an issue is complex, it may not be resolved quickly and neatly. For a while, you might need to say, "I don't know" and be comfortable with that answer until more is known.
- *Seek situations where good thinking is practiced.* Attend conferences in clinical or educational settings that support open examination of all sides of issues and respect opposing viewpoints.
- *Create environments that support critical thinking.* Nurses in leadership positions must be particularly aware of the climate for thinking that they establish. They should create a stimulating environment that *encourages* differences of opinion and fair examination of ideas and options. As leaders, nurses should encourage colleagues to examine evidence carefully before they come to conclusions and to avoid *group think*, the tendency to defer unthinkingly to the will of the group.
- *Practice critical thinking.* Everyone can achieve at least some level of critical thinking skill. Although critical thinking is not easy, with practice you can develop a critical attitude and good thinking skills. You are taking the first steps on the path to critical

thinking when you realize that understanding is more important than memorizing, and when you trust your own ability to make sense of information and principles. The Think About It questions in this book and the case study at the end of each chapter help you to practice critical thinking and clinical reasoning. At Pearson Nursing Student Resources, the nursing process exercises promote clinical reasoning, and a Critical Thinking Practice exercise in each chapter explains a particular critical thinking skill and asks you to apply it. As you develop habits of critical thinking, you will find that your thinking is no longer limited by the influences of your unexamined beliefs, feelings, and values. This will help you in your efforts to bring about good outcomes for your clients.

Take-away point: Critical thinking does not "come naturally," but it can be developed with practice.

2-4 WHAT DO YOU KNOW?

List five guidelines to help you develop your critical thinking abilities.

See answer to #2-4 What Do You Know? in Appendix A.

SUMMARY

Nurses:

- Must be critical thinkers because of the nature of their work.
- Use critical thinking skills in each step of the nursing process.
- Use five types of knowledge: nursing science, nursing art, nursing ethics, personal knowledge, and practice wisdom.

Critical thinking:

- Involves both attitudes (feelings) and cognitive thinking skills.
- Is rational and reasonable.
- Involves creative thinking.
- Involves cognitive skills, such as using language, perceiving, believing and knowing, clarifying, comparing, judging and evaluating, and reasoning.
- Includes complex intellectual activities, such as problem solving, nursing process, decision making, clinical reasoning, reflective judgment, clinical judgment, and critical analysis.
- Can be improved with practice.

Critical thinkers:

- Consider issues before forming an opinion.
- Believe in their ability to think things through and make decisions.
- Apply knowledge and principles to specific situations.

- Think for themselves and are not easily manipulated.
- Are aware of the limits of their knowledge.
- Have an attitude of inquiry.

CRITICAL THINKING AND CLINICAL REASONING: A CASE STUDY

Mrs. Lutz is a 78-year-old woman who has undergone radiation therapy and three surgeries for cancer. She is not progressing well, cannot eat, and is losing weight. The physician has decided to place a subclavian catheter in order to administer total parenteral nutrition. The nurse takes the informed consent form to Mrs. Lutz for her signature and explains to her that "the doctor will place a small tube in your vein, about here, so we can give you more nutrients and help you regain your strength and heal." Mrs. Lutz says, "I'm so tired of all this pain. I'm not sure I want anything else done, and I surely don't want to be hurt again."

1. What factors does the nurse need to assess that might affect Mrs. Lutz's *ability* to consent?
2. Before Mrs. Lutz signs the consent form, how can the nurse be certain that her consent was truly "informed"? (Informed consent means that the client has been informed about and understands the treatment, including its risks and benefits.)

The nurse replies to Mrs. Lutz: "Now, now, your doctor has prescribed this to make you well. Don't worry, we'll make sure you don't feel a thing. Your doctor will be here soon, and he will expect this permit to be signed. Won't you please sign it now?"

3. Evaluate the nurse's approach to Mrs. Lutz in regard to this invasive procedure. (What do you think about it, and why?)
4. Which phase of the nursing process is the nurse using in Items 1 and 2?
5. In Items 1 and 2, which standard(s) of reasoning is/are involved (see Table 2–3).

See suggested responses to Critical Thinking and Clinical Reasoning: A Case Study in Appendix A

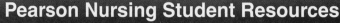

Pearson Nursing Student Resources

Find additional review materials at **www.nursing.pearsonhighered.com**
Prepare for success with additional NCLEX®-style practice questions, interactive assignments and activities, Web links, animations and videos, and more!

Assessment

3

Assessment: The First Phase of the Nursing Process

Assessment, the first phase in the nursing process, is the systematic gathering of relevant and important patient data. **Data** are information or facts about the patient. Nurses use data to (a) identify health problems, (b) plan nursing care, and (c) evaluate patient outcomes. During the assessment phase, the nurse collects, validates, records, and organizes data into predetermined categories (Box 3–1 and Figure 3–1).

Standards of Practice

American Nurses Association (ANA) and Canadian Nurses Association *standards of practice* outline nurses' accountability for assessment. Adhering to the standards in Box 3–2 will help you to collect data in a professional manner. Keep these standards of practice in mind as you work through this chapter. A revision of the ANA standards will probably be available at about the same time this book is published. However, major changes to the assessment standard are not expected. To be sure you have the most recent standards, Go to the ANA website at http://www.nursingworld.org.

Purpose of Nursing Assessment

The purpose of nursing assessment is to get a total picture of the patient and how he can be helped. This requires data about patient, family, and community patterns of health and illness, deviations from normal, strengths, coping abilities, and risk factors for health

BOX 3–1

OVERVIEW OF ASSESSMENT PHASE

1. Collect data
   Interview
   Observation
   Physical examination
2. Validate data with client and significant others
   Compare subjective with objective data
   Validate conflicting data
3. Organize and record data
   Initial assessment: Use printed form (admission database)
   Ongoing assessment: Use nursing model to organize; record on care plan
      or nursing progress notes
   Special-purpose assessments: Perform as needed

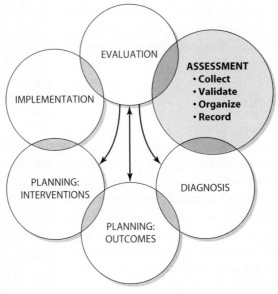

FIGURE 3–1

The assessment phase

problems. The nursing assessment focuses on patient responses—unlike the medical assessment, which focuses on disease processes and pathology. The nurse may gather data about a medical diagnosis, but this is not the focus of the assessment. For example, when admitting a patient to the hospital for surgery, the nurse is interested in the disease symptoms and the nature of the surgery but focuses primarily on how the symptoms affect the patient's ability to care for himself, what he expects from the surgery, how his recovery period will affect his life, and what his main concerns are at this time.

BOX 3–2

STANDARDS OF PRACTICE

American Nurses Association Standard I: Assessment

The registered nurse collects comprehensive data pertinent to the patient's health and/or the situation.

Competencies

The registered nurse:

1. Collects comprehensive data including but not limited to physical, functional, psychosocial, emotional, mental, sexual, cultural, age-related, environmental, spiritual/transpersonal, and economic assessments in a systematic and ongoing process while honoring the uniqueness of the person.
2. Elicits patient values, preferences, expressed needs and their knowledge of the healthcare situation.
3. Involves the patient, family/support system, other healthcare providers, and environment, as appropriate, in holistic data collection.
4. Identifies barriers (such as psychosocial, financial, cultural, etc.) to effective communication and makes appropriate adaptations.
5. Recognizes impact of personal attitudes, values and beliefs when assessing patients with diverse backgrounds or situations.
6. Assesses family dynamics and impact on patient health and wellness.
7. Prioritizes data collection activities based on the patient's immediate condition, or anticipated needs of the patient or situation.
8. Uses appropriate evidence-based assessment techniques and instruments and tools.
9. Synthesizes available data, information and knowledge relevant to the situation to identify patterns and variances.
10. Documents relevant data in a retrievable format.
11. Applies ethical, legal, and privacy guidelines and policies to the collection, maintenance, use, and dissemination of data and information.
12. Recognizes the person as the authority on his/her own health and honors their preferences in regards to their care.

Note: This material is from the draft for public comment (ANA, 2010, in press); its wording may be somewhat changed in the final published version (August 2010). For that version of the ANA standards, visit http://www.nursingworld.org.

Source: Reprinted with permission from American Nurses Association (2010, in press). In *Nursing: Scope and standards of practice* (2nd ed.). (Public Comment draft, January). Silver Spring, MD. Available at http:/nursebooks.org.

Canadian Standards of Practice (Example)

In Canada, nursing practice standards are set by individual provincial/territorial regulatory bodies. The following is one example of a portion of a Canadian standard of practice addressing assessment.

(continued)

BOX 3–2

STANDARDS OF PRACTICE *continued*

Province of Alberta

Standard 2. Knowledge-Based Practice

The registered nurse continually strives to acquire knowledge and skills to provide competent, evidence-based nursing practice. The registered nurse:

2.3   Demonstrates critical thinking in **collecting and interpreting data**, planning, implementing and evaluating all aspects of nursing care.

2.6   Documents timely, accurate reports of **data collection**, interpretation, planning, implementing and evaluating nursing practice

---

Source: College & Association of Registered Nurses of Alberta. *Nursing practice standards* (2005). Nursing Practice Standards approved March 2003; Effective November 30, 2005; Canadian Nurses Association Code of Ethics for Registered Nurses (2005) effective Oct. 1, 2005. Available at http://www.nurses.ab.ca/Carna-Admin/Uploads/new_nps_with_ethics.pdf.

Take-away point: A nursing assessment focuses on patient responses, not on disease processes and pathology.

Relationship to Other Phases of the Nursing Process

Recall from Chapter 1 that even though the steps of the nursing process are discussed separately to help you understand them, they are actually interrelated and overlapping. This is especially true of the assessment phase. Assessment data must be accurate and complete because they form the basis for the decisions made in the remaining steps of the nursing process. The usefulness and validity of the nursing diagnoses depend greatly on thorough, accurate data collection. In the planning phase, the nurse uses patient data to decide which goals are realistic and which nursing orders will be most effective.

In effect, assessment is a continuous process carried out during all phases of the nursing process. For example, you may begin to formulate a tentative problem in your mind (diagnosis phase) while still collecting data. Assessment overlaps with implementation and evaluation in that you will continue to collect patient data while carrying out these steps.

EXAMPLE: As the nurse is bathing a patient (implementation), she is observing his skin condition and joint mobility. After the nursing orders have been carried out, during the evaluation phase, the nurse collects data to determine patient progress toward goal achievement (e.g., she observes the skin to see if turning and positioning the patient have prevented pressure sores).

Take-away point: Assessment is continuous and is carried out in all phases of the nursing process.

Critical Thinking in Assessment

Assessment is more than just writing information on an assessment form. You will need critical thinking skills and a good knowledge base to decide which assessments to make, how much information you need, and where and how to get that information. When performing assessments, you will apply principles and theories about basic human needs, anatomy and physiology, disease processes, human growth and development, human behavior, socioeconomic patterns and trends, and various cultures and religions.

You must make reliable observations, distinguish relevant and important data from irrelevant and unimportant data, and recognize when information is missing. All of this requires critical thinking, as does organizing and categorizing data in a useful manner. To check the quality of your thinking in the assessment phase, review the standards of reasoning in Table 2–3 and ask yourself the questions in Table 3–1.

3-1 THINK & REFLECT!

Think about the measurement criteria in Box 3–2 (ANA Standard I). Which of the standards of reasoning (in Table 3–1) are implied by each criterion? For example, Competency 1 implies "breadth" because comprehensive data collection helps ensure that data will be complete. What other standards are implied by Competency 1? By the other criteria?

See suggested responses to #3-1 Think & Reflect! in Appendix A.

Reflective Practice

Recall from Chapter 2 that critical thinking requires reflection. In the assessment phase, the core question for reflection is: What information do I need to care for this person, family, or community? This will require you to reflect more deeply, asking such questions as:

- Who is this person?
- What is this person's story (e.g., what health event caused the person to seek care)?
- How has this person's life been changed by this illness or event?
- Who and what are this person's supports?
- How is this person feeling?

Collecting Data

Data collection is the process of gathering information about client, family, or community health status. The following are examples of client, family, and community data:

Client data: Blood pressure reading, urine color, lab test results

Family data: Genogram, family income, home safety data

Community data: Environment (air, water), morbidity and mortality rates

This section will help you develop your data-collection skills.

TABLE 3–1 Assessment: Think About Your Thinking

Standard of Reasoning	Questions to Ask Yourself	Discussion and Examples
Clarity—A statement must be clear in order for someone to know whether it is accurate, relevant, and so on.	■ Did the patient express herself clearly in the interview? ■ Are the data recorded clearly?	*Unclear:* "Patient states he has been sick for a long time." *Clearer:* Nurse should ask for and record more details: How does patient describe "sick," and exactly how long is "a long time"?
Accuracy—A statement can be clear but not accurate.	■ Are my measurements correct? ■ Is there reason to believe that the patient gave me incorrect information? ■ Did I validate data when necessary (e.g., compare subjective and objective data)?	*Example:* If the blood pressure was difficult to hear, you would ask another nurse to check it. Also, data may be inaccurate if instruments need to be calibrated (e.g., meters for checking blood glucose, heart monitors). *Example:* A patient might not feel comfortable enough to be frank with the nurse, might be embarrassed if family members are present, or might have mental deficits.
Precision—A statement can be both clear and accurate, but not precise.	■ What details can I provide to make these data more exact? ■ Would someone else know exactly what I mean by this?	*Imprecise:* "Patient states he has a headache." *More precise:* "Patient states he has a mild, throbbing pain in his left temple, which began about an hour ago."
Relevance—A statement can be clear, accurate, and precise but not relevant to the issue.	■ Do I have data that relate to this nursing diagnosis or problem? ■ Do I have data about factors that are contributing to the problem?	In the admission (comprehensive) assessment, almost anything may be relevant. Focus assessments are more selective (e.g., to evaluate the status of a decubitus ulcer, the appearance of the ulcer is relevant; you also need data about the patient's mobility and nutrition; it is irrelevant that the patient is coughing).
Depth—A statement can be clear, accurate, precise, and relevant—but superficial.	■ Did I cover all areas on the assessment form? ■ Are there any other data that would shed some light on the problem? ■ In the interview, did I follow up on patient leads with probing questions?	*Example:* A nurse was to obtain a patient's signature on a surgery consent form. She first checked the patient's chart and noted that the patient had a designated power of attorney for health care. This alerted the nurse that she needed more data in order to determine whether the patient was actually competent to sign the form.

TABLE 3–1 Assessment: Think About Your Thinking (*continued*)

Standard of Reasoning	Questions to Ask Yourself	Discussion and Examples
Breadth—A line of reasoning can meet all the other standards, but be one-sided.	▪ Did I get data about patient and family concerns, as well as my own? ▪ Did I see only what I expected to see?	*Example:* A nurse who expects patients to be anxious preoperatively might be inclined to "see" signs of anxiety: to see normal moving about as restlessness.
Logic—Reasoning brings various thoughts together in some kind of order. When the thoughts make sense in combination, thinking is logical.	▪ Do these data make sense? ▪ How can both of these "facts" be true?	See "Validating the Data."
Significance—Related to relevance: What is *most* important?	▪ Which of the facts are most important? ▪ Are there abnormal findings that I need to report to someone immediately?	As a student, you should report abnormal data to your instructor or an experienced nurse as soon as possible. Be prepared in advance; know the norms for relevant data.

Source: Based on Paul, R. (1996). *Critical thinking workshop handbook.* Dillon Beach, CA: Foundation for Critical Thinking. See http://www.Criticalthinking.org.

Subjective and Objective Data

Subjective data are sometimes called *covert data* or *symptoms*; objective data are sometimes called *overt data* or *signs.* Both types of data are needed for a thorough assessment.

Subjective data are not measurable or observable. They can be obtained only from what the client tells you. Subjective data include the client's thoughts, beliefs, feelings, sensations, and perceptions of self and health (e.g., pain, dizziness, nausea, sadness, happiness). Although you will usually obtain subjective data from the client, data from significant others and other health professionals may also be subjective if they consist of opinion and perception rather than fact. You may not always be able to obtain subjective data. Some people, such as infants, unconscious people, or those who are cognitively impaired, may not be able to provide subjective data, or their data may be unreliable. See Table 3–2 for approaches to use when it is difficult to obtain subjective data.

Objective data can be detected by someone other than the client. You will usually obtain it by observing and examining the client. Examples of objective data include pulse rate, skin color, urine output, and results of diagnostic tests or radiographs.

When used in the nursing process, the terms *subjective* and *objective* have the special meanings just described. *Subjective* does not suggest biased information or personal interpretation of meaning, as it does in common use, and *objective* does not necessarily carry the common meaning of *impartial.* See Table 3–3 for examples of subjective and objective data.

TABLE 3–2   Nursing Actions to Use When It Is Difficult to Obtain Subjective Data

Contributing Factor	Symptoms	Nursing Activities
Language barrier (e.g., not fluent in English)	Patient is unable to communicate information clearly.	Use simple, clear language; obtain an interpreter.
Severe illness or pain	Short responses; patient's main concern is to obtain relief; impatient with "questioning."	Provide needed intervention (e.g., give pain medication) before interviewing. Ask closed-end questions; obtain only essential data. Ask family or friends.
Anxiety	Patient has rapid, incoherent speech. He provides distorted or inaccurate information.	Speak slowly and quietly to the person. Emphasize that you need accurate information to give appropriate help.
Fear of incapacitating effects of illness	Patient denies certain symptoms or deliberately gives misleading facts.	Explore discrepancies between client statements and physical findings or data from other sources (see "Validating the Data").
Limited mental capacity	Patient may give inaccurate, unreliable information.	Encourage client to provide as much information as possible; then use secondary sources to fill in gaps and validate data.
Previous negative experience with health-care professionals; lack of trust	Patient is reluctant to provide data. She believes, "It won't help me anyway. It didn't do any good before."	Acknowledge previous experience and the imperfection of health professionals. Request another chance to help. Demonstrate competence. Convey respect for client's thoughts and feelings.

TABLE 3–3   Examples of Subjective and Objective Data

	Subjective	Objective
Description	*Covert data; symptoms.* What the patient says. Data can be perceived and verified only by the patient.	*Overt data; signs.* Data can be observed by others or measured against a standard.
Examples	Itching Pain Anxiety "I'm afraid." "I feel weak all over."	Pulse rate 100 bpm Blood pressure 120/80 mm Hg Skin pale and cool to touch Urine output 350 mL Radiography results Skin turgor Posture

Primary and Secondary Data Sources

Data sources fall into two broad categories: primary and secondary. You should use the most reliable source of data, whether it is the patient or a significant other, and indicate the source on the patient's record. The client is the **primary data** source; all other data sources are secondary. Both primary and secondary source data can be subjective or objective; that is, they can both be obtained from what the client tells you or by observation and examination. **Secondary data** are obtained from sources other than the client (e.g., other people, client records).

Significant others, such as family or friends, are especially valuable sources when the client is a child or has difficulty communicating. When possible, you should get the client's consent before collecting data from significant others.

Other healthcare providers, such as the physician, social worker, and respiratory therapist, can provide information about the areas of client functioning with which they are involved. Sharing information among disciplines is especially important when the client is being transferred from one institution to another (e.g., from a nursing home to a hospital) or discharged from the institution for follow-up care at home.

The client's written record from present and past hospitalizations is a secondary source. The client's record should be reviewed early in the data-collection process to help you plan the initial nursing assessment and to confirm the other data.

Information from nursing and other literature is especially important for students and beginning practitioners. For example, if you have never cared for a client with trigeminal neuralgia, you should read a textbook in order to know what signs and symptoms to expect. The literature also provides helpful information about developmental norms, cultural differences, and spiritual practices to use as a guide during data collection. Table 3–4 provides examples of primary and secondary data sources.

Take-away point: Data collection is the process of gathering information about client, family, or community health status. Data may be subjective or objective as well as primary or secondary.

TABLE 3–4   Examples of Primary and Secondary Data Sources

	Primary	Secondary
Description	Subjective or objective data obtained directly from the patient	Information about the patient obtained from family and friends, verbal reports from other healthcare professionals, information from patient records
Examples	Itching Patient statement of pain Patient statement of anxiety Pulse rate Skin color Posture	Statements from records (e.g., radiography results; nurse's note that "Client refused dinner.") Verbal report from caregivers (e.g., "Needed pain medication at 8 A.M.") Family statement, "He has been in pain all day."

TABLE 3–5   Initial Versus Ongoing Assessment

Initial	Ongoing
Admission assessment	Focus assessment
Database assessment	Focuses on specific problems, activities, or behaviors
Comprehensive assessment	Focuses on identified problems (can also be used to identify new problems)
Can include focus assessment	
Data are used to make initial problem list.	Data are used to evaluate outcomes achievement and problem resolution.

Initial versus Ongoing Assessment

Assessment begins with the nurse's first contact with the client and continues throughout all subsequent encounters. Initial and ongoing assessment differs in purpose and, usually, in scope.

The **initial assessment** is made during the first nurse–client encounter and is usually comprehensive, consisting of all subjective and objective data pertinent to the client's health status. When the initial assessment is performed on the client's arrival at a healthcare agency, it is called the **admission assessment**. Each client should have an initial assessment to determine the need for care and further assessment.

Ongoing assessment consists of data gathered after the database is completed—ideally, during every nurse-patient interaction. These data are used to identify new problems and to evaluate the status of problems that have already been identified. See Table 3–5 for a summary comparison of initial and ongoing assessment.

Comprehensive versus Focus Assessment

A **comprehensive assessment** provides an overall picture of the client's health status. The nurse obtains data about all the client's body systems and functional abilities without necessarily having a particular health problem in mind. A nursing database usually follows the agency's printed assessment form (e.g., Figure 3–2).

Information obtained from the comprehensive assessment makes up the **nursing database**. In fact, the initial (admission) assessment is also called "database assessment." Figure 3–3 illustrates the place of the database in the assessment phase. The complete database consists of the nursing history and physical examination, as well as data from the patient's records, consultations, and sometimes a review of the literature.

In a **focus assessment**, the nurse gathers data about a *specific condition*: an actual, potential, or possible problem that has been identified (Alfaro-LeFevre, 2010). The assessment focuses on a specific topic or particular area of the body instead of the client's overall health status. Data from focus assessments are used to evaluate the status of existing problems and to identify new problems.

EXAMPLE: *Evaluation of an existing problem.* The care plan for Hassim Asad included the problem of Deficient Fluid Volume. When performing ongoing assessment during Mr. Asad's bath, the nurse noted that his oral mucous membranes were moist and that he had good skin turgor—signs that his fluid volume problem was resolving.

Name: _Luisa Sanchez_   Age: _28_   Phone #: _641-1212_   Date: _7/16/11_   Time: _1515_
Primary Physician: _R. Katz_   Phone #: _643-7690_
Chief Complaints/Procedure: _"chest cold x 2 wks. s.o.b. on exertion"_   Height: _5 ft 2 in_   Weight (lbs.): _125_
Historian: _Patient_   Temp: _103°_   Pulse: _92 weak_   Resp: _18 shallow_   BP: _122/80_
Religious Affiliation: _Catholic. Would want Last Rites_   Hospitalized within 30 days: Yes ☐   No ☒

UNABLE TO OBTAIN HISTORY .... ☐	GASTROINTESTINAL	Pregnant .... ☐
Reason:_____	Dysphagia .... ☐	Lactating .... ☐
NEUROLOGICAL/SENSORY PERCEPTION	Hiatal Hernia .... ☐	LMP/Date: _7-1-11_
Glaucoma .... ☐	Liver Disease/Jaundice .... ☐	**VACCINATION/DATE**
Hearing Loss/Deaf .... Right ☐ Left ☐	Pancreatitis .... ☐	Flu:_____ Hepatitis B:_____
Motion Sickness .... ☐	Gall Stones .... ☐	Pneumonia:_____
Paresthesia .... Right ☐ Left ☐	Ostomy .... ☐	**BEHAVIORAL HEALTH**
Fibromyalgia/Migrane .... ☐	Last Bowel Movement: _7-15-11_	Anxiety Disorder .... ☐
Spina Bifida .... ☐	Other:_____	Depression .... ☐
Stroke/CVA/TIA .... ☐	**GENITOURINARY/RENAL**	Suicide (thoughts/attempts) .... ☐
Altered Mental Status .... ☐	Kidney Disease/Urogenital .... ☐	Patient is a Baker Act .... ☐
Other:_____	Prostate Problems .... ☐	Other:_____
CARDIOVASCULAR/HEMATOLOGY	Voiding Problems .... ☐	**CANCER**
Bleeding Problems .... ☐	Other: _↓ amt. & frequency x 3 days_	Type:_____ ☐
Blood transfusion in the past 3 months ... ☐	**MUSCULOSKELETAL**	Radioactive Seeds/Implant .... ☐
Chest Pain/Angina _on caughing_ ...... ☒	Arthritis .... ☐	Date:_____
Heart Attack/Date:_____ ☐	Back/Disc Problem .... ☐	Other:_____
Heart Disease .... ☐	Fractures .... ☐	**SOCIAL HISTORY**
High Blood Pressure .... ☐	Other: _"I feel weak"_	Tobacco .... _No_ .... ☐
Irregular Beats/Pacemaker/AICD .... ☐	**ENDOCRINE**	Number of years:_____
Mitral Valve Prolapse .... ☐	Diabetes/type:_____ ☐	# of packs per day:_____
Murmur .... ☐	Thyroid Disease _Partial thyroidectomy_ ☐	Year Quit:_____
Peripheral Vascular Disease .... ☐	Other:_____	Would you like smoking cessation info?
Sickle Cell Disease .... ☐	**INFECTIOUS DISEASE**	☒ No ☐ Yes ☐ information provided
Venous Access Device/Type_____ ☐	Fevers ... _"Usual colds"_ .... ☒	Alcohol .... ☐
Other:_____	Hepatitis/type/active .... ☐	Drinks per day: _None_
RESPIRATORY	HIV/AIDS .... ☐	Amount:_____
Asthma .... ☐	Recent Cold .... ☒	Type:_____
Bronchitis .... ☐	Sexually Transmitted Disease/type ... ☐	Recreational Drug ... _No_ .... ☐
COPD/Emphysema .... ☐	Tuberculosis/Active: .... ☐	Amount:_____
Post Nasal Drip/Rhinitis/Sinusitis ...... ☐	Other:_____	Type:_____
Pneumonia _current diagnosis_ ...... ☑		Year Quit:_____
Tracheostomy .... ☐		Detoxification Protocol Initiated .... ☐
Other:_____		

ALLERGIES & REACTION	None Known ☐	Allergy Bracelet on ☒
Medications:	**Symptoms:**	
Penicillin	_Rash, nausea_	Blood Reaction: ☐
Food/Shellfish/other allergies: _No_		Latex: ☐
Contrast/Dye:		Latex Allergy Protocol Initiated: ☐

PAST HOSPITAL/PROCEDURE (Surgical/Medical/Behavioral Health)		**CURRENT MEDICATIONS** (include ASA/Anticoagulant, over the counter medications, ointments, patches, eye drops, herbal, vitamins and nutritional supplements)			
		Medication	**Dose**	**Frequency**	**Last Dose**
Appendectomy	_1982_	_Synthroid_	_0.1 mg_	_daily_	_7/16/11_
Partial thyroidectomy	_1995_				
		Food/Drug Interaction information provided ☐			
Initiate Social Service Consult		(Note: Additional medication can be listed on last page)			

ADDRESSOGRAPH

✳
North Broward Hospital District

NURSING ADMISSION DATA

FIGURE 3–2
Assessment for Luisa Sanchez (*Source:* Adapted from "Nursing Assessment Tool," Broward General Medical Center, Broward County, FL. Reprinted with permission.)

PAIN HISTORY

Have you been experiencing pain? ☒ Yes
If yes, when _Now_ ___ Intensity (0-10): _6_ ___ Goal (0-10): _1_
Location: _Chest_
Radiation: ___
Duration: _when coughing_
Quality: ___
Aggravating factors _coughing_

What medications/interventions are effective in relieving your pain?
sitting very still

Acute Pain Management - It is Your Right brochure provided ☒

PSYCHOSOCIAL ASSESSMENT

☐ Lives alone ☒ Lives with spouse/SO ☐ Nursing Home/ALF
☐ Homeless ☐ Rehab Facility ☐ Other: ___
Marital Status ☐ Single ☒ Married ☐ Divorced ☐ Widowed ☐ Separated
Next of Kin: _Michael Sanchez_ ___ **Phone #:** _641-1212_
Supportive Adult: _same_ ___ **Phone #:** _same_
Has anybody threatened/hit/abused you within the last year?
☐ Yes (refer to policy RA 004015 mauve manual) ☒ No

EDUCATIONAL LEARNING ASSESSMENT

Learner ☒ Patient ☐ Family ☐ Significant Other
Readiness to learn ☐ Eager to learn ☒ Asks questions
☒ ~~Extremely~~ anxious ☐ Denies need for Education
Knowledge of current health status ☐ No knowledge
☒ Partial understanding ☐ Full understanding
Barriers to learning ☐ Physical ☒ Emotional (anxiety)
☐ Language ☐ Religious ☐ Cultural
☐ Reading Ability ☐ Changes in Short Memory
☐ None
Preferred Learning Method ☐ Reading ☐ Lecture
☐ Video ☒ Demo/Practice
Communication ☒ English ☐ Spanish ☐ Creole
☐ Sign Language ☐ Other: ___
Do you have any religious/cultural practices that are important to you or may alter your care or education? ☒ No ☐ Yes ___

☒ Patient Handbook provided ☒ Patient safety information provided
☒ Patient's Bill of Rights and Responsibilities information provided
Other Educational Materials: ___

PERSONAL EFFECTS: Do you use the following: _NO_

	YES	WITH PT.	FAMILY/SO
Wheelchair	☐	☐	☐
Braces	☐	☐	☐
Cane/Crutches	☐	☐	☐
Walker	☐	☐	☐
Prosthesis	☐	☐	☐
Medications	☐	☐	☐
Dentures: (Full)	☐	☐	☐
Upper	☐	☐	☐
Lower	☐	☐	☐
Glasses	☐	☐	☐
Contacts	☐	☐	☐
Hearing Aids	☐	☐	☐
Other:			

Initiate Social Service Consult

ADVANCE DIRECTIVES

Do you have an Advance Directive?
(must check one)
☐ **No** Information provided to patient
☐ **No** Patient elects not to receive information
☒ **Yes** (check advance directive patient states he/she has)
☒ **Living Will** ☐ **Health Care Surrogate** ☐ **State DNAR form**
☐ **Durable Power of Attorney** ☐ **Organ Donation**
(If patient has an Advance Directive, inform patient to provide copy within 24 hours or they may complete a new advance directive or verbalize their wishes)
Do you have a guardian? ☐ Yes name _No_
(Inform patient to provide guardianship form within 24 hours)
☐ **Patient unable to respond/family not available**

FALL SCREEN: *If any of the following are checked, initiate*
Safety/Protective Intervention Protocol
Inability to understand or follow instructions .... ☐
Impaired mobility, visual impairment, drug therapy, surgical procedure, unsteady gait, incontinence .... ☐
Unable to use call light .... ☐
Altered mental status .... ☐
Nocturnal/urgency/frequency in elimination .... ☐
Dizziness .... ☐
History of falls .... ☐
No Criteria Met .... ☒

NUTRITIONAL SCREEN: *If any of the following are checked, enter in the computer request for **Nutritional Consult***
Nausea/vomiting > 5 days _Nausea past 3 days_ .... ☐
No food/drink for 3 days _No food past 2 days_ .... ☐
Recent unexplained weight loss > 10 lbs. .... ☐
Difficulty swallowing/dysphagia .... ☐
Evidence of Stage III - IV pressure ulcer .... ☐
Feeding tube .... ☐
New onset diabetes .... ☐
TPN .... ☐
Pregnant/lactating .... ☐
Surgical patients > 70 years of age .... ☐
Ethnic diet/special needs **(include in diet order and order for Preference consult)** .... ☐
Difficulty chewing **(include in diet order and order for Preference consult)** .... ☐
No Criteria Met .... ☒

FUNCTIONAL SCREEN: *If any of the following are checked, please request physician order for physical therapy consult.*
New onset of paralysis .... ☐
New onset stroke/CVA .... ☐
New amputation .... ☐
Unsteady gait .... ☐
Decreased mobility .... ☐
Dysphagia .... ☐
No Criteria Met .... ☒

FIGURE 3–2

(continued)

OUTPATIENT PRE-ADMISSION NOTE: Date of Call/Visit _NA_ Date of Surgery:_____ | **Pre-op Work Up:**
Autologous Blood ☐   Direct Donor ☐   Confirmed with Blood Bank ☐   # of Units Available_____ | BGMC☐   NBMC☐   IPMC☐   CSMC☐
Parent Present Induction ☐ | Other:_____

ANESTHESIOLOGIST EVALUATION: ASA class I II III IV   NPO:_____ | **INITIAL EVALUATION EXCEEDING 48 HOURS:**
Anesthesia Plan   Gen☐   MAC☐   Regional☐   Type_____ | No Change in Assessment ☐
Airway:_____   Dentition: Good☐ Fair☐ Poor☐   EKG_____ | Changes in Assessment   ☐
Neck_____   Natural☐ Caps☐   CXR _NA_ | Comments:_____
Previous Anesthesia ☐   Dentures/Bridges☐   H & H_____
Past anesthesia problems_____   Malampati score 1 2 3 4   Platelets _____
OTHER: _____

Comments:_____

Anesthesiologist_____ Date_____ Time_____ | Anesthesiologist:_____
| Date/Time: _____

| **NURSING DIAGNOSIS** | **NURSING INTERVENTIONS** | **PLANNED OUTCOME/EVALUATION** |

NURSING DIAGNOSIS
Potential/actual knowledge deficit
Pre-op preparation/
planned surgical intervention.

_NA_

Anxiety

Psycho/Social

Actual/Potential
Individual Needs
Self Care/Discharge Planning

NURSING INTERVENTIONS
☐ Patient/family learning needs/level of understanding assessed.
☐ Clear explanation of pre-operative routine given.
☐ Instructions on turning, coughing, deep breathing, leg exercises given.
☐ Procedure specific instructions _____
☐ Pain management modalities and scale explained.
  Modality preference_____
  Pain scale goal _____
☐ Written copy of pre-op instructions and patient responsibility provided.
☐ Allow to express feelings, ask questions.
☐ Emotional support given.
☐ Sense of wellness promoted.
☐ Cultural/Spiritual Needs: _____
☐ Discharge planning initiated/home care assessed.
☐ Needs identified/Action:

PLANNED OUTCOME/EVALUATION
☐ Patient verbalizes understanding of pre-op preparation,
  pre-op routine and procedure specific information.
☐ Patient copes with anxiety, shows relaxed affect.
☐ Demonstrates understanding of explanations.
☐ Patient verbalizes understanding of pain management and
  plan of care.
☐ Needed referrals/arrangements made.
☐ Care individualized to meet patients needs.
☐ Patient verbalizes understanding of discharge plan.

Standard of Care/Protocol: ☐ Yes

R.N. Signature:_____ Date:_____

Nurse Signature: _____ Unit: _____ Date: _____ Time: _____
Nurse Signature: _____ Unit: _____ Date: _____ Time: _____

DATE & TIME	**INTERDISCIPLINARY NOTES/ADVANCE DIRECTIVES INFORMATION**
7-16-11	
1545	S— States "chest cold x2 weeks." c/o sharp chest pain when coughing, and dyspnea on exertion. States unable to do her daily exercises for the past week. Cough relieved "if I sit up and sit still." Nausea associated with coughing. Having occasional "chills." States, "I get so scared when I can't breathe." Well groomed, but "too tired to mess with hair and make-up."
	States her supports are good (eg, relationship with husband). States, "worried about my daughter" because husband is out of town until tomorrow. Left 3-y.o. daughter with neighbor. Also states concern about her work (is attorney). "I'll never get caught up."
	O— Chest expansion < 3 cm no nasal flaring or use of accessory muscles. Breath sounds and inspiratory crackles in right upper and lower chest. Slow capillary refill.
	Informed of need to save urine for 24-hr. specimen. IV of D5W-LR 1000 mL started in right arm, 100 mL/hr. Head of bed elevated to facilitate breathing.

Nurse Signature: _Mary Medina_ Unit: _2 east_ Date: _7/6/11_ Time: _1545_
Nurse Signature: _____ Unit: _____ Date: _____ Time: _____

Anticipated Discharge Needs

☐ Transportation ☐ Placement needed
Medical Equipment: ☐ Oxygen ☐ CPAP ☐ Nebulizer ☐ Blood Glucose Meter Other:_____
Community Services: (Home Health, Reach to Recovery, Meals On Wheels, etc.): _____

Nurse Signature: _____ Unit: _____ Date: _____ Time: _____
Nurse Signature: _____ Unit: _____ Date: _____ Time: _____

FIGURE 3–2
(*continued*)

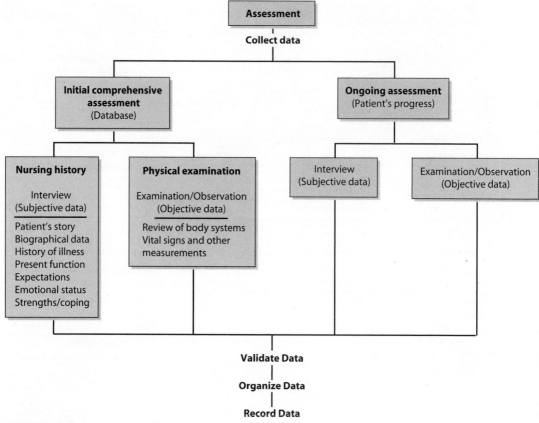

FIGURE 3–3
Overview of assessment.

EXAMPLE: *Identification of a new problem.* During his bath, Mr. Asad mentioned that his head was beginning to hurt. He had not mentioned headaches before. The nurse took his blood pressure and questioned him about the nature and onset of the pain. Mr. Asad's blood pressure was elevated, and his vision was blurred. The nurse elevated the head of the bed, relieving his pain somewhat, and notified the physician of this new development.

A focus assessment is not limited to ongoing data collection; it can also be used in the initial assessment when the client reports a symptom or other unusual findings. Any symptom or difficulty the client reports should be expanded on by asking further questions about it (e.g., When did it begin? What makes it worse? What relieves it?). When a client needs repeated in-depth assessment of a particular problem area, most agencies have special assessment forms for recording the ongoing focus assessment (e.g., a flow sheet for hourly neurologic assessments).

3-1 WHAT DO YOU KNOW?

1. What is the difference between subjective and objective data?
2. What is the difference between primary and secondary data sources?

See answer to #3-1 What Do You Know? in Appendix A.

Use of Computers in Assessment

Many healthcare agencies use computerized information systems to facilitate data collection. In some automated assessment systems, patients respond directly to interview questions on the computer screen. In other systems, the nurse interviews the patient and enters the data into a bedside terminal. Nurses may also use bedside terminals to prompt them through a systematic and complete physical examination of a patient. And finally, nurses use computers to record the interview and examination data. Figure 3–4 is an example of a computer screen showing a portion of a flowsheet on which nurses record ongoing assessments at a bedside computer.

In addition, a variety of monitors can be programmed to make continuous or periodic patient assessments. Examples are digital thermometers, digital scales, pulse oximeters, electrocardiography machines, telemetry and hemodynamic monitors, apnea monitors, fetal heart monitors, and blood glucose analyzers. Most of these instruments

			10/12 08:00	12:00	16:00	20:00	10/13 00:00	04:00	08:00	12:00
NEURO	Behavior		Anxious	Cooperat	Restless	Calm	Sleeping	Anxious	Calm	Cooperat
	Level of Consciousness	Orientation	x3 P-P-T	No Change	No Change	x3 P-P-T	Reorients	x3 P-P-T	x3 P-P-T	No Change
		LOC	Alert	No Change	No Change	Alert		Alert	Alert	No Change
	Mentation		Normal	No Change	No Change	Normal	Normal	Normal	Normal	No Change
	Speech		Clear	No Change	No Change	Clear	Clear	Clear	Clear	No Change
	Movement	RA	Normal	No Change	No Change	Normal	No Change	No Change	Normal	No Change
		LA	Normal	No Change	No Change	Normal	No Change	No Change	Normal	No Change
		RL	Normal	No Change	No Change	Normal	No Change	No Change	Normal	No Change
		LL	Normal	No Change	No Change	Normal	No Change	No Change	Normal	No Change
	Pupil Size(mm)/Reaction	R	5 Brisk	4 Brisk	4 Brisk	4 Brisk	3 Brisk	4 Brisk	5 Brisk	4 Brisk
		L	5 Brisk	4 Brisk	4 Brisk	4 Brisk	3 Brisk	4 Brisk	5 Brisk	4 Brisk
CV	Heart Sounds		Murmur	No Change	No Change	Murmur	No Change	No Change	Murmur	No Change
			Irregular	No Change	No Change	Irregular	No Change	No Change	Regular	No Change
	Edema Assessment	Edema	Dependent	No Change	No Change	Dependent	No Change	Dependent	Dependent	No Change
		Type	2+Pitting			1+Pitting		2+Pitting	1+Pitting	
		Location	BilAnkles			BilAnkles		BilAnkles	BilAnkles	
	Femoral	R	PalpStrng			PalpStrng			PalpStrng	
		L	PalpStrng			PalpStrng			PalpStrng	
	Popliteal	R	PalpWeak			PalpWeak			PalpWeak	
		L	PalpWeak			PalpWeak			PalpWeak	
	Posterior Tibialis	R	PalpWeak	No Change	No Change	PalpWeak	No Change	No Change	PalpWeak	No Change
		L	PalpWeak	No Change	No Change	PalpWeak	No Change	No Change	PalpWeak	No Change
	Dorsalis Pedis	R	PalpWeak	No Change	No Change	PalpWeak	No Change	No Change	PalpWeak	No Change
		L	PalpWeak	No Change	No Change	PalpWeak	No Change	No Change	PalpWeak	No Change
RESP	Breath Sounds	R	Decreased	FineRales	InspWheez	FineRales	FineRales	No Change	Crackles	Crackles
			Clear		ExpWheez		ExpWheez			ExpWheez
		L	Decreased	FineRales	InspWheez	FineRales	FineRales	No Change	Crackles	Crackles
			Clear		ExpWheez		ExpWheez			ExpWheez
		RXL							bases	
GI	Abdomen		Rounded	No Change	No Change	Soft	No Change	No Change	Rounded	No Change
			NonTender	No Change	No Change	NonTender	No Change	No Change	NonTender	No Change
	Bowel Sounds	R	Present	No Change	No Change	Present	No Change	No Change	Hypo	Present
			Present	No Change	No Change	Present	No Change	No Change	Hypo	Present
		L	Present	No Change	No Change	Present	No Change	No Change	Hypo	Present
			Present	No Change	No Change	Present	No Change	No Change	Hypo	Present
		Flatus	Present			Present				
GU	Urine	Route	Foley	No Change	Foley	Foley	No Change	Foley	Foley	Foley
		Color	Yellow	No Change	Amber	Yellow	No Change	Amber	Amber	Yellow
		Character	Sediment	No Change	Sediment	Sediment	No Change	Cloudy	Cloudy	Sediment
SKIN	Skin Vitals	Color	Pale	No Change	Pale	Pale Pink	No Change	Pale Pink	Pale Pink	No Change
		Temp	Warm	No Change	Cool	Warm	No Change	Cool	Warm	No Change
		Moisture	Dry	No Change	Clammy	Dry	No Change	Dry	Dry	No Change
		Cap Refill	< 3 sec	No Change	< 3 sec	< 3 sec	No Change	< 3 sec	< 3 sec	No Change
		Nailbeds	Pink	No Change	Dusky	Pink	No Change	Pink	Pink	No Change
		Turgor	Elastic	No Change	Elastic	Elastic	No Change	Elastic	Elastic	No Change

FIGURE 3–4

Computer screen showing portion of assessment flowsheet (*Source*: Courtesy of Shore Memorial Hospital, Somers Point, NJ.)

keep a record of the most recent values. Some can transmit their data to a more sophisticated computer or print out a paper record. Some have digital displays that "talk" to the user, giving instructions or results. Most have alarms to indicate either that the instrument is malfunctioning or that the assessed value is outside predetermined parameters. These devices, with their tiny but powerful computer chips, make it possible to extend the nurse's observations and provide valid and reliable data.

Data-Collection Methods

Take-away point: Three methods of collecting data are used in both comprehensive and focus nursing assessments: observation, physical examination, and interview.

Observation

Observation is the conscious, deliberate use of the physical senses to gather data from the patient and the environment. It occurs whenever the nurse is in contact with the client or support persons. Examples of data observed through use of the senses are found in Table 3–6. Nursing observations must be systematic so that no significant data are missed. At each patient contact, try to develop a sequence of observation, such as the following:

1. As you enter the room, *observe the patient for signs of distress* (e.g., pallor, labored breathing, behaviors indicating pain or emotional distress).
2. *Scan for safety hazards* (e.g., Are the side rails up? Are there spills on the floor?).
3. *Look at the equipment* (e.g., urinary catheter bag, intravenous [IV] pumps, oxygen, monitors). Is the equipment working? Do any of the alarms or screens indicate a need for immediate attention? Is the IV running? Is the urinary catheter draining?
4. *Scan the room.* Who is there, and how do those people interact with the patient?
5. *Observe the patient more closely for data* such as skin temperature, breath sounds, drainage odors, condition of dressings, condition of bed linens, and need for repositioning.

Physical Examination

The **nursing physical examination** is a systematic assessment of all body systems. It is concerned with identifying strengths and deficits in the client's functional abilities rather than identifying pathology. Physical examination provides objective data that can be used

TABLE 3–6   Examples of Observation Data

Sense	Examples of Data Obtained
Touch	Pulse rate and rhythm; lesions (e.g., masses, nodules); firmness of uterine fundus in post-partum woman; skin temperature
Vision	General appearance (e.g., estimate of height and weight, posture, grooming), skin color, facial expression, body movements, personal articles in room (e.g., religious books, icons, beads, family pictures), equipment (e.g., IV pump, electrocardiogram monitor)
Smell	Body, breath, or urine odors; wound secretions
Hearing	Blood pressure, breath sounds, bowel sounds, heart sounds, spoken words (e.g., to indicate thoughts, feelings, ability to communicate, and orientation)

to validate the subjective data obtained in the interview or to clarify the effect of the patient's disease on her ability to function. Data from the initial physical examination serve as a baseline. After providing nursing and medical interventions, the nurse can compare that data with the baseline data to assess the client's responses to nursing and medical interventions.

One approach is to proceed from *head to toe*. That is, first examine the head and neck and then the shoulders, chest (including heart and lungs), and back. Another approach is to examine each of the *body systems* in a predetermined order—for example, respiratory, neurologic, cardiovascular, musculoskeletal, and so on. Whatever approach you choose, follow the same order for every exam to prevent omission of data.

You will use the techniques of inspection, auscultation, percussion, and palpation when performing a physical examination. Refer to a fundamentals of nursing or physical assessment text for in-depth discussion of these techniques and other aspects of the physical examination.

Inspection is done visually either with the naked eye or with instruments such as an otoscope, which is used in examining the ears. Abdominal distension and skin pallor are examples of data found on inspection.

Auscultation uses the nurse's hearing. Using direct auscultation with the unaided ear, you can hear sounds such as the client's coughing. A stethoscope is used for indirect auscultation to amplify the sounds made within the client's body, such as crackles and wheezes in the lungs.

Percussion is the striking of a body surface, usually with the tip of the finger, to elicit sound or vibration. Different sounds are produced, depending on whether the finger strikes over a solid, fluid-filled, or air-filled area. It is useful, for instance, in determining whether a patient's abdomen is distended with air or fluid.

Palpation uses the sense of touch. The finger pads are usually used because they are the most sensitive to tactile stimulation. You will use palpation, for example, to check for bladder distension and to obtain the patient's pulse rate and strength.

3-2 WHAT DO YOU KNOW?

1. Give three examples of data you could obtain from physical examination.
2. Give two examples of data you could obtain from observation.

See answer to #3-2 What Do You Know? in Appendix A.

Interview

A **nursing interview** is purposeful, structured communication in which the nurse questions a patient to obtain subjective data. An admission interview is formal and planned. During ongoing assessment, interviews may be informal, brief, narrowly focused interactions between nurse and patient, but they are still purposeful, structured communication.

Take-away point: Nursing interviews may be formal or informal, but they are always purposeful, structured communication.

Purpose of the Interview During the initial assessment, the main purpose of the interview is to obtain subjective data for the nursing history. The **nursing history** contains data about the effects of the illness on the patient's daily functioning and ability to cope. It considers the whole person, including data about all the patient's basic needs, not just the biological ones. The specific content of a nursing history varies in different settings but usually includes the general content areas shown in Box 3–3.

At the time of the initial interview, you will usually also orient the patient to the room and provide some information about the hospital stay (e.g., how to call for help, where to put belongings). Although the focus is on obtaining data, you should provide enough teaching and counseling to relieve some of the patient's anxieties. This is important because impressions gained in the initial interview form the basis for the beginning of the nurse-patient relationship.

Preparing for the Interview As a rule, you should begin by reviewing the chart so you will know who the patient is and what you want to accomplish. This will prevent you from covering topics already assessed by someone else, which can be tiring and annoying for patients. Be careful, though, not to form preconceived ideas about the patient. Failure to approach the person with an open mind can cause you to miss some data. Your preparation should also include the following the guidelines in Box 3–4.

BOX 3–3

COMPONENTS OF A NURSING HEALTH HISTORY

Component	Example or Explanation
Biographical information	Age, sex, marital status
Chief complaint or reason for visit	Specifically, what initiated the patient to seek help (e.g., chest pain, weight loss, check-up)
History of current illness	Includes usual health status, chronology of the illness, and effect of the illness on the client's daily life
Past health status	Previous hospitalizations or surgeries, childhood diseases
Review of systems and their effect on client's functioning	Subjective data regarding body systems such as respiratory system (e.g., cough, shortness of breath) or related to difficulties with activities such as dressing, grooming, eating, and elimination
Social and family history	Family relationships, friendships; ethnic affiliation; occupational history; economic status; home and neighborhood conditions; exposure to toxic materials
Lifestyle, including usual habits and patterns of daily living	Personal habits such as alcohol and tobacco use; usual diet; sleep and rest patterns; exercise
Spiritual well-being	Client's source of strength or hope
Psychological data	Major stressors; usual coping pattern; available supports; communication style; self-concept
Client's perception of health status and illness	Does the client realize the implications of the illness (e.g., does he think his arthritis can be cured)?
Client's expectations of caregivers	What the client thinks will be done for him; what he wants the nurses to do to help

BOX 3–4

GUIDE FOR INTERVIEWING

1. **Prepare for the interview.**
   - *Read the chart.*
   - *Form goals for the interview and think of some initial questions.*
   - *Provide privacy.* Ask visitors to leave; pull the bed curtain.
   - *Don't rush.* Schedule a block of time for the interview when you will not be interrupted—not too close to mealtime, treatments, or visiting hours.
   - *Reduce distractions* (e.g., turn off the television).
   - *Be sure the client is comfortable* (e.g., offer bedpan, drink of water).
   - *Consider the patient's emotional state.* If he is very anxious or frightened, you may need to relieve his anxiety before proceeding with the interview.

2. **Set the stage.**
   - *Call the patient by name.* Ask what name the patient prefers you to use.
   - *Introduce yourself,* including your position and the purpose of the interview.
   - *SOLER*
   - *Set a time limit* at the beginning of the interview.

3. **Obtain the data.**
   - *Start with the client's main complaint* ("Why are you here?").
   - *Ask about nonthreatening subjects and symptoms.* Introduce personal or threatening material later in the interview when you are both more at ease.
   - *Don't mechanically fill out the form.* Follow patient leads for expanding on or introducing a new topic.

4. **Use good communication techniques.**
   - *Say "I," not "we"* ("We need some information from you"). "We" indicates lack of personal involvement and creates psychological distance between you and the patient.
   - *Don't use endearing names,* such as "grandma," "dear," or "sweetie." Many people feel belittled by this.
   - *Use language the patient can understand.* Many patients do not know the meaning of "void" or "vital signs." Check the patient's understanding of a word by saying, for example, "Explain what happens when you have diarrhea."
   - *Don't talk down to the patient* (e.g., "I need to feel your tummy").
   - *Don't ask too many questions*—you may seem curious rather than concerned. Instead, use neutral statements and reflection to obtain information (e.g., instead of, "Where do you work?" say, "Tell me about your job").
   - *Use an appropriate balance of closed and open-ended questions.*
   - *Avoid asking "why" questions* (e.g., "Why have you been unable to stop smoking?"). For many people, "why" connotes disapproval and may provoke a defensive response.
   - *Don't put words in the patient's mouth.* Avoid leading questions such as, "Are you worried about your surgery tomorrow?"

(continued)

BOX 3–4

GUIDE FOR INTERVIEWING *continued*

- *Don't give advice.*
- *Encourage the patient to continue* by nodding or saying, "Um-hm," "Yes . . .," or "Go on."
- *Don't interrupt.* If the patient is rambling, allow him to finish a sentence and then try to redirect the conversation by saying something like, "You hadn't finished telling me about . . ."
- *Use and accept silence.* Give the patient time to search for and organize her thoughts.
- *Validate your understanding* of the content and feeling of the patient's message. Summarize the meaning of what you have heard and ask for feedback (e.g., "Did I understand you to say . . ." or "I hear you saying . . . Do I have it right?").

Types of Interviews There are two basic types of interview: directive and nondirective. A **directive interview** is highly structured. The nurse controls the subject matter and asks questions in order to obtain specific information. This is an efficient way to obtain factual, easily categorized information, such as age, gender, and analysis of symptoms.

During a **nondirective interview** the nurse allows the patient to control the purpose, subject matter, and pacing. The nurse clarifies, summarizes, and uses open-ended questions and comments to encourage communication. Nondirective interviewing is time consuming and can result in obtaining a great deal of irrelevant data; however, it is useful in helping a patient to express feelings, promoting communication, and building rapport.

Kinds of Interview Questions Questions are classified as closed or open ended (see Table 3–7 for examples). **Open-ended questions**, associated with the nondirective interview, invite patients to discover and explore (elaborate, clarify, or illustrate) their thoughts and feelings. An open-ended question may specify the topic of discussion, but it is broad and requires elaboration from the patient.

TABLE 3–7   Closed and Open-Ended Questions

Closed-Ended Questions	Open-Ended Questions
When was the accident?	Tell me about your accident.
Are you in pain?	Describe your pain to me.
Was this a planned pregnancy?	What were your thoughts or feelings when you found out you were pregnant?

Closed questions, used in the directive interview, generally require only "yes," "no," or short factual answers giving specific information. Thus, the amount of information gained is limited. Closed questions often begin with "when," "where," "who," "what," "do (did, does)," "is (are, was)" and sometimes "how." Closed questions are especially effective in emergency situations or when a patient is highly stressed or anxious or has difficulty communicating.

The nursing interview requires a combination of directive and nondirective techniques. Use closed questioning to obtain the more specific information on the nursing history (e.g., biographical information, previous surgeries, childhood diseases). Then use broad statements to guide the patient to talk about other topics, such as sleep patterns, pain, and usual routines. Finally, follow up or clarify those responses with specific, closed questions.

EXAMPLE:

(Closed question)	*Nurse:*	How many times have you been pregnant?
	Patient:	Four.
(Closed question)	*Nurse:*	Were there any problems with your other deliveries?
	Patient:	Yes, with my last one.
(Open-ended question, directing topic)	*Nurse:*	What happened?
	Patient:	I was in labor a long time, and then something happened to the baby's heart rate. They did an emergency cesarean section.
(Open-ended question)	*Nurse:*	What plans have you made for this delivery?

The last, broad question seeks information about a topic of the nurse's choice. A more directive, closed question along the same lines would be, "Do you plan to have a cesarean birth again this time?" If the nurse wanted to explore the patient's feelings, she might have said, "What are your concerns for *this* delivery?"

Take-away point: Closed questions can be answered with a "yes" or "no." Broadly stated open-ended questions encourage the patient to talk and explore her thoughts and feelings.

Table 3–8 lists some common interviewing problems along with some suggestions for handling them. Along with Box 3–4, these suggestions should help you improve the quality of your interviews.

Active Listening When first learning to interview, students tend to focus on what questions to ask and how to phrase them. However, the most important communication strategy is active listening. Most people think they are listening, but often they are focusing on preparing a response to what they are hearing rather than trying to understand what they are hearing. Active, empathic listening is done with the ears, eyes, and heart. It means being attentive to the patient's verbal and nonverbal messages, listening for feelings, and conveying acceptance and respect. The following acronym will help you to remember behaviors of active listening (Townsend, 2009):

TABLE 3–8 Common Interviewing Problems

Source of Problem	Explanation	Suggested Nursing Actions
Interviewer's own discomfort	■ You may feel you are imposing on the patient, perhaps because you do not clearly know how the information will be used (especially true for students).	■ Do your homework. Be sure you understand the purpose of the interview; explain it to the patient during the introduction phase.
	■ You may feel uncomfortable asking personal questions of a stranger.	■ Remember that nurses are concerned with the whole person and that data are needed in order to give comprehensive care. Early in the interview, tell the patient to respond only as he feels comfortable. Remember that patients can choose what they wish to tell you, so they have some power to preserve their own privacy. Remind yourself that patients are usually at ease if you are at ease. Also, it may be that the patient has felt the need to talk about the subject, did not know how to bring it up, and is relieved that you have done so.
	■ Knowing that patients may respond to some questions with tears or anger, you may be afraid to ask such questions.	■ It may be hard to accept another's expressions of feelings, but it is important that you learn to do so. Avoiding potentially upsetting topics can leave large gaps in the database. Remember that the patient usually feels better after expressing emotions—even though you may be uncomfortable.
Interviewer's curiosity	■ There is a fine line between interest and curiosity. Patients appreciate interest but resent curiosity. This may cause them to be less inclined to talk to you.	■ Don't become too enmeshed in the details of the patient's story. Focus on getting the information you need for planning care.
Patient's family and visitors inhibit responses	■ The client may be embarrassed to discuss personal information in front of others, or it may be information clients do not wish others to know (e.g., a wife may not want her husband to know that she was treated for a sexually transmitted disease before they were married).	■ Unless the visitor is an important source of information (e.g., when the patient is a small child), ask the visitor to step out for a few minutes or postpone the interview until the visitor leaves.
Patient's family and visitors inhibit responses	■ Spouses often answer the questions you address to patients.	■ Thank the spouse for the information but remind him or her that it is important for you to get the information from the patient's perspective.
Nurse is not culturally sensitive	■ There are cultural variations in communication (e.g., in some cultures, social courtesies must be established before personal topics are discussed).	■ Be aware of differences in the meaning of phenomena such as touch, facial expressiveness, use of silence, and need for physical space. For example: —In some cultures, strangers do not make direct eye contact. —As a rule, men of all cultures require more space than women.

S   Sit or stand facing the patient to indicate that you are interested in what
     he is saying.
O   Open posture: arms and legs uncrossed.
L   Lean forward toward the patient.
E   Establish and maintain eye contact.
R   Relax to convey a sense of connection with the patient.

3-2 THINK & REFLECT!

1. Observe a conversation between peers or family members. What nonverbal behaviors did you see? Did the speakers (a) put words in each other's mouth, (b) interrupt, or (c) make value judgments or give advice?
2. Recall a recent conversation between a nurse and a patient. Did the nurse do (a), (b), or (c)? Did the nurse make eye contact? Use silence as a technique?

See suggested responses to #3-2 Think & Reflect! in Appendix A.

Interviewing Older Adults Interview techniques in this chapter focus on patients with normal cognitive and communication abilities. However, some patients, such as older adults, require special communication techniques. Older adults make up an ever-growing proportion of the U.S. population, and most nurses will care for at least some of these patients. In addition to the general interview guidelines in Box 3–4, consider the following when interviewing older adults:

1. *Proceed slowly.* Speak slowly and clearly, giving the client plenty of time to form an answer.
2. *Check for sensory deficits at the beginning of the interview.* Don't wait until you come to that area of the assessment form. Until you have checked the patient's hearing, look at him as you speak to allow for lip reading.
3. *Don't assume all elderly people are deaf or unable to understand your meaning.* The fact that you need to speak slowly does not mean that you need to speak loudly.
4. *Be aware that appropriate affect and articulate speech do not always go together.* Likewise, inappropriate affect and incoherent speech do not necessarily indicate a lack of understanding. A patient may speak coherently and make sense as she tells you about her loss of appetite and then begin crying for no apparent reason. Nevertheless, the information about her appetite may be credible. Another patient may laugh appropriately at something funny and yet be unable to speak clearly or find the words to express what he means.
5. *Rely more than usual on body language.* Be aware of nonverbal communication, such as quivering of the lips, tears in the eyes, or movements of the hands and feet. As noted above, some older patients have difficulty finding the words to express their ideas and feelings.
6. *Be alert for intermittent confusion.* Some older clients are confused at one time and not another. A client may be giving you credible information and then, as the

interview progresses, begin to lose track of the topic or introduce irrelevant material. When the patient seems confused, use focus assessment to determine his mental status. If you conclude that his answers are unreliable, you can finish the interview later when he is no longer confused.

7. *When possible, try to get data directly from the client.* Some clients are reluctant to answer questions. Also, families are sometimes very protective of clients and tend to answer for them. Explain to them that it is important for you to hear what the client has to say.

These suggestions apply in some degree to people of all ages, but they are especially important in meeting the challenges that occur when the aging process is superimposed on a disease process.

3-3 THINK & REFLECT!

Imagine you are a patient and the nurse says to you: "Lab will be here STAT to do a stick for gases, lytes, and enzymes. Then you'll go down for a CAT scan and an ECG. Meanwhile, I need to take your vitals. Also, do you take any OTC meds?"

- Would you understand what the nurse means?
- How would patients feel about these statements?
- Which terms are jargon that should be clarified?

See suggested responses to #3-3 Think & Reflect! in Appendix A.

Cognitive Deficits In addition to the normal changes of aging, many older people have mild to severe problems with memory and at least one other ability (e.g., judgment, thinking, language, or coordination). This is referred to as **dementia**. Nearly 50% of people older than age 85 are affected by Alzheimer's disease, a type of dementia. People with dementia have difficulty speaking and comprehending. Consult gerontology journals and texts for help in communicating with patients affected by dementia because the techniques vary from those discussed in this chapter. The following are a few examples of such variations:

- *Repeat the words exactly if the patient does not respond to your comment or question.* Usually when someone does not understand, you would try a new word, hoping it will be in her vocabulary. For patients with dementia, giving new information only adds to their confusion.
- *If you do not understand, ask the patient to repeat.*
- *Use simple, short, direct sentences.* Do not give more than one instruction or question at a time. Ask, "Where does it hurt?" not "What does it feel like, and when did it start?"
- *Do not use vague comments such as "Um-hmm" and "I see" to show attentive listening.* The patient will not be able to interpret such responses. Echo the patient's comment and bluntly state your response: "You are thirsty. I will bring you a drink."
- *Use words the person can understand.*
- *It may aid conversation to ask "yes" or "no" questions.*
- *Don't press for an answer if it makes the person anxious.*

- *Don't constantly correct the patient's statements if they include wrong information.*
- *Understand that the patient's reality is confused, and he cannot behave differently.* This is easy to forget because when the patient is smiling and conversing superficially, he may seem competent.
- *If conversation is not successful, try again later.*

Take-away point: When interviewing older adults, keep the normal changes of aging in mind. Also be aware of the possibility of cognitive deficits.

Validating the Data

Validation is the act of double-checking or verifying data. Critical thinkers validate data in order to:

- Ensure that assessment information is complete, accurate, and factual.
- Eliminate their own errors, biases, and misperceptions of the data.
- Avoid jumping to faulty conclusions about the data.

To collect data accurately, you must be aware of your own biases, values, and beliefs and be able to separate fact from interpretation and assumption. The unthinking acceptance of assumptions is called **premature closure**. For example, a nurse seeing a man holding his arm to his chest might assume that he is experiencing chest pain, when in fact he has a painful hand. To avoid premature closure, the nurse should ask the man why he is holding his arm to his chest. His response may validate the nurse's assumption (of chest pain) or prompt further questioning. Not all data require validation, though. For example, data such as height, weight, birth date, and most laboratory studies can be accepted as factual. As a rule, you should validate data when any of these four conditions apply:

1. Subjective and objective data (or interview and physical examination data) do not agree.

   EXAMPLE: Ms. Dolan states she has never had high blood pressure. However, the nurse obtains a reading of 190/100 mm Hg.

2. The client's statements differ at different times in the assessment.

   EXAMPLE: A labor patient initially stated that this was her first pregnancy. Later, when the nurse asked about prior hospitalizations, she said, "Once, in 1994, to have my appendix removed, and in 1998 when I had a miscarriage." The nurse realized that a miscarriage is counted as a pregnancy, making this the patient's second pregnancy.

3. The data seem odd or very unusual.

   EXAMPLE: The client has a resting pulse of 50 bpm and a blood pressure of 190/100 mm Hg.

4. Factors are present that interfere with accurate measurement.

   EXAMPLE: A crying infant will have a higher than normal respiratory rate and should be quieted in order for assessment data to be correct.

Table 3–9 contains suggestions for ways to validate data.

TABLE 3–9   Suggestions for Validating Data

Nursing Activities	Examples
Clarify vague or ambiguous statements by asking the patient more questions.	*Client:* "My son has been acting strange this week." *Nurse:* "What, exactly, did your son do when he started 'acting strange'?"
Always compare subjective and objective data to verify the patient's statements with your observations.	■ Compare pain behaviors with the patient's statements about the pain. ■ Take the patient's temperature when he complains of "feeling hot."
Recheck your measurement to be sure it is accurate.	Take the blood pressure a second time in the opposite arm.
Ensure that your measuring device is working correctly or use a different piece of equipment.	■ Calibrate the glucose monitor. ■ Take the patient's temperature with two different thermometers. ■ Palpate the pulse rate and compare with electronic monitor reading.
Ask someone else to verify your findings.	Ask a more experienced nurse to listen to the patient's lungs. Ask a nursing assistant to retake the blood pressure.
Use references (e.g., journals, the Internet, textbooks) to explain findings.	When the nurse discovered tiny purple swollen areas under an elderly client's tongue, she considered it abnormal. When she consulted a text about physical changes of aging, she discovered that such varicosities are common among the elderly.

3-3 WHAT DO YOU KNOW?

1. State four conditions that require you to validate data.
2. Define *validation*.

See answer to #3-3 What Do You Know? in Appendix A.

Organizing Data

ANA Standard I requires, in part, that data collection be systematic (see Box 3–2). This means that in addition to collecting and validating data, nurses organize related cues into predetermined categories. Most healthcare agencies have standardized forms for the comprehensive nursing assessment (e.g., Figure 3–2). Such forms help to ensure that no data are missed. They are also efficient, enabling you to organize data at the same time you collect and record it. For ongoing and focus assessment, you will not always have a data-collection form, so you will need to organize (cluster) the data *after* you collect it. Chapter 4 explains data clustering more fully.

The content of assessment forms (tools) is determined by two factors:

1. *The requirements of various agencies.* Government agencies (e.g., Medicare), insurance companies, and accrediting agencies, such as the Community Health Accreditation Program (CHAP), have different requirements.

2. *The type of patients seen on the unit or the agency.* For example, nurses working in a hospital maternity unit need different information about their patients than do nurses working in a long-term care facility.

Regardless of the content of the form, the agency determines the framework that will be used to organize the information. A **framework** is, very simply, a way of looking at something.

   EXAMPLE: A patient is trembling. A nurse using a psychological framework might conclude the patient is frightened; a nurse using a biological framework might conclude that the patient is cold.

Some frameworks focus on body systems, human needs, adaptive responses, self-care abilities, and so on. A framework indicates which data are significant and guides the nurse in selecting which patient characteristics to observe. A framework groups related data, helping the nurse to find the patterns necessary for identifying client strengths, problems, and risk factors.

Nursing Models

A **nursing model (theoretical framework)** is a set of interrelated concepts that represents a particular way of thinking about nursing, clients, health, and the environment. Such models are also called *theories, frameworks,* or *conceptual frameworks.* Those terms differ in meaning, depending on the extent to which the set of concepts has been used and tested in practice, and on the level of detail and organization of the concepts. For the purposes of this chapter, you do not need to know whether a theorist's ideas are a framework, a model, or a theory. You can use any level of organized concepts to guide data collection.

A nursing model tells you what to assess and why. The major concepts of the framework provide the categories for collecting and organizing data. Whereas a medical, or body systems, model provides data that are useful for medical diagnoses and treatments, a nursing model produces data that are useful in planning nursing care. The following are some examples:

- *Gordon's Functional Health Patterns Framework* directs nurses to collect data about common patterns of behavior that contribute to health, quality of life, and achievement of human potential (Gordon, 1994). Using this framework, you would note emerging patterns and determine whether the client's functioning in each of the patterns is functional or dysfunctional (Table 3–10).
- *Orem's Self-Care Model* focuses on the patient's abilities to perform self-care to maintain life, health, and well-being. Using this framework, you would identify self-care deficits that require nursing intervention (Box 3–5).
- *Roy's Adaptation Model* describes patients as biopsychosocial beings, constantly adapting to external and internal demands. Using this model, you would note patterns indicating the patient's inability to adapt in one of four modes: physiological, self-concept, social role, and interdependence (Table 3–11).
- *NANDA International Taxonomy II (2009)* provides a framework for assessing and diagnosing. Strictly speaking, though, it is not a nursing theory. It classifies data and nursing diagnoses into 13 domains (Table 3–12).

TABLE 3–10   Using Gordon's 11 Functional Health Patterns to Organize Data

Functional Health Pattern	Describes	Examples
Health perception/ health management	Client's perception of health and well-being and how health is managed	Compliance with medication regimen; use of health-promotion activities, such as regular exercise, annual check-ups
Nutritional/ metabolic	Pattern of food and fluid intake relative to metabolic need indicators of local nutrient supply	Condition of skin, teeth, hair, nails, mucous membranes; height and weight; fluid and electrolyte balance
Elimination	Patterns of excretory function (bowel, bladder, and skin); includes client's perception of "normal" function	Frequency of bowel movements, voiding pattern, pain on urination, appearance of urine and stool
Activity/ exercise	Patterns of exercise, activity, leisure, and recreation	Exercise, hobbies; may include cardiovascular and respiratory status, mobility, and activities of daily living
Cognitive/ perceptual	Sensory-perceptual and cognitive patterns	Vision, hearing, taste, touch, smell, pain perception and management; cognitive functions such as language, memory, and decision making
Sleep/rest	Patterns of sleep, rest, and relaxation	Client's perception of quality and quantity of sleep and energy, use of sleep aids, routines client uses
Self-perception/ self-concept	Client's self-concept pattern and perceptions of self; emotional patterns	Body comfort; body image; feeling state; attitudes about self; perception of abilities; objective data such as body posture, eye contact, voice tone
Role/relationship	Client's pattern of role engagements and relationships	Perception of current major roles and responsibilities (e.g., father, husband, salesman); satisfaction with family, work, or social relationships
Sexual/ reproductive	Patterns of satisfaction and dissatisfaction with sexuality; reproductive pattern and stage	Histories of pregnancy and childbirth; difficulties with sexual functioning; satisfaction with sexual relationships
Coping/ stress tolerance	General coping pattern and effectiveness of the pattern in terms of stress tolerance	Client's usual manner of handling stress, available support systems, perceived ability to control or manage situations
Value/belief	Patterns of values, beliefs (including spiritual), and goals that guide clients' choices or decisions	Religious affiliation, what client perceives as important in life, value or belief conflicts related to health, special religious practices

Source: Adapted with permission from Gordon, M. (1994). *Nursing diagnosis: Process and application* (3rd ed.). St. Louis: C.V. Mosby, p. 70.

BOX 3–5

USING OREM'S SELF-CARE MODEL TO ORGANIZE DATA

Group data into the following categories of what Orem termed "universal self-care requisites."

1. Maintaining an adequate intake of oxygen
2. Maintaining an adequate fluid intake
3. Maintaining sufficient food intake (adequate nutrition)
4. Providing care associated with elimination (e.g., bowel, bladder)
5. Achieving a balance between activity and rest
6. Achieving a balance between the amount of time spent alone and with others
7. Taking actions to avoid hazards to life, functioning, and well-being
8. Developing human functioning and development within social groups, taking into account one's potential, limitations, and desire for "normality" (as determined by science, culture, and social values)

Source: Adapted from Orem, D. E. (1991). *Nursing: Concepts of practice* (4th ed.). St. Louis: Mosby-Year Book.

TABLE 3–11   Using Roy's Adaptation Model to Organize Data

Categories (Adaptive Modes)	Explanation
Physiological needs Activity and rest Nutrition Elimination Fluid, electrolytes, and acid–base balance Oxygenation Protection Temperature regulation Regulation of the senses Regulation of neurologic function Regulation of endocrine function	Balance must be maintained in each of the subcategories.
Self-concept Physical self Personal self	Adaptation means developing a positive self-concept, including the physical self, moral-ethical self, and self-ideal. Includes self-esteem, coping strategies, effective sexual function, and psychological integrity.
Role function	Ability to function in various roles, such as parent, spouse, worker, and so on.
Interdependence	Balance between dependence and independence is achieved in relationships and achieving needs through interdependence with others. Includes giving and receiving love, respect, and value.

Source: Adapted from Roy, C. (2009). *The Roy adaptation model* (3rd ed). Upper Saddle River, NJ: Pearson, pp. 69–71.

TABLE 3–12   Using NANDA International Taxonomy II to Organize Data

Domains	Definitions	Classes
Health Promotion	The awareness of well-being or normality of function and the strategies used to maintain control of and enhance that well-being or normality of function	***Health Awareness*** Recognition of normal function and well-being ***Health Management*** Identifying, controlling, performing, and integrating activities to maintain health and well-being
Nutrition	The activities of taking in, assimilating, and using nutrients for the purposes of tissue maintenance, tissue repair, and the production of energy	***Ingestion*** Taking food or nutrients into the body ***Digestion*** The physical and chemical activities that convert foodstuffs into substances suitable for absorption and assimilation ***Absorption*** The act of taking up nutrients through body tissues ***Metabolism*** The chemical and physical processes occurring in living organisms and cells for the development and use of protoplasm and the production of waste and energy, with the release of energy for all vital processes ***Hydration*** The taking in and absorption of fluids and electrolytes
Elimination and Exchange	Secretion and excretion of waste products from the body	***Urinary System*** The process of secretion, reabsorption, and excretion of urine ***Gastrointestinal System*** Excretion and expulsion of the end products of digestion ***Integumentary System*** Process of secretion and excretion through the skin ***Respiratory System*** The process of exchange of gases and removal of the end products of metabolism
Activity/ Rest	The production, conservation, expenditure, or balance of energy resources	***Sleep/Rest*** Slumber, repose, ease, relaxation, or inactivity ***Activity/Exercise*** Moving parts of the body (mobility), doing work, or performing actions often (but not always) against resistance ***Energy Balance*** A dynamic state of harmony between intake and expenditure of resources

TABLE 3–12 Using NANDA International Taxonomy II to Organize Data (*continued*)

Domains	Definitions	Classes
		Cardiovascular/Pulmonary Responses Cardiopulmonary mechanisms that support activity and rest ***Self-Care*** Ability to perform activities to care for one's body and bodily functions
Perception/ Cognition	The human information processing system including attention, orientation, sensation, perception, cognition, and communication	***Attention*** Mental readiness to notice or observe ***Orientation*** Awareness of time, place, and person ***Sensation/Perception*** Receiving information through the senses of touch, taste, smell, vision, hearing, and kinesthesia and the comprehension of sense data resulting in naming, associating, or pattern recognition ***Cognition*** Use of memory, learning, thinking, problem solving, abstraction, judgment, insight, intellectual capacity, calculation, and language ***Communication*** Sending and receiving verbal and nonverbal information
Self-Perception	Awareness about the self	***Self-Concept*** The perception(s) about the total self ***Self-Esteem*** Assessment of one's own worth, capability, significance, and success ***Body Image*** A mental image of one's own body
Roles/ Relationships	The positive and negative connections or associations among persons or groups of persons and the means by which those connections are demonstrated	***Caregiving Roles*** Socially expected behavior patterns by persons providing care who are not healthcare professionals ***Family Relationships*** Associations of people who are biologically related or related by choice ***Role Performance*** Quality of functioning in socially expected behavior patterns
Sexuality	Sexual identity, sexual function, and reproduction	***Sexual Identity*** The state of being a specific person in regard to sexuality, gender, or both ***Sexual Function*** The capacity or ability to participate in sexual activities

(*continued*)

TABLE 3–12   Using NANDA International Taxonomy II to Organize Data (*continued*)

Domains	Definitions	Classes
		Reproduction Any process by which human beings are produced
Coping/ Stress Tolerance	Contending with life events and life processes	*Post-Trauma Responses* Reactions occurring after physical or psychological trauma *Coping Responses* The process of managing environmental stress *Neurobehavioral Stress* Behavioral responses reflecting nerve and brain function
Life Principles	Principles underlying conduct, thought, and behavior about acts, customs, or institutions viewed as being true or having intrinsic worth	*Values* The identification and ranking of preferred modes of conduct or end states *Beliefs* Opinions, expectations, or judgments about acts, customs, or institutions viewed as being true or having intrinsic worth *Value/Belief/Action Congruence* The correspondence or balance achieved between values, beliefs, and actions
Safety/ Protection	Freedom from danger, physical injury or immune system damage; preservation from loss; and protection of safety and security	*Infection* Host responses after pathogenic invasion *Physical Injury* Bodily harm or hurt *Violence* The exertion of excessive force or power so as to cause injury or abuse *Environmental Hazards* Sources of danger in the surroundings *Defensive Processes* The processes by which the self protects itself from the nonself *Thermoregulation* The physiologic process of regulating heat and energy within the body for the purposes of protecting the organism
Comfort	Sense of mental, physical, or social well-being or ease	*Physical Comfort* Sense of well-being or ease or freedom from pain *Environmental Comfort* Sense of well-being or ease in or with one's environment

TABLE 3–12 Using NANDA International Taxonomy II to Organize Data (*continued*)

Domains	Definitions	Classes
Growth/ Development	Age-appropriate increases in physical dimensions, maturation of organ systems, or progression through the developmental milestones	*Social Comfort* Sense of well-being or ease with one's social situations *Growth* Increases in physical dimensions or maturity of organ systems *Development* Progression or regression through a sequence of recognized milestones in life

Source: Adapted from NANDA International (2009). *NANDA International nursing diagnoses: Definitions and classification 2009–2011.* Oxford: Wiley-Blackwell, pp. 370–380.

Nonnursing Models

Frameworks from other disciplines may also be helpful for clustering data. **Maslow's Hierarchy of Needs** organizes data according to basic human needs that are common to all people. This model theorizes that a person's basic needs (e.g., physiological) must be met before their higher needs (e.g., self-esteem) can be met. See Table 3–13 for examples.

A **body systems (medical) model** is useful for identifying data that may indicate a medical problem. Most assessment forms have at least a section that is organized by body systems (Box 3–6). A form that combines body systems with other models

TABLE 3–13 Using Maslow's Basic Human Needs to Organize Data

Data Categories (Needs)	Examples of Data
Physiological (Basic survival needs)	Oxygen, nutrition, fluids, body temperature regulation, warmth, elimination, shelter, sex
Safety and Security (Need to be safe and comfortable)	Physical safety (infection, falls, drug side effects); psychological security (knowledge of procedures, bedtime rituals, usual routines, fear of isolation dependence needs); pain
Love and Belonging (Need for love and affection)	Information about family and significant others, social supports
Esteem and Self-Esteem (Need to feel good about self)	Changes in body image (e.g., puberty, surgery); changes in self-concept (e.g., ability to perform usual role in family); pride in capabilities
Self-Actualization (Need to achieve one's maximum potential; need for growth and change)	Extent to which goals are being achieved, autonomy, motivation, problem-solving abilities, ability to give and accept help, feelings about accomplishments, roles

Source: Adapted from Maslow, A. H. (1970). *Motivation and personality* (2nd ed.). New York: Harper & Row.

BOX 3-6	
BODY SYSTEMS MODEL	
Integumentary	Musculoskeletal
Respiratory	Gastrointestinal
Cardiovascular	Genitourinary
Nervous	Reproductive
Endocrine	Immune

(e.g., Maslow's Hierarchy of Needs or a nursing model) provides a holistic approach that enables the nurse to identify both medical and nursing problems.

No matter which model you use, it is important to use it consistently in order to become familiar with it. Even if you do not use a form to collect data, you will still classify related cues according to your framework. Remember that a framework gives you a special way to view the patient; helps you to make thorough, systematic assessments; and makes the data more meaningful.

3-4 THINK & REFLECT!

Does your school provide a nursing assessment form for you to use in clinical? What model(s) does it use to organize data? What are the major categories? How is it different from the forms used by the nurses on your clinical unit?

See suggested responses to #3-4 Think & Reflect! in Appendix A.

Recording Data

ANA Standard I (see Box 3–2) requires that assessment data be *documented* in a retrievable format. The nursing database becomes a part of the client's permanent record. Therefore, you should record the assessment in ink on the form provided by the agency on the same day the client is admitted. Write neatly and legibly using only the abbreviations approved by the agency. Do not try to write everything the client says word for word because this is likely to interfere with the communication between you and the client.

Record subjective data in the client's own words, when possible, using quotation marks. Alternatively, you may paraphrase or summarize what the client says and omit the quotation marks. Be sure to record the data, not what you think they mean. Record **cues** (what the client tells you and what you see, hear, feel, smell, and measure), not **inferences** (your judgment or interpretation of what the cues mean). Table 3–14 compares cues with conclusions (inferences).

Avoid vague generalities such as *good, normal, adequate,* or *tolerated well.* These words mean different things to different people. Suppose a nurse writes, "Vision adequate." Does this mean the client can read newsprint without eyeglasses? Or when she is

TABLE 3–14 Comparison of Data and Conclusions (Cues and Inferences)

	Cues (Data)	Inferences
Subjective	**Objective**	
"My back really hurts." (Paraphrase: Patient states his back hurts.)	Lying rigidly in bed. Facial grimacing is observed.	Patient is in pain.
"My armband is too tight, and my arm is really sore." (Paraphrase: Patient says his armband is too tight and his arm is sore.)	Left arm is hot, red, and swollen in a 4″ 4″ area around IV insertion site.	Left arm is infected at IV site.
"I'm not sure I should have this surgery. It might not even help, and it is very dangerous. I guess I'm scared."	Tearful. Facial muscles tense. Pulse rate 100 bpm. Hands trembling.	Patient is afraid of having surgery.
Remember: You should record cues, not inferences.		

wearing glasses? Or that she can see well enough to ambulate without assistance? It would be better to record, "Able to read newsprint at 24 in while wearing glasses."

Take-away point: Record data, not conclusions. Use concrete, specific terms; avoid vague generalities such as "tolerated well."

3-5 THINK & REFLECT!

Scenario: You are making a focused assessment for Disturbed Sleep Pattern. Your patient says, "Well, of course, I'm tired! I didn't sleep a bit last night. My roommate snores like a freight train, and the night nurse was in here making noise all night long. If she'd get organized, she wouldn't have to disturb us so much."

1. In this case, what do you think of your text's directions to "record subjective data in the client's own words?"
2. What would you write when recording these data? Why?

See suggested responses to #3-5 Think & Reflect! in Appendix A.

Special-Purpose Assessments

You may wish to perform an in-depth assessment of certain areas of a client's functioning. Most agencies have developed forms for special assessments. For example, you may gather in-depth data about a client's nutritional status using a form provided by your school. Or you may use a special form to monitor the level of consciousness, pupil reaction, and limb movement of a comatose patient. This section discusses functional, home health, cultural, spiritual, wellness, family, and community assessments.

Home Care and Functional Assessment

Reimbursement and accrediting agencies mandate patient education and discharge planning to aid patients in the transition from acute care to self-care. Data about the patient's knowledge and self-care abilities enable the nurse to develop an individualized teaching plan. However, nurses have less time than ever to focus on the patient as an individual. One way to overcome this obstacle is to have the patient complete a self-assessment checklist. For example, a tool might assess patients' self-care (or functional) abilities. Examples of functional abilities include the patient's ability to feed, bathe, dress, groom and toilet herself; to transfer from a bed or chair; and to safely walk or use a wheelchair.

Accreditation and managed care companies also require outcomes data from home care agencies. For example, Medicare uses the Outcomes Assessment Information System (OASIS). A comprehensive home healthcare assessment includes data about the home environment, family, psychosocial status, education, physiologic status, and functional abilities. Functional assessment (activities of daily living, or ADLs) data are important because they are part of the OASIS data and because they help the nurse determine a client's rehabilitative prognosis. To continue to provide home-care services to the client, you must include in your documentation (a) evidence of homebound status and (b) evidence of continued need for skilled care (Centers for Medicare and Medicaid Services, 2009). To see the entire OASIS assessment form, go to the Pearson Nursing Student Resources.

Three functional assessment tools—PULSES, the Barthel Index, and the Functional Independence Measure—are summarized in Table 3–15. These tools measure only basic activities of daily living. They do not measure "instrumental" activities of daily living, such as cooking, driving, and shopping. Therefore, a high score indicates that a patient should not require attendant care but does not necessarily mean that the patient can live alone (Neal, 1998).

Cultural Assessment

Because nurses are expected to provide individualized care, they must understand how clients' cultural beliefs and practices can affect their health and illness (ANA, 1991, p. 1). **Cultural sensitivity** begins in the first phase of the nursing process when you obtain culturally specific information for the client's health history. **Cultural competence** requires knowledge of the values, beliefs, and practices of various cultures along with an attitude of awareness, openness, and sensitivity. Figure 3–5 is a heritage assessment that analyzes the degree to which a person identifies with the dominant culture and with a traditional culture (Spector, 2000). You may wish to use this tool with clients or as a self-assessment to discuss with your peers. The remainder of this section provides an overview of phenomena that must be assessed in order to provide culturally competent nursing care (Wilkinson & Treas, 2011).

Ethnicity/Race/Cultural Affiliation Ethnicity may include race, but it is not the same as race. The U.S. Census Bureau has defined the following categories for race:

- American Indian and Alaska Native
- Asian American (including Asian Indian, Chinese, Filipino, Japanese, Korean, and Vietnamese, and Other Asian)
- Black or African American
- Native Hawaiian

TABLE 3–15 Functional (Self-Care) Assessment Tools

Instrument	Description	Categories Assessed
PULSES (Moskowitz and McCann, 1957)	Expands functional assessment to include the client's physical condition and support system. The patient is scored 1 to 4 on each item, with 1 representing independence.	**P**hysical condition **U**pper limb functions **L**ower limb functions **S**ensory components **E**xcretory functions **S**upport factors
Barthel Index (Mahoney and Barthel, 1965)	Assesses independence with basic ADLs. The patient is scored "independent" or "with help" on each category.	Feeding Moving from wheelchair to bed and returning Performing personal toilet (e.g., wash face, shave) Getting on and off toilet Bathing Walking on level surface Propelling wheelchair Going up and down stairs Dressing and undressing Bowel continence Bladder control
Functional Independence Measure	Measures basic ADLs in a bit more detail than the Barthel Index and has been used primarily with children (Neal, 1998).	Self-care Sphincter control Mobility Locomotion Communication Social cognition (e.g., problem solving)

- Pacific Islander (including Guamanian or Chamorro, Samoan, and Other)
- White
- Two or more races

In addition, the Census Bureau identifies two categories for describing ethnicity: (a) Hispanic, Latino, or Spanish origin and (b) *not* Hispanic, Latino, or Spanish origin. Hispanics and Latinos may be of any race (U.S. Census Bureau, 2010). Any of the races can be found in the Hispanic/Latino or not Hispanic/Latino categories because the Census Bureau does not include Hispanic/Latino as a race but as a sociocultural category. The terms *race* and *ethnicity* overlap somewhat because race can be a characteristic of a specific ethnic group.

Race is important information because of biological variations, such as lactose intolerance, and susceptibility to specific disease process, such as sickle cell anemia or Tay-Sachs disease. Be aware that skin color is not necessarily an indicator of either race or culture. Do not assume ethnic or racial affiliation; allow patients to self-report these data. You might ask an open-ended question such as: "I want to learn about your cultural heritage. Can you tell me about your cultural group?"

Heritage Assessment

I. Demographic Data

1. Location_____
2. (a) Age _____
   (b) Date of Birth _____
   (c) Place of Birth _____
3. Sex
   (1) Female   (2) Male
4. What is the highest grade
   completed in school? _____
5. Are you
   (1) Married   (2) Widowed
   (3) Divorced   (4) Separated
   (5) Never married

II. Heritage Assessment: Your Ethnic, Cultural, and Religious Background

1. Where was your mother born?

   _____

2. Where was your father born?

   _____

3. Where were your grandparents born?:
   a. Your mother's mother?

      _____

   b. Your mother's father?

      _____

   c. Your father's mother?

      _____

   d. Your father's father?

      _____

4. How many brothers do you
   have?_____ sisters?_____
5. In what setting did you grow up?
   Urban   Rural   Suburban
6. In what country did your parents
   grow up?
   Father _____
   Mother_____
7. How old were you when you came
   to the United States?
8. How old were your parents when
   they came to the U.S.?
   Mother_____
   Father _____
9. When you were growing up, who
   lived with you?_____

   _____

10. Have you maintained contact with:
    a. Aunts, uncles, cousins Yes No
    b. Brothers and sisters?   Yes No
    c. Parents?   Yes No
    d. Your own children?   Yes No

11. Did most of your aunts, uncles,
    cousins live near to your home?
    Yes   No
12. Approximately how often did you
    visit your family members who lived
    outside of your home?
    (1) Daily (2) Weekly (3) Monthly
    (4) Once a year or less (5) Never
13. Was your original family name
    changed?
    Yes   No
14. What is your religious preference?
    (1) Catholic   (2) Jewish
    (3) Protestant   (4) Denomination
    (5) Other   (6) None
15. Is your spouse the same religion as
    you?
    Yes   No
16. Is your spouse the same ethnic back-
    ground as you?
    Yes   No
17. What kind of school did you go to?
    (1) Public   (2) Private
    (3) Religious
18. As an adult, do you live in a neigh-
    borhood where the neighbors are
    the same religion and ethnic back-
    ground as yourself?
    Yes   No
19. Do you belong to a religious institu-
    tion?
    Yes   No
20. Would you describe yourself as an
    active member?
    Yes   No
21. How often do you attend your reli-
    gious institution?
    (1) More than once a week
    (2) Weekly   (3) Monthly
    (4) Special holidays only (5) Never
22. Do you practice your religion in your
    home?
    Yes   No
    (if yes, please specify)
    (1) Praying   (2) Bible reading
    (3) Diet
    (4) Celebrating religious holidays
23. Do you prepare foods of your ethnic
    background?
    Yes   No
24. Do you participate in ethnic activities?
    Yes   No
    (if yes, please specify)
    (1) Singing
    (2) Holiday celebrations
    (3) Dancing   (4) Festivals
    (5) Costumes   (6) Other

25. Are your friends from the same reli-
    gious background as you?
    Yes   No
26. Are your friends from the same eth-
    nic background as you?
    Yes   No
27. What is your native language?

    _____

28. Do you speak this language?
    (1) Prefer   (2) Occasionally
    (3) Rarely
29. Do you read your native language?
    Yes   No

III. Beliefs and Practices Regarding Personal Health and Illness

(Note: Use a separate sheet of paper for long answer questions.)

1. How do you describe "health"?

2. How do you rate your health?
   (1) Excellent   (2) Good
   (3) Fair   (4) Poor

3. How do you describe "illness"?

4. What do you believe causes illness?
   (1) Poor eating habits?   Yes No
   (2) Incorrect food
       combinations?   Yes No
   (3) Viruses, bacteria, "germs?"   Yes No
   (4) God's punishment for sin?   Yes No
   (5) The "Evil Eye?"   Yes No
   (6) Other people's hexes
       or spells?   Yes No
   (7) Witchcraft?   Yes No
   (8) Changes in environment,
       i.e., cold/hot weather?   Yes No
   (9) Exposure to drafts   Yes No
   (10) Overwork?   Yes No
   (11) Underwork?   Yes No
   (12) Grief and loss?   Yes No
   (13) Other

5. What did your mother do to keep
   you from getting sick?

6. How do you keep yourself from getting sick?

7. What home remedies did your
   mother use to treat illness?

8. What home remedies do you use?

9. Describe in 200–300 words an incident in your nursing practice when
   cultural differences (religious, ethnic,
   or lay nursing) caused a problem for
   you.

FIGURE 3–5

Heritage assessment (*Source*: Spector, R. E. (2004). *Cultural diversity in health and illness* (6th ed.). Upper Saddle River, NJ: Prentice-Hall.)

Birthplace and Place of Residence Patients who have lived in this society only a short time may not have assimilated Western healthcare practices. This information may provide an idea of the degree to which the patient may be able to adhere to a prescribed regimen. Part II of Figure 3–5 covers this category thoroughly.

Communication Abilities Gestures, touch, eye contact, and body language are culturally related (e.g., some Asian Americans may avoid direct eye contact as a show of respect). Determine which nonverbal cues given by the client or the nurse facilitate or hinder communication. Assess the client's language fluency and obtain an interpreter if needed. Be aware that from the client's point of view, if the interpreter is too young, of the opposite gender, or of a different sociocultural background, the client may not wish to share personal information. When assessing communication, identify the patient's native language, note regional dialect, listen for speech volume and emotional tone, and be alert that the same word may have more than one meaning.

Food Sanctions or Restrictions Food choice and selection have more than just nutritional value and may be closely related to religious practices and health beliefs. Ask, "What kind of foods do you eat to maintain health? What foods do you eat during illness? Do they require special preparation?" Ask about religious restrictions on eating (e.g., is the client required to fast or to avoid certain foods?). Consult a nutritionist as needed for making culturally acceptable food substitutions.

Religious and Spiritual Beliefs and Practices The nurse should facilitate patients' observance of spiritual beliefs. Some cultures rely on spiritual healers; others may require the presence of a religious representative during delivery of health care; still others sanction the use of mood-altering substances during ceremonies. For more information, refer to Figure 3–5 and the section on Spiritual Assessment.

Health Beliefs, Theories of Illness, Folk Practices Western health practices are based on the *scientific perspective* (all diseases have a measurable cause and effect). The *holistic model* of illness emphasizes a balance between mind-body-spirit and the universe (e.g., "hot-cold theory," "Yin-Yang theory"). The *magicoreligious model* holds that the supernatural forces of good and evil cause disruptions in health. People often hold a combination of these beliefs. Part III of Figure 3–5 provides questions for assessing health beliefs. In addition, ask, "What are you considering now, and how can we help?"

Family and Support System In some families, decisions are made by one dominant authority; in others, the collective community makes decisions, and the patient must abide by them. Ask questions such as: "Who are the members of your family? What family duties do women and men usually perform in your culture? Whom do you consult when making healthcare decisions (e.g., family member, cultural or religious leader)? Who will be able to help you during and after treatment?"

Space Orientation The relationship between one's body and objects and persons in the environment is learned. People in Western societies tend to be more territorial (e.g., "You are in my space"). The patient may withdraw if the nurse is perceived as being too close (e.g., to assess the lungs, a nurse needs to move into the patient's intimate space).

Time Orientation Time may have a different meaning and value to people of different cultures. Time orientation also refers to the person's focus on the past, the present, or the future. Most cultures combine all three orientations, but one is more likely to dominate. Healthcare workers tend to value time and an orientation toward the future (e.g., medication schedules, appointment times).

Pain Responses There are both cultural and individual differences in pain perception and responses. In some cultures, pain may be considered a punishment for bad deeds, so the patient is expected to tolerate pain without complaint. In other cultures, tolerance of pain suggests strength and endurance; in still others, the expression of pain elicits attention and sympathy.

Spiritual Assessment

A holistic assessment includes information about the client's spiritual well-being. For healthy clients, the spiritual dimension is important to overall well-being. For those who are ill, spirituality can be a source of either support or difficulty. Nurses usually elicit spiritual data as a part of the general history. It is best to do the spiritual assessment at the end of the interview after you have developed a relationship with the client. The following questions may be helpful when working with clients who indicate a religious affiliation:

- Please tell me about any particular religious practices that are important to you.
- Has being here (or being ill) interfered with your religious practices?
- Do you feel that your faith is helpful to you? In what ways is it important to you right now?
- How can I help you carry out your faith? For example, would you like me to read your prayer book to you?
- Would you like a visit from your spiritual counselor, a minister, or the hospital chaplain?

Nurses sometimes hesitate to ask questions about spirituality because they are afraid they may impose their own ideas of spirituality on the client or because they fear that using "religious language" would alienate a client who does not express spirituality in such language (e.g., "Do you pray regularly?" or "Are you saved?"). It may help to think of spirituality in a broad sense, not as limited to religion. The following are some questions and observations that may help you to assess the client's spiritual status without asking direct, spiritual questions (Cathell, 1991; Stoll, 1979):

1. *The patient's concept of "God."* Most people are religious in the sense that they need something to give meaning to their lives. For some, "God" is the religious meaning of God; for some, it is their work; for others, it is their lifestyle, their children, and so on. Listen to what the patient says about how he spends his time and energy. Observe the books at his bedside and the programs he watches on television. Does the patient's life have meaning, value, and purpose? Does he seem to be at peace with himself?

2. *The patient's source of hope and strength.* This might be God in the traditional sense, a family member, or the client's "inner source" of strength. Notice who the client talks about most often or ask, "Who is important to you?" "Where do you go to feel

loved and understood?" or "What helps you when you feel afraid or in need of special help?"

3. *The significance of religious practice and rituals.* In addition to asking specific questions, notice whether the client seems to be praying when you enter the room, before meals, or during procedures. Observe whether a clergy member visits. Look for such items as religious literature, pictures, rosaries, church bulletins, and religious get-well cards at the bedside. These provide clues to the kinds of spiritual support that are meaningful to the client.

4. *The patient's thoughts about the relationship between spiritual beliefs and state of health.* Is the client questioning the meaning of his illness: "Why did God let this happen to me?" Some people believe illness is a punishment for some wrong they have done. Others may see illness as a test of their faith. Still others may see their faith as therapy for their illness: "If I have faith, I will get well." You might ask questions such as, "What has bothered you most about being sick?" or "What is most frightening or meaningful about your illness?"

5. *The patient's fear of alienation, loneliness, or solitude.* This can take many forms. Instead of appearing lonely, patients may use distancing behaviors such as joking. Some patients are overly sophisticated about their illness. They talk about it in terms of lab values, pathophysiology, and medications, but they do not say how they feel about it or what it means in their lives. Other clients may pace the halls; have sleep disturbances; or seem angry, apathetic, or preoccupied.

Take-away point: Be aware of spiritual needs:

- Look for visual cues (e.g., Bible, prayer beads)
- Listen for verbal cues (e.g., references to God or church)
- Assess for spiritual distress (e.g., crying, anger, wishing to die)

3-4 WHAT DO YOU KNOW?

List the phenomena to be assessed in a cultural assessment.

See answer to #3-4 What Do You Know? in Appendix A.

Wellness Assessment

A thorough assessment of the client's health status is basic to health promotion. **Health promotion** is more than avoidance or prevention of disease. It includes activities undertaken for the purpose of improving well-being and achieving a higher level of health (e.g., stress management and physical fitness). See Table 3–16 for a summary of the components of a wellness assessment.

Health promotion assumes that people can identify their own health needs. In this framework, assessment involves active listening and a dialogue between the nurse and the client. The nurse and client collaborate to achieve a deeper understanding of the client's health experiences. The nurse may ask questions in order to make the client more aware of factors that may be influencing his condition, and the client asks

TABLE 3–16 Components of a Wellness Assessment

Assessment Categories	Explanation and Examples
Physical fitness evaluation	Because of sedentary lifestyles, this is a critical component. Includes cardiovascular tolerance (e.g., step test), general appearance, muscle strength (e.g., sit-ups), joint flexibility, body proportions, percent of body fat.
Nutritional assessment	Poor eating habits and dietary risk factors are widespread in all socioeconomic groups. Includes muscle mass, 24-hour recall of food intake, knowledge of nutrition, effect of sociocultural beliefs on diet, use of MyPyramid and Recommended Daily Intakes of essential nutrients, and comparison of weight with body build and height.
Health risk appraisal	Assessment of a client's risk of disease or injury over the next 10 years by comparing the client's characteristics with those of corresponding age, sex, and racial group. A **risk factor** is anything that increases a person's chance of acquiring a specific disease, such as cancer (e.g., exposure to the sun is a risk factor for skin cancer). Risk factors may be categorized according to age, genetic factors, biologic characteristics, personal health habits, lifestyle, and environment. Many health risk tools are available. They commonly assess five categories of risk: cardiovascular disease, cancer, automobile accidents, suicide, and diabetes.
Lifestyle assessment	Categories generally assessed are physical activity, nutritional practices, stress management, safety practices, healthcare practices (e.g., last Pap smear, last chest x-ray), and such habits as smoking, alcohol consumption, and drug use. Figure 3–6 is an example of a lifestyle assessment.
Health beliefs	Healthcare beliefs provide an indication of how much the person believes he/she can influence or control health through personal behaviors (e.g., breast self-examination). Assess clients' beliefs about such things as exercise benefits and barriers, social support for exercise, the definition of health, and health locus of control (i.e., whether the person, chance, or powerful others influences the person's health).
Life stress review	People who have high levels of stress are more prone to illness and less able to cope with illness. Various tools have been developed that assign numerical values to recent life events (e.g., divorce, pregnancy, retirement). High scores are associated with an increased likelihood of illness.
Social support systems review	Social support is the subjective feeling of belonging and being accepted; being valued for oneself. The *natural support system* is the family; this is usually the primary support group. *Peer support systems* are people who function informally to meet the needs of others (e.g., a group of widows and widowers). *Organized religious support systems* (e.g., churches) provide support through shared values. *Professional supports* consist of helping professionals with a specific set of skills and services (e.g., financial counselor, bereavement counselor). *Organized support systems not directed by health professionals* include voluntary service groups and mutual help groups, such as Alcoholics Anonymous.
Spiritual health assessment	Because spiritual beliefs affect the client's interpretation of life events, they are a critical component of health assessment. Spiritual assessment goes beyond religious affiliation to explore feelings about the meaning of life, love, hope, forgiveness, life after death, and connectedness. Refer to "Spiritual Assessment," in the preceding pages.

Sources: Andrews, M., & Boyle. J. (2007) *Transcultural concepts in nursing care* (5th ed.). Philadelphia: Lippincott; Giger, J., & Davidhizar, R. (2008). *Transcultural nursing: Assessment and intervention* (5th ed.). St Louis: Mosby; Leininger, M., & McFarland, M. (2002). *Transcultural nursing: Concepts, theories, research and practices.* (3rd ed.). New York: McGraw-Hill; Purnell, L., & Paulanka, B. (2008). *Transcultural health nursing: A culturally competent approach* (3rd ed.). Philadelphia: F. A. Davis; Suzuki, L., & Ponterotto, J. (2007). *Handbook of multicultural assessment: Clinical, psychological, and educational applications.* (3rd ed.). San Francisco: Jossey-Bass; Wilkinson, J., & Treas, L. (2011). *Fundamentals of nursing* (2nd ed). Philadelphia: F. A. Davis.

Physical Activity Section

1. I engage in sweat-producing physical activity for 20–30 minutes at least three times per week.

   Almost Never   Occasionally   Often   Very Often   Almost Always

2. My physical activity includes stretching, aerobic activity and strength conditioning.

   Almost Never   Occasionally   Often   Very Often   Almost Always

3. I walk or bicycle as a means of transportation whenever possible.

   Almost Never   Occasionally   Often   Very Often   Almost Always

4. An integral part of my leisure time includes physical activity instead of TV viewing or surfing the Internet.

   Almost Never   Occasionally   Often   Very Often   Almost Always

5. If I am not in shape, I avoid sporadic (once per week or less) strenuous exercise. (If you are in shape answer "Almost Always.")

   Almost Never   Occasionally   Often   Very Often   Almost Always

Nutrition Section

6. I eat at least five servings of fruits and vegetables every day (one serving equals one piece of fruit or 1/2 cup).

   Almost Never   Occasionally   Often   Very Often   Almost Always

7. I avoid eating at fast-food restaurants.

   Almost Never   Occasionally   Often   Very Often   Almost Always

8. I intentionally include foods that are high in fiber in my diet on a daily basis (i.e., whole grain breads and cereals, beans, etc.).

   Almost Never   Occasionally   Often   Very Often   Almost Always

9. I maintain my weight within the recommendations for my height and gender.

   Almost Never   Occasionally   Often   Very Often   Almost Always

10. I avoid eating foods that are high in fat (whole-milk dairy products, fried foods, hot dogs, desserts, gravies, and fatty meats).

    Almost Never   Occasionally   Often   Very Often   Almost Always

Self-Care Section

11. I avoid the use of tobacco products (cigarettes, smokeless tobacco, cigars, pipes).

    Almost Never   Occasionally   Often   Very Often   Almost Always

12. I examine my breasts or testes on a monthly basis.

    Almost Never   Occasionally   Often   Very Often   Almost Always

13. I protect my skin from sun damage by using sunscreen, wearing hats, and/or avoiding tanning booths and sun lamps.

    Almost Never   Occasionally   Often   Very Often   Almost Always

FIGURE 3–6

TestWell Individual Assessment (Part 2) (*Source:* All material copyright © 2000 by the National Wellness Institute—All Rights Reserved. Used by permission. Available at http://www.TestWell.org/part2.asp. Accessed 3/1/03.)

14. I maintain my blood pressure within the range recommended by my doctor. (If you do not have your blood pressure checked, answer "Almost Never.")

    Almost Never   Occasionally   Often   Very Often   Almost Always

15. I floss my teeth every day.

    Almost Never   Occasionally   Often   Very Often   Almost Always

Safety Section

16. I wear a seat belt when traveling in a vehicle.

    Almost Never   Occasionally   Often   Very Often   Almost Always

17. I stay within five miles per hour of the speed limit.

    Almost Never   Occasionally   Often   Very Often   Almost Always

18. I avoid riding with drivers who are under the influence of alcohol or other drugs.

    Almost Never   Occasionally   Often   Very Often   Almost Always

19. I avoid the use of alcohol and other drugs.

    Almost Never   Occasionally   Often   Very Often   Almost Always

20. I use the recommended safety equipment (pads, mouthguards, goggles, life jacket, etc.) for any activity I participate in.

    Almost Never   Occasionally   Often   Very Often   Almost Always

Social and Environmental Wellness Section

21. I regularly recycle my paper, plastic, glass or aluminum.

    Almost Never   Occasionally   Often   Very Often   Almost Always

22. My behavior reflects fairness and justice.

    Almost Never   Occasionally   Often   Very Often   Almost Always

23. I take time to play with my family and friends.

    Almost Never   Occasionally   Often   Very Often   Almost Always

24. When I notice something that is dangerous to others I take action to correct it.

    Almost Never   Occasionally   Often   Very Often   Almost Always

25. I contribute time and/or money to at least one organization that strives to better the community where I live.

    Almost Never   Occasionally   Often   Very Often   Almost Always

Emotional Awareness and Sexuality Section

26. My sexual relationships and behaviors are maintained in a manner that is healthy for me and for others.

    Almost Never   Occasionally   Often   Very Often   Almost Always

27. I am able to develop close intimate, personal relationships.

    Almost Never   Occasionally   Often   Very Often   Almost Always

FIGURE 3–6
(*continued*)

28. I am tolerant of others who have different sexual orientations.

| Almost Never | Occasionally | Often | Very Often | Almost Always |

29. If I engage in sexual behavior I take action to avoid unwanted pregnancy. (If you do not engage in sexual intercourse, answer "Almost Always.")

| Almost Never | Occasionally | Often | Very Often | Almost Always |

30. I feel positive about myself as a sexual person.

| Almost Never | Occasionally | Often | Very Often | Almost Always |

Emotional Management Section

31. I express my feelings of anger in ways that are not hurtful to others.

| Almost Never | Occasionally | Often | Very Often | Almost Always |

32. I set realistic objectives for myself.

| Almost Never | Occasionally | Often | Very Often | Almost Always |

33. When I make mistakes, I learn from them.

| Almost Never | Occasionally | Often | Very Often | Almost Always |

34. I do not feel unreasonably hurried in my daily routine.

| Almost Never | Occasionally | Often | Very Often | Almost Always |

35. I accept responsibility for my own actions.

| Almost Never | Occasionally | Often | Very Often | Almost Always |

Intellectual Wellness Section

36. I keep informed about social, political and/or current issues.

| Almost Never | Occasionally | Often | Very Often | Almost Always |

37. I watch educational programs on television every week (news, political discussions, documentaries, public TV, or the Discovery channel).

| Almost Never | Occasionally | Often | Very Often | Almost Always |

38. I accept responsibility for my own actions.

| Almost Never | Occasionally | Often | Very Often | Almost Always |

39. Before making decisions, I gather facts.

| Almost Never | Occasionally | Often | Very Often | Almost Always |

40. I participate in activities such as visiting museums, exhibits, and zoos, or attending plays and concerts at least three times a year.

| Almost Never | Occasionally | Often | Very Often | Almost Always |

Occupational Wellness Section

41. I enjoy my work.

| Almost Never | Occasionally | Often | Very Often | Almost Always |

FIGURE 3–6
(*continued*)

42. I am satisfied with the balance between my work time and leisure time.

   Almost Never   Occasionally   Often   Very Often   Almost Always

43. I am satisfied with my ability to manage and control my workload.

   Almost Never   Occasionally   Often   Very Often   Almost Always

44. My work is consistent with my values.

   Almost Never   Occasionally   Often   Very Often   Almost Always

45. At work my level of authority is consistent with my level of responsibility.

   Almost Never   Occasionally   Often   Very Often   Almost Always

Spirituality and Values Section

46. I feel that my life has a positive purpose.

   Almost Never   Occasionally   Often   Very Often   Almost Always

47. My leisure time activities are consistent with my values.

   Almost Never   Occasionally   Often   Very Often   Almost Always

48. My actions are guided by my own beliefs, rather than the beliefs of others.

   Almost Never   Occasionally   Often   Very Often   Almost Always

49. I spend a portion of every day in prayer, meditation, and/or personal reflection.

   Almost Never   Occasionally   Often   Very Often   Almost Always

50. I am tolerant of the values and beliefs of others.

   Almost Never   Occasionally   Often   Very Often   Almost Always

FIGURE 3–6
(*continued*)

questions of the nurse. This type of assessment promotes mutual input into decision making and planning to improve the client's health (Pender et al, 2006).

Family Assessment

Nurses assess the health of individuals, families, and communities. When a family is the client, the nurse determines the health status of the family and its individual members, as well as the level of the family's functioning, interaction patterns, and strengths and weaknesses. Even if the client is an individual, data about the family enable the nurse to reflect more holistically on the client's story. Nurses assess families in a variety of settings (e.g., mental health clinics, schools, community health, home care, inpatient maternity units). See Box 3–7 for a guide to making family assessments.

Community Assessment

Community assessment is not limited to public health nurses. Acute care nurses use knowledge of community resources to make referrals and coordinate clients' transition from hospital to home care. Clients also benefit if their home care nurse is aware of groups and services available for continuing support.

BOX 3-7

FAMILY ASSESSMENT GUIDE

Family Structure

- Family type: traditional, nuclear, blended, extended, single-parent, or other
- Age, sex, and number of family members

Lifestyle

- Level of knowledge of sexual and marital roles (e.g., teenage pregnancy and marriage)
- Child, spouse, or elder abuse
- Chemical dependency, including alcohol and nicotine
- Safety of the home environment

Psychosocial Factors

- Adequacy of income
- Adequacy of child care when both parents work
- Availability of support persons (e.g., friends, church groups)
- Work or social pressures that create stress

Developmental Factors

- Older adults, especially if living alone
- Adolescent parents
- Families with new babies

Family Roles

- Persons working outside the home; type of work; satisfaction with work
- Division of household responsibilities; family members' satisfaction with this arrangement
- Person who makes the major decisions; person making day-to-day decisions
- Most significant family member in each person's life

Communication and Interaction

- Openness and honesty in communication among family members
- Ways of demonstrating love, sorrow, anger, and other feelings
- Degree of emotional support given to each other
- Methods of handling conflict and stressful situations among family members

Physical Health

- Current health status of each member
- Ways the family obtains health services
- Preventive measures (e.g., immunizations, dental hygiene, visual examinations)
- Genetic predisposition to disease (e.g., cardiovascular disease, diabetes)
- Health practices (e.g., foods eaten, bedtime, exercise)

(continued)

BOX 3–7

FAMILY ASSESSMENT GUIDE *continued*

Family Values

- Views about importance of education, teachers, and school
- Cultural affiliation and degree to which cultural practices are followed
- Religious orientation; degree of importance in family life
- Use of leisure time and whether shared or individual
- Extent to which health is valued (e.g., preventive care, exercise, diet)

EXAMPLE: An elderly woman has fallen and has a lacerated foot that is healing slowly. A nurse visits her daily to make dressing changes. Because she has diabetes and poor circulation, the client needs to be treated by wound care specialists. However, she is not able to drive. Is there a wound care clinic in the community? Are there transportation services that she could use?

A community assessment answers these kinds of questions. In addition, the data can be analyzed to determine the overall health status of a particular group (e.g., pregnant adolescents, home health clients with diabetes) or community (e.g., a neighborhood,

BOX 3–8

MAJOR ASPECTS OF A COMMUNITY ASSESSMENT

Category	*Examples*
Physical environment	Geographic size, types of housing, density, crime rate
Population and health status	Includes census data about characteristics of the population such as race, ethnicity, and homelessness; as well as the prevalence of various illnesses in the population
Education	School lunch programs, parental involvement in schools, health services handled by the schools
Safety and transportation	Police, fire, ambulance, and sanitation services; public transportation; air quality
Politics and government	Type of government, influential people and organizations, recent election issues
Health and social services	Hospitals, clinics, home care, long-term care, accessibility of healthcare services
Communication	Newspapers, radio stations, postal services
Economics	Major employers in the community, income levels, employment rate
Recreation	Number and types of churches, playgrounds, parks, sports facilities, and theaters

the city government, the American Diabetes Association). Major aspects of a community assessment are shown in Box 3–8. The best way to assess a community is to live in it. However, you can get an overview of the community with a "windshield survey"—by traveling through the area and observing the surroundings (e.g., types of buildings, condition of roads, people walking about). This provides only superficial data, so you will need to network with other professionals who live or work there.

> **3-5 WHAT DO YOU KNOW?**
>
> List six types of special-purpose assessment.
>
> **See answer to #3-5 What Do You Know? in Appendix A.**

Ethical and Legal Considerations

As in all aspects of care, nurses must be aware of their ethical responsibilities when assessing clients. According to Provision 1 of the ANA *Code of Ethics for Nurses* (2001):

> The nurse, in all professional relationships, practices with compassion and respect for the inherent dignity, worth, and uniqueness of every individual, unrestricted by considerations of social or economic status, personal attributes, or the nature of health problems.

Issues of honesty and confidentiality are frequently encountered during assessment.

Honesty

The principle of **veracity** (honesty) holds that we should tell the truth and not lie. In assessing patients, this means that you should be honest about how you will use the data—to plan the patient's care, for research, for a student paper, and so forth. When you introduce yourself to patients, tell them what to expect from the interview and how the information will be used.

Truthfulness also affects the patient's autonomy. The moral principle of **autonomy** holds that a person has the right to be independent and to decide for himself what is to happen to him. A patient who does not know how the data will be used cannot make a truly informed choice about whether to participate in the interview and thereby loses some autonomy.

Confidentiality

Treat assessment data as confidential. Failure to do so robs the patient of his autonomy because it removes his control over how data are used and shared. Among other things, confidentiality means that assessment notes should be kept in the patient's chart, not lying about where others can read them. It also means that you should not use the patient's name on any written learning assignments, and you should not talk about patient data at the desk, in the halls, or in the lunchroom, where casual observers might overhear.

A client may tell you something in confidence that you feel you must tell in order to protect her; for example, a client might tell you of her plans for suicide. If you believe you cannot keep the information confidential, then you are obligated (by the principle of veracity) to tell the client that, in her best interest, you must share the information with other caregivers. A similar situation arises when a client tells you something that you believe you must reveal in order to protect someone else. There is no rule about when to tell and when not to tell. You will, each time, have to balance the need to preserve autonomy against the need to protect the client or others.

In both instances, it is better from an ethical standpoint to stop the client from telling you something you cannot keep confidential. Of course, this is not always possible, but often you can pick up clues from the client that she is about to disclose this kind of information. If you do, you might say something like, "This sounds like something I may not be able to keep confidential. Are you sure you want to go on with it?"

Malpractice Suits

Monitoring is frequent, ongoing assessment often done at specified intervals. It is focused assessment; for example, you might monitor the reflexes of a patient receiving magnesium sulfate or the fluid intake and output of a patient with burns. Monitoring is sometimes ordered by a primary care provider, but some monitoring can also be ordered by a nurse (e.g., monitoring the mental status of a patient who has had episodes of disorientation and confusion). Failure to monitor is a common cause of malpractice suits. If a physician orders frequent monitoring for a patient, be sure to do the following:

1. Have the physician specify the frequency or follow the frequency specified in your agency's policies and protocols.
2. Perform the monitoring as specified.
3. Thoroughly document the monitoring (and all interventions).

> **EXAMPLE:** (Actual case) An infant was admitted to a hospital for heart surgery. After surgery, a nurse allegedly failed to monitor the infant's urinary output and delayed obtaining blood gas analysis, which were ordered by the physician. The infant's injuries resulted in cerebral palsy, and the case was settled for $2.2 million (Eskreis, 1998, p. 38).

An unreasonable delay in a comprehensive admission assessment could also create a risk for malpractice because the patient might be harmed by a delay in treatment. If you are unable to perform a timely admission assessment, inform your supervisor. When you have time, document your conversation and request in writing that your unit be given additional staff. As soon as possible, assess the patient fully.

SUMMARY

Assessment:

- Is the collection, validation, organization, and recording of data using interview, observation, and examination.
- Requires critical thinking skills, a good knowledge base, and an awareness of ethical issues.

- Uses directive and nondirective interviewing techniques, adapting to the special needs of the client.
- May be comprehensive or focused.
- May involve various conceptual frameworks to collect and organize data.
- May include in-depth assessment for special purposes (e.g., wellness, spiritual, and cultural assessment).
- May be performed for individuals, families, or communities.
- Should consider the moral issues of honesty and confidentiality.
- Should meet professional and legal standards.

CRITICAL THINKING AND CLINICAL REASONING: A CASE STUDY

As needed to work with this case, discuss with classmates, and look up unfamiliar terms (e.g., *fractured hip, senile dementia*) in a textbook. Steven Brown is an 82-year-old man who has been admitted to an extended-care facility because he is no longer able to live at home alone. He has a medical diagnosis of senile dementia. On admission, he states his name and knows you are a nurse, but he thinks he is at his daughter's house.

1. What information do you need to gather when planning *safety* measures for Mr. Brown?
2. How is that information different from the information you'd need if everything in the case was the same except that instead of senile dementia, the medical diagnosis is fractured hip 1 week postoperatively?
3. Refer to Question 1. What data collection method will you use to get each piece of information? What data sources will you use?
4. What special techniques will you use to communicate with Mr. Brown? Write at least three questions (or statements) you would use when obtaining information from him.
5. What critical thinking attitudes or skills did you use in this exercise? Refer to Chapter 2, if necessary, to refresh your memory.

See suggested responses to Critical Thinking and Clinical Reasoning: A Case Study in Appendix A

Diagnostic Reasoning

4

Introduction

This chapter will (a) discuss diagnosis as a step of the nursing process; (b) define *patient health status*; (c) help you begin to differentiate between a problem and other phenomena, such as symptoms; and (d) explain the diagnostic reasoning process. It will help you to identify and describe client health status, including problems, more precisely. The diagnostic process is not just a matter of choosing labels from a list. The labels must accurately reflect the client's health status. This chapter deals with the broad concepts of *problems* and *health status*, not just with nursing diagnoses. Standardized NANDA International terminology will be introduced in Chapter 5.

Both students and practicing nurses tend to see diagnosis as the most difficult aspect of the nursing process. One of the difficulties is that diagnosis is both a process and a product:

1. *Diagnosis* names a phase of the nursing process.
2. *Diagnosis* (or *diagnostic reasoning*) is a reasoning process that nurses use to interpret patient data.
3. The end product of that reasoning process is a statement of health status that is called a *nursing diagnosis*.
4. In order to write the diagnostic statement, nurses refer to a standardized list of terms that are called *nursing diagnoses* (e.g., see Table 3–12 and the inside front cover of this text).

In the literature, you will see diagnosis used in all those ways. To minimize confusion, this text uses the terms as they are shown in Figure 4–2.

LEARNING OUTCOMES

After completing this chapter, you should be able to do the following:

- Explain how diagnosis is related to the other phases of the nursing process.
- Explain what is meant by present health status.
- Identify patient strengths, wellness diagnoses, nursing diagnoses, medical diagnoses, and collaborative problems.
- Recognize actual, potential, and possible nursing diagnoses.
- Compare the advantages and disadvantages of computer-aided diagnosis.
- State ways in which nursing diagnoses can be used with critical pathways.
- Describe a process for diagnostic reasoning.
- Use standards of reasoning to evaluate your diagnostic thinking.
- Describe common diagnostic errors and explain how to prevent them with critical thinking.
- Discuss the ethical implications of the diagnostic process.

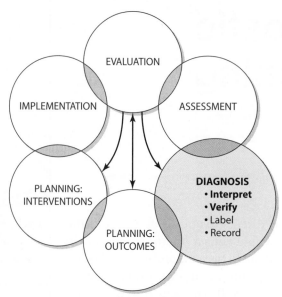

FIGURE 4–1

The diagnosis phase: interpreting data and verifying the diagnoses

Diagnosis: Second Phase of Nursing Process

In the second phase of the nursing process, nurses use diagnostic reasoning to analyze data and draw conclusions about the client's health status. They verify these conclusions with the client, select standardized labels, and record them on the plan of care.

Recall from Chapter 1 that the steps of the nursing process are interdependent and overlapping. Diagnosis is a pivotal step. All activities preceding this step are directed toward formulating the nursing diagnoses. All the care-planning activities following this step are based on the nursing diagnoses (Figure 4–3).

Diagnosis depends on the assessment phase because the quality of the data acquired during assessment affects the accuracy of the nursing diagnoses. Also, the two stages

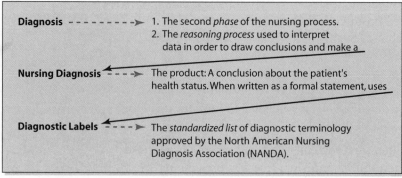

FIGURE 4–2

Diagnosis terminology

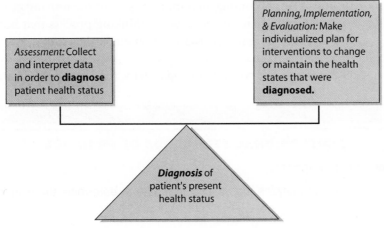

FIGURE 4–3
Diagnosis: a pivotal step in the nursing process

overlap. Like most nurses, the nurse in the following example begins to interpret some of the data (diagnosis) at the same time she is collecting it (assessment).

EXAMPLE: While interviewing Keisha Mandela, the school nurse notices that the child is speaking hesitantly and softly, giving brief answers, and avoiding eye contact. She wonders if Keisha is shy, withdrawn, anxious, or perhaps having difficulty with her self-concept. The nurse continues to gather data to confirm or deny these possibilities. In the diagnosis step, she will critically examine all the data she has gathered and draw a firmer conclusion about its meaning.

Diagnosis also affects the planning, implementation, and evaluation steps. When specifically and accurately stated, the problems and strengths identified during diagnosis guide the nurse in developing appropriate goals and nursing orders for the plan of care (planning). The diagnosis and implementation phases sometimes occur almost simultaneously. For example, in an emergency situation, a nurse may take action (implementation) as soon as the urgent problem is recognized—before consciously making a plan or identifying the rest of the problems or even before completely assessing the patient. Diagnosis also overlaps with the evaluation phase. During evaluation, the nurse determines whether the patient's health status has changed. If not, nursing diagnoses are reexamined to be sure they were diagnosed correctly and completely.

History of Nursing Diagnosis

The term *nursing diagnosis* began to appear in the nursing literature in the 1950s to describe the functions of a professional nurse (McManus, 1951). Fry (1953) stated that nursing diagnosis is based on the client's needs for nursing, rather than medical, care. Until that time nursing had been seen as a set of tasks, and nursing care was planned around those tasks. Nurses assisted physicians in treating diseases. They gathered data about patients to ensure that doctors could make medical diagnoses, not to plan nursing care.

In the 1960s, diagnosis was becoming an important part of the nursing process, but it was still necessary to establish that diagnosis was a thinking process that nurses could and should use and that they were not encroaching on medical territory.

In 1973, the American Nurses Association (ANA) Standards of Nursing Practice included nursing diagnosis as an important nursing activity, making it a legitimate function

---

BOX 4–1

PROFESSIONAL STANDARDS OF PRACTICE

ANA Standard 2: Diagnosis

The registered nurse analyzes the assessment data to determine the diagnoses or issues.

Competencies

The registered nurse:
1. Derives the diagnoses or issues based on assessment data.
2. Validates the diagnoses or issues with the patient, family, and other healthcare providers when possible and appropriate.
3. Documents diagnoses or issues in a manner that facilitates the determination of the expected outcomes and plan.
4. Identifies actual or potential risks to the patient's health and safety or barriers to health which may include but are not limited to interpersonal, systematic, or environmental circumstances.
5. Uses standardized classification systems, when available, in naming diagnoses.

Note: This material is from the draft for public comment (ANA, 2010, in press); its wording may be somewhat changed in the final published version (August 2010). For that version of the ANA standards, visit http://www.nursingworld.org.

Source: Reprinted with permission from American Nurses Association (2010, in press). In *Nursing: Scope and standards of practice* (2nd ed.). (Public Comment draft, January). Silver Spring, MD. Available at http:/nursebooks.org.

Canadian Standards (Example)

In Canada, practice standards are set by individual provinces. The following is an example of Canadian standards of practice addressing diagnosis.

2. Knowledge-Based Practice

The registered nurse continually strives to acquire knowledge and skills to provide competent, evidence-based nursing practice.

2.3 The registered nurse demonstrates critical thinking in collecting and interpreting data, planning, implementing, and evaluating all aspects of nursing care.

2.6 The registered nurse documents timely, accurate reports of data collection, interpretation, planning, implementing, and evaluating practice.

Source: Quoted from College & Association of Registered Nurses of Alberta (2005). *Nursing Practice Standards*. Available at http://www.nurses.ab.ca/pdf/Nursing%20Practice%20Standards.pdf.

of professional nurses. During the 1970s and 1980s, the term *nursing diagnosis* was incorporated into nearly all state nurse practice acts, and diagnosis became a nursing obligation as well as a legal right. Diagnosis is now taught in most schools of nursing, commonly used in the literature, and frequently used by nurses to describe their practice. Refer to Box 4–1 for current standards of practice.

Importance of Nursing Diagnosis

Nursing diagnosis can benefit both nurses and healthcare consumers in the following ways:

- **Nursing diagnoses facilitate individualized care.** Driven by cost considerations, today's healthcare organizations emphasize standardized care as a way to promote efficiency and decrease cost. But even though patients with identical medical conditions may need similar nursing interventions, the priorities of care may differ for each (e.g., see Box 4–2). Nursing diagnoses focus attention on a patient's unique needs, which may not be met by standardized plans of care.
- **Nursing diagnoses promote professional accountability and autonomy by defining and describing the independent area of nursing practice.** Nursing diagnosis language makes it clear that nurses do far more than simply carry out orders for medical treatments. It will help you to communicate to legislators, consumers, and insurance providers the unique care you deliver and the specific nature of the health conditions you treat.
- **Nursing diagnoses provide an effective vehicle for communication among nurses and other healthcare professionals.** Because a nursing diagnosis consolidates a great deal of information into a concise statement, it provides a shorthand means of communicating client status. For example, imagine you have collected the following data: Patient states his mouth is painful; his tongue is coated and mucous membranes are dry; there are vesicles and ulcerations in his mouth; and his mouth has a strong odor. The nursing diagnosis Impaired Oral Mucous Membrane gives you the same

---

BOX 4–2

PRIORITIZED NURSING DIAGNOSES FOR TWO PATIENTS WITH THE SAME MEDICAL DIAGNOSIS (MYOCARDIAL INFARCTION)

For Mary Chinn
1. Risk for Deficient Fluid Volume related to nausea and vomiting associated with pain and stress
2. Chest Pain related to reduced oxygenation of myocardium
3. Activity Intolerance related to decreased cardiac output

For Donald Schulz
1. Anxiety related to anticipation of financial difficulties because of absence from his business
2. Ineffective Breathing Pattern related to depressant effects of medications
3. Constipation related to decreased mobility, narcotics, and fear that straining will cause another heart attack

picture of the patient as that entire set of data. ANA *Scope and Standards of Practice* and competencies set by the Quality and Safety Education for Nurses (QSEN) group stress the importance of effective communication.

- **Nursing diagnoses help determine assessment parameters.** Using the preceding example, after you have grasped the concept of Impaired Oral Mucous Membrane, the term will alert you to other cues related to this diagnosis. For example, when you see that a patient is mouth breathing, you would check to see if his mucous membranes are dry and if he is drinking sufficient fluids.

4-1 WHAT DO YOU KNOW?

1. When did nursing diagnosis become incorporated into most nurse practice acts?
2. State three reasons why nursing diagnosis is important.

See answer to #4-1 What Do You Know? in Appendix A.

Human Responses

Nurses diagnose **human responses**—reactions to an event or stressor such as disease or injury. The following are some characteristics of human responses.

- **Human responses occur in several dimensions**. They can be biological (physical), psychological, interpersonal/social, or spiritual.

4-1 THINK & REFLECT!

For each of the dimensions (physical dimension, psychological dimension, interpersonal/social dimension, or spiritual dimension), think of some ways a person might respond to the stressor of having a hysterectomy (removal of the uterus).

See suggested responses to #4-1 Think & Reflect! in Appendix A.

- **Human responses occur at different levels.** They can be cellular, systemic, organic, or whole person (organismic). A cellular response occurs at the level of individual cells; for example, the ability of a cell to use glucose may change. Systemic responses occur in body systems, such as the circulatory or respiratory system (e.g., peripheral vasodilation, increased respiratory rate). Localized skeletal muscle fatigue—in a runner's calves, for instance—is an example of organic response. Nursing occurs at and affects all levels, but nursing diagnosis is usually at the whole person or the systemic level. A single stressor can cause multilevel responses.

EXAMPLE: A person who is severely burned loses large amounts of body fluids. If the fluids are not replaced, she responds by losing water from the cells into the bloodstream (cellular level). The sympathetic nervous system responds to the trauma by decreasing the activity of the gastrointestinal system (systemic level). The person may respond by perceiving pain (whole-person level) or, later, by social isolation (social level).

■ **Responses to stressors can be helpful as well as harmful.** Human responses may be adaptive, helping to restore health, or they may be maladaptive and damaging to health. In fact, the same response can be helpful at one time and harmful at another.

EXAMPLE: Mrs. Mason has a "chest cold" and a severe cough. She feels very ill. Her psychological response is fear (that she may have pneumonia). The fear motivates her to see her physician for treatment—an adaptive response.

EXAMPLE: At a later time, Mrs. Mason has an episode of postmenopausal bleeding. Her psychological response is again fear (that she may have cancer). This time she is overwhelmed by her fear. She avoids seeing a physician because she is afraid he will tell her she has cancer, thereby making it real. This time the fear was a maladaptive response because it immobilized her instead of motivating her to act.

Refer to Table 4–1 for some examples of stressors and various types and levels of human responses. Notice that a response can become a stressor that produces still another response (e.g., Mrs. Mason's fear produced avoidance).

You can recognize a **health problem** (maladaptive or harmful response) by the following characteristics. A health problem:

■ is a human response to a life process, event, or stressor.
■ is a health-related condition that both the patient and the nurse wish to change.

TABLE 4–1   Examples of Stressors and Human Responses

Stressor	Human Response	Dimension	Level	Effect
Blocked coronary artery causing decreased oxygen to heart muscle	Damage to heart muscle (ischemia)	Physical	Cellular and organic	Maladaptive
	Pain	Psychological and physical	Whole person (organismic)	Adaptive, if causes decreased activity, conserving oxygen; maladaptive, if causes fight-or-flight response, increasing demand for oxygen
	Fear of death	Psychological	Whole person	Can be adaptive or maladaptive (see above)
Fear of death from heart attack	Increased heart rate	Physical	Systemic	Probably maladaptive
	Praying	Spiritual	Whole person	Probably adaptive

- requires intervention in order to prevent or resolve illness or to facilitate coping.
- results in ineffective coping, adaptation, or daily living that is unsatisfying to the patient.
- is an undesirable state.

While learning, you may confuse problems with various phenomena that are related but not the same. Table 4–2 provides examples of things that are *not* problems but that act as stressors to cause a human response that *is* a problem.

TABLE 4–2 Misunderstandings about Problems

A Problem Is NOT:	Examples (Incorrect)	The Problem (Human Response) Is:
A nursing goal or a nursing problem	Urinary drainage device will be kept patent and draining freely.	Bladder distention
	Patient is noisy and disturbs other patients.	Anxiety; confusion, disorientation
Implications for the nurse: View the problem from the patient's perspective. The "problem" is the response (a) that will occur if the nurse's goal is not met or (b) that is causing the nurse's problem.		
A nursing action or routine	Give emotional support.	Anxiety; fear; grief; powerlessness
	Check urinary catheter hourly for patency.	Risk for urinary tract infection
Implications for the nurse: Get the right focus. The incorrect examples focus on *the nurse* (activities to be performed). Problems are statements of client health status—focus is on *the client*.		
A diagnostic test, medical treatment, or equipment	Patient is having a barium enema.	Risk for constipation; embarrassment
	New colostomy.	Lack of knowledge and skill in caring for the appliance; fear of social contact; impaired skin integrity around the stoma
	Must stay on a salt-free diet.	Lack of motivation to change eating habits; lack of knowledge of high-sodium foods
	Patient has cast on leg.	Decreased mobility; itching
	Has new dentures.	Change in body image; speech distortion
Implications for the nurse: Patients may respond in many ways to the same treatment. A list of treatments does not provide enough direction for individualizing care. Remember that the problem is the patient's *response* to the test or treatment.		
A patient need	Needs more sleep.	Fatigue; sleep-pattern disturbance; depression
	Needs emotional support.	Grief; poor self-concept; anxiety
Implications for the nurse: An unmet need may be the *cause* of a problem, but it is not the same thing as a problem. As a rule, do not use the word "need" in stating problems.		

Take-away point: Human responses can occur in several dimensions and on several levels (e.g., cells, systems, organs, whole person). They may be helpful or harmful.

Diagnosing Health Status

The purpose of diagnosing is to identify the patient's *present health status*. A comprehensive plan of care includes diagnostic statements describing patient health status in terms of strengths; wellness, actual, potential, and possible nursing diagnoses; collaborative problems; and medical problems. Nurses analyze data for all types, although their responsibility is different for each type. Nurses cannot legally make definitive medical diagnoses, but they are expected to recognize and refer situations that are beyond their diagnostic and treatment expertise (i.e., medical problems). Remember, all problems belong to the *patient*. No one profession "owns" any of the problems. Nursing, collaborative, and medical diagnoses are all addressed, to at least some extent, by all members of the multidisciplinary health team.

Identifying Patient Strengths

It is important to integrate patient (family, community) strengths into the plan of care. **Strengths** are those areas of normal, healthy functioning that will help the patient to achieve higher levels of wellness or to prevent, control, or resolve problems. Strengths can occur in the same dimensions as responses, discussed previously:

- Physical—e.g., good nutritional status enables a client to heal faster after surgery
- Psychological—e.g., good coping and problem-solving skills
- Psychosocial—e.g., a strong family support system
- Spiritual—e.g., strong personal values

Other examples of strengths include the following:

- Sense of humor
- Motivation to change
- Supportive extended family
- Good knowledge of disease process
- History of successful coping
- Good cardiovascular and respiratory reserve
- Strong religious faith

When identifying spiritual strengths, you might ask questions such as: "What is the most important and powerful thing in your life? Is faith important in your life?" and "What can you do to show love for yourself?" (Burkhardt, as cited in Dossey, 1998, p. 45). You can find strengths in the health examination data and the nursing database (e.g., information about health practices, home life, education, recreation, exercise, work, friends, and religious beliefs).

Recognizing Nursing Diagnoses

A nursing diagnosis is a statement about the patient's present health status. It describes an actual, potential (risk), or possible problem that nurses can legally diagnose and for which they can prescribe the primary treatment and prevention measures (Table 4–3).

TABLE 4–3   Comparison of Nursing Diagnoses, Collaborative Problems, and Medical Diagnoses

Category	Nursing Diagnoses	Collaborative Problems	Medical Diagnoses
Example	Activity Intolerance related to decreased cardiac output	Potential complication of myocardial infarction (heart attack): congestive heart failure	Myocardial infarction
Description	Describe human responses to disease process or stressors; written as one-, two-, or three-part statements	Describe potential physiologic complications of disease, tests, or treatments; written as two-part statements	Describe disease and pathology; do not consider other human responses; usually written in three words or less
Problem status	Actual, potential, or possible	Always potential	Actual or possible ("rule out")
Duration	Can change frequently; not associated with a particular medical diagnosis	Present when the disease (or medical diagnosis) is present	Remains the same while the pathology exists
Orientation	Oriented to the individual	Oriented to pathophysiology (potential complications)	Oriented to pathology and medical procedures
Responsibility for diagnosing	Nurses are responsible for diagnosing	Nurses are responsible for diagnosing	Physicians are responsible for diagnosing; diagnosis is not within scope of nursing practice
Nursing focus	Treat and prevent	Prevent and monitor for onset or status of the complication	Implement medical orders for treatment; monitor status of condition
Treatment orders	Nurse can order most interventions to prevent and treat	Requires medical orders for definitive prevention and treatment; nurse may order some preventive measures	Physician orders primary interventions to prevent and treat
Nursing actions	Independent	Some independent actions but primarily for monitoring	Dependent (primarily)
Classification system	Classification systems (e.g., NANDA-I) are developed and being used but not universally accepted	No classification system	Well-developed classification universally accepted by the medical profession

Source: Adapted with permission from Kozier, B., Erb, G., Berman, A., et al. (2000). *Fundamentals of nursing* (6th ed.). Upper Saddle River, NJ: Prentice Hall Health, p. 295.

The key term here is *primary.* Nurses may not prescribe *all* the care for a nursing diagnosis (e.g., most patients with a nursing diagnosis of Pain have medical orders for analgesics), but if it is a nursing diagnosis, the nurse can prescribe most of the interventions needed to prevent or resolve the problem. Usually the nurse does not need to confer with a physician about treatments for nursing diagnoses.

Because human responses vary, you cannot predict with certainty which nursing diagnoses will occur with a particular disease or treatment. Any number of nursing diagnoses may—or may not—occur with a particular medical diagnosis (e.g., see Box 4–2). You cannot assume, for example, that someone with diabetes will have Fear of Injections or Deficient Knowledge about a diabetic diet.

Take-away point: "A nursing diagnosis is a clinical judgment about individual, family, or community responses to actual or potential health problems/life processes. A nursing diagnosis provides the basis for selection of nursing interventions to achieve outcomes for which the nurse is accountable" (NANDA International, 2009, p. 41).

Examples of nursing diagnoses include the following:

- Impaired Skin Integrity (excoriation) related to incontinence
- Risk for Infection (of abdominal incision) related to poor nutritional status
- Dysfunctional Grieving related to unresolved guilt feelings

---

Take-away point: Nursing diagnoses can be wellness diagnoses or actual, potential (risk), or possible nursing diagnoses.

Wellness Diagnoses

Wellness diagnoses describe areas in which a healthy client is functioning normally—there is no problem, but the person wishes to achieve a higher level of wellness. For example, a client may be within normal weight limits but may wish to increase the fiber content of his diet. Or perhaps the client has no apparent problems but wants to begin an exercise program. In such cases, you would make a wellness diagnosis. **A wellness diagnosis** is a statement reflecting a client's healthy responses in areas where the nurse can intervene to promote growth or maintenance of the healthy response.

NANDA International (NANDA-I) defines wellness as "the quality or state of being healthy," and a wellness diagnosis as describing "human responses to levels of wellness in an individual, family, or community that have a readiness for enhancement" (2009, p. 45). Examples of NANDA-I wellness diagnoses include the following:

- Effective Therapeutic Regimen Management
- Readiness for Enhanced Nutrition
- Readiness for Enhanced Sleep
- Readiness for Enhanced Parenting
- Readiness for Enhanced Community Coping

Take-away point: *Wellness diagnoses* are used to develop care plans to support a healthy patient's change to a higher level of wellness. *Strengths* are characteristics that help patients overcome problems or reach wellness goals. No plan of care is made to change patient status (e.g., motivation, knowledge).

Actual Nursing Diagnoses

An **actual nursing diagnosis** is a problem that is actually present at the time you make the assessment. You would recognize it by the presence of associated signs and symptoms (defining characteristics). Nursing care is directed toward relieving, resolving, or coping with actual problems.

> **EXAMPLE:** The Crain family is experiencing many stressors. The parents, Todd and Dana, are caring for their son, Billy, who has leukemia, and Dana has had to quit her job. While making a family visit, the nurse observes that when Todd tries to discipline Billy, Dana interferes to protect him. In a later conversation, Todd tells the nurse, "I mostly just stay out of it. She can take care of Billy better than I can anyway." Dana confirms that Todd has withdrawn from contact with his son. The nurse diagnoses an *actual problem,* Compromised Family Coping related to family disorganization and role changes.

Potential (Risk) Nursing Diagnoses

A **potential** (or **risk**) **nursing diagnosis** is one that is likely to develop if the nurse does not intervene. You will diagnose this by the presence of risk factors that predispose a patient to developing a problem. Nursing care is directed toward preventing the problem by reducing the risk factors or toward early detection of the problem to lessen its consequences.

> **EXAMPLE:** Marianne Akiba is a single parent whose child, Janelle, has a new medical diagnosis of leukemia. The nurse knows that Marianne has only one or two people she can turn to for emotional or other support. In an interview, Marianne indicates, "I don't know anything about this disease or how to take care of my child." Although the nurse sees no signs of ineffective coping, she realizes that lack of knowledge and support place this family at risk, so she makes a *potential nursing diagnosis* of Risk for Compromised Family Coping related to limited support system and lack of knowledge.

A potential (risk) nursing diagnosis should be used only for patients who have a higher than normal risk for developing a problem—those who have more risk factors than the general group to which they belong. NANDA-I says that a **risk nursing diagnosis** "describes human responses to health conditions/life processes that may develop in a vulnerable individual, family or community. It is supported by risk factors that contribute to increased vulnerability" (2009, p. 25).

For those who have the same risk as the general population, a collaborative problem (potential complication) can be used (refer to Table 4–3). For example, *all* patients receiving a general anesthetic are at risk for respiratory problems. However, for those who have no risk factors in addition to the surgery, routine postoperative "turn, deep breathe, cough" treatment is adequate; their care planning could be based on the collaborative problem Potential Complications of Surgery (Respiratory). By contrast, if a patient is a smoker and is given general anesthesia for a high abdominal incision, his respiratory status merits special attention. He is at higher risk than the general population of surgery patients, so the nurse should write a nursing diagnosis of "Risk for Ineffective Airway Clearance related to high abdominal incision and smoking."

TABLE 4–4   Differentiating among Actual, Potential, and Possible Nursing Diagnoses

Actual Nursing Diagnosis	Potential (Risk) Nursing Diagnosis	Possible Nursing Diagnosis
▪ Problem present ▪ Signs and symptoms present	▪ Problem may develop ▪ Risk factors present	▪ Unsure if problem is present ▪ Some signs or symptoms present but not definitive ▪ Data incomplete

Possible Nursing Diagnoses

A **possible nursing diagnosis**, similar to a physician's *rule-out diagnosis,* is one that you tentatively believe to exist. You have enough data to suspect a problem but not enough to be sure. A possible problem directs nursing care toward gathering focus data to confirm or eliminate the diagnosis. Using possible problems can help you avoid:

1. Omitting an important diagnosis.
2. Making an incorrect diagnosis because of insufficient data.

> **EXAMPLE:** A patient who has had abdominal surgery has no history of smoking and has been adhering to the schedule of turning, coughing, and deep breathing every 2 hours. Still, she is slightly pale and reports that she feels "a little short of breath." The nurse auscultates and finds no abnormal breath sounds. There are no other signs of respiratory distress, but the nurse wants to be sure the situation is carefully evaluated by other shifts, so she diagnoses a *possible problem*: Possible Ineffective Airway Clearance.

For a side-by-side comparison of actual, potential, and possible nursing diagnoses, see Table 4–4.

Recognizing Collaborative Problems

Collaborative problems are predictable physiological complications of medical diagnoses or treatments that nurses manage by using both physician-prescribed and nursing-prescribed interventions. Independent nursing interventions for collaborative problems focus on monitoring for onset or changes in status and minimizing complications. Definitive treatment of the condition requires *both* medical and nursing interventions (see Table 4–3) (Carpenito, 1997).

Because there are a limited number of physiological complications for a given disease, the same collaborative problems—unlike nursing diagnoses—tend to be present any time a particular disease or treatment is present. That is, each disease or treatment has particular complications that are always associated with it. For example, all postpartum patients have similar collaborative problems (potential complications), such as postpartum hemorrhage and thrombophlebitis. But not all new mothers have the same nursing diagnoses. Some might have Risk for Impaired Attachment (delayed bonding), but most will not. Some might have a Deficient Knowledge problem; others will not.

Collaborative problems (potential complications) are *potential* problems. The patient's medical diagnosis, treatments, and medications are the risk factors (or stressors). The following guidelines will help you to predict and detect potential complications:

1. **Look up the patient's medical diagnosis.** What are the most common complications associated with it? You can find this information in textbooks, journals, and patient records (e.g., diagnostic studies, medical history). Appendix C is a comprehensive list of collaborative problems that are commonly associated with various diseases and pathophysiologies. Appendix D is a list of collaborative problems associated with surgical treatments.
2. **Look up all the patient's medications.** Serious side effects, toxicity, drug interactions, and other adverse reactions are potential complications (e.g., Potential Complication of Magnesium Sulfate Therapy: Hypermagnesemia).
3. **Look up the most common complications associated with the patient's surgery, treatments, or tests.** Again, you may need to refer to a text or other references. Appendix C lists complications associated with various surgeries. Table 4–5 lists examples of collaborative problems associated with various tests and treatments.
4. **Be sure you know the signs and symptoms of the potential complications so you will know what assessments are needed.** For example, the early symptoms of Potential Complication of Magnesium Sulfate Therapy: Hypermagnesemia are profound thirst, depressed reflexes, sedation, confusion, and muscle weakness. Thus, in addition to monitoring lab results of plasma magnesium levels, you would regularly assess for those symptoms. Review agency procedures, protocols, and critical paths for your patient's condition (e.g., the agency may have a protocol for peritoneal dialysis or oxygen administration).

4-2 WHAT DO YOU KNOW?

1. If there are no signs or symptoms present, is the problem an actual diagnosis, a potential diagnosis, or a possible diagnosis?
2. A collaborative problem is a physiological complication of a disease or treatment that nurses can treat independently. True or false?

See answer to #4-2 What Do You Know? in Appendix A.

Recognizing Medical Diagnoses

Although both medical and nursing diagnoses are made by using a diagnostic reasoning process, they are quite different. A **medical diagnosis** identifies a disease process or pathology and is made for the purpose of treating the pathology. It does not necessarily consider the human responses to the pathology.

TABLE 4–5   Multidisciplinary (Collaborative) Problems Associated with Tests and Treatments

Test or Treatment	Potential Complications (Collaborative Problems)	
Arteriogram	Allergic reaction	Paresthesia
	Embolism	Renal failure
	Hemorrhage; hematoma	Thrombosis at site
Bone marrow studies	Bleeding	Infection
Bronchoscopy	Airway obstruction or bronchoconstriction	Hemorrhage
Cardiac catheterization	Cardiac arrhythmias	Infarction, perforation
	Embolism, thrombus	Paresthesia
	Hypervolemia	Site hemorrhage or
	Hypovolemia	hematoma
Casts and traction	Bleeding	Misalignment of bones
	Edema	
	Impaired circulation	Neurological compromise
Chemotherapy (antineoplastic drugs)	Anaphylactic reaction	Hemorrhagic cystitis
	Anemia	Leukopenia
	Central nervous system toxicity	Necrosis at intravenous (IV) site
	Congestive heart failure	Pneumonitis
	Electrolyte imbalance	Renal failure
	Enteritis	Thrombocytopenia
Chest tubes	Bleeding leading to hemothorax	Septicemia
	Blockage or displacement leading to pneumothorax	
Foley catheter	Bladder distention (tube not patent)	Urinary tract infection
Hemodialysis	Air embolism	Transfusion reactions
	Bleeding	Shunt clotting; fistulas
	Dialysis dementia	Infection or septicemia
	Electrolyte imbalance	Hepatitis B
	Embolism	Fluid shifts
IV therapy	Fluid overload	Phlebitis
	Infiltration	
Medications	Allergic reactions (specify)	Toxic effects/overdose
		Side effects (specify)
Nasogastric suction	Electrolyte imbalance	
Radiation therapy	Fistulas, tissue necrosis	Radiation burns
	Hemorrhage	Radiation pneumonia
Tracheal suctioning	Bleeding	Hypoxia
Ventilation (assisted)	Acid–base imbalance	Pneumothorax
	Airway obstruction (tube plugged or displaced)	Respirator dependence
	Ineffective oxygen–carbon dioxide exchange	Tracheal necrosis

Source: Wilkinson, J. M., & Ahern, N. R. (2009). *Nursing diagnosis handbook* (9th ed.). Upper Saddle River, NJ: Prentice Hall Health.

EXAMPLE: The primary care provider diagnoses hypertension and prescribes antihypertensive medications and a low-salt diet. The nurse will diagnose and treat the patient's and family's responses to the medical diagnosis. Is the patient motivated to change his diet? What changes will the family need to make to incorporate the diet change into their menu plan? Does the patient understand the importance of taking his medications even though they may have unpleasant side effects? If the patient is hospitalized, the nurse will give the medications prescribed by the primary provider.

As long as the disease process is present, the medical diagnosis does not change. Nursing diagnoses, by contrast, change as the client's responses change. In the preceding example, the nursing diagnosis might initially be "Risk for Noncompliance with medication regimen related to lack of understanding of therapeutic and side effects of the drug." However, as the patient shows knowledge of the drug and takes it as prescribed, this diagnosis would no longer apply. If the patient found the side effects unpleasant and continued to skip doses of the drug, the diagnosis might change to actual "Noncompliance with medication regimen. . . ." Remember that clients who have the same medical diagnosis may have very different nursing diagnoses. Consider the example of Mary Chinn and Donald Schulz, in Box 4–2, who both have a medical diagnosis of myocardial infarction (heart attack) but who have very different nursing diagnoses.

Nurses make observations pertinent to patients' medical diagnoses and perform treatments delegated by the physician. Although nurses do not diagnose or prescribe treatments for medical problems, nursing judgment is required. Nurses must know the pathophysiology of the disease and understand why the medications or treatments are being given.

See Figure 4–4 for a decision tree to help you determine whether a problem is a nursing diagnosis, a collaborative problem, or a medical problem.

4-2 THINK & REFLECT!

Refer to Figure 4–4. Each of the following patients has undergone major abdominal surgery. Determine whether each set of cues represents a nursing diagnosis, a medical diagnosis, or a collaborative problem.

Patient A. Four days after surgery, incision is red, oozing pus, and not healing—symptoms of an infection.

Patient B. Two days after surgery, the patient's vital signs are normal, but he is breathing shallowly and not moving very much. These cues represent risk factors for postoperative pneumonia.

Patient C. The patient has just returned from surgery. The surgical dressing is dry but must be monitored to ensure that surgical hemostasis was obtained and that no excessive bleeding will occur.

See suggested responses to #4-2 Think & Reflect! in Appendix A.

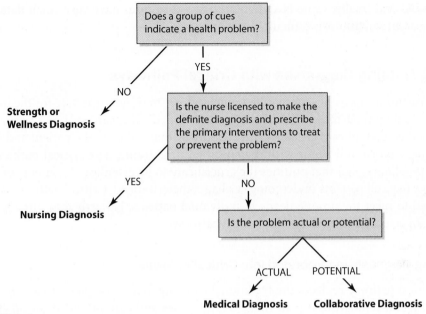

FIGURE 4–4
Decision tree for nursing diagnoses and collaborative problems

Computer-Assisted Diagnosis

In some agencies, nurses use computers to classify and interpret assessment data. Such application programs, called **expert** (or **knowledge-based**) **systems,** are a kind of artificial intelligence that uses reasoning to infer conclusions from stored facts. After the nurse enters the assessment data, the software compares the cues to those associated with each nursing diagnosis in its database.

1. The computer then generates a list of abnormal cues or a list of possible diagnoses. The nurse chooses which diagnoses to accept or reject or add to the list.
2. When the nurse chooses a diagnostic label, the next screen shows that label with all its associated signs and symptoms. The nurse compares them with the actual patient data and accepts or rejects the diagnostic label.
3. If the nurse accepts the diagnostic label, the next screen will list possible etiologies for the diagnosis. The nurse completes the problem statement by choosing the appropriate etiologies (causes) of the problem.

The advantages of computer-assisted diagnosis are that computers are consistent, systematic, and organized. They do not experience fatigue, distraction, or other human weaknesses; therefore, they are able to identify patterns the nurse might overlook. You must use professional judgment in evaluating the computer-generated diagnoses, though. The computer will assume that all the patient data are true, correct, and current. You must be sure this is so. Furthermore, patients respond to health problems in infinite ways, so it is impossible to predict all combinations of cues and all possible diagnoses. And finally, some NANDA-I nursing diagnoses have very small databases, making accurate diagnosis difficult.

Using Nursing Diagnoses with Critical Pathways

Many organizations use a system called *managed care* to standardize care for the medical diagnoses they treat most often. Each common medical diagnosis has a preprinted, standardized plan of care called a **critical pathway** that indicates the patient and family outcomes that should occur within a specified time frame. The critical pathway is a multidisciplinary plan that outlines the crucial care to be given for all patients of a certain type (e.g., all patients undergoing cardiac catheterization). Critical pathways are not designed to meet the unique needs of individual patients. Nevertheless, nursing diagnoses can be used successfully with critical pathways.

Nursing Diagnosis Incorporated into Critical Pathway

The critical pathway replaces the traditional (nursing diagnosis) plan of care for many clients. It is a standardized plan that lists outcomes and care intended for *all* clients. However, nursing diagnoses are unique to the individual and cannot really be predicted to occur in the presence of particular diseases and treatments. Some agencies do include in the critical pathway the nursing diagnoses most often seen with the medical diagnosis (e.g., a critical pathway for total knee replacement might include nursing diagnoses of Pain and Impaired Mobility).

Nursing Diagnosis Used to Name Variance

Some agencies use nursing diagnoses to name variances from the predicted outcomes and time frames and to develop an individualized plan for achieving revised outcomes. A **variance** occurs when the patient does not achieve a goal in the time predicted by the critical pathway.

> **EXAMPLE:** The critical pathway for a patient with newly diagnosed type 1 diabetes would not include a nursing diagnosis but instead would list teaching needs for each day. On day 5, if the patient is unable to meet the predicted outcome of self-injection, the nurse would identify and analyze this variance. The nurse would then write a nursing diagnosis of "Ineffective Management of Therapeutic Regimen . . ." to individualize the nursing care and hasten outcome achievement.

4-3 WHAT DO YOU KNOW?

1. What is a critical pathway?
2. What is a variance?

See answer to #4-3 What Do You Know? in Appendix A.

Nursing Diagnosis Used for Problems Not on the Critical Pathway

You should use nursing diagnoses to individualize care to meet unique patient needs that are not addressed by the standardized critical pathway.

Take-away point: If only the standardized care is given, that care can probably be given by someone other than a nurse.

EXAMPLE: Al Collins has had a myocardial infarction. He is also blind. The critical pathway outlines care only for his heart condition. The nurse writes a separate nursing diagnosis to provide information about the amount of help Mr. Collins needs with eating, ambulating, and other activities of daily living.

Critical pathways can improve care by indicating the most important care for a specific condition (e.g., for a patient with pneumonia). However, they can impede care if task-oriented nurses use them in place of thinking. Busy caregivers who know the "routine" care on the pathway may rush through assessments and outcomes evaluation.

Take-away point: Do not let the critical pathway, or any standardized approach, make a robot of you. Be alert for patient care needs that are not addressed by the critical pathway.

Diagnostic Reasoning

Diagnosing is an intellectual activity in which nurses use critical thinking skills to identify patterns and draw conclusions about data. It is the same reasoning process that experts of any discipline use to draw conclusions about their phenomena of concern (i.e., what they work on). Speech therapists diagnose speaking problems, teachers diagnose learning problems, and automobile mechanics diagnose engine problems. Diagnostic reasoning can be divided into three broad stages: (a) interpreting the data, (b) verifying the diagnosis, and (c) labeling (and recording) the diagnosis. Refer to Box 4–3 for an overview of these processes.

Use of Nursing Models

How you define and recognize patient problems depends somewhat on the nursing model you use. For example, using the Roy (1984) model in Chapter 3, you would recognize a problem as a failure to adapt. In the Gordon (1994) model, you would recognize it as a dysfunctional health pattern (i.e., a group of related cues that do not meet expected norms). The theory you use also helps determine problem etiologies—the "causes" of the problem.

Using a physiology theory, the cause of infant colic is swallowed air and intestinal gas. Using a psychology theory, the cause of colic might be excessive parental anxiety and tension. The concepts of a framework help you to recognize relationships among isolated pieces of data. Concepts cause clusters to stand out for your attention. For example, the concept of *deficient fluid volume* would help Luisa Sanchez's nurse (see Figure 3–2) to notice that Luisa's decreased urine output, poor skin turgor, and elevated temperature were somehow related. This chapter will use Gordon's

---

BOX 4–3

OVERVIEW OF DIAGNOSTIC REASONING

Interpret the Data

Level I—Identify significant cues.

1. *Organize data* in a concise format using a nursing framework.
2. *Compare individual data with standards and norms* to identify significant cues.

Level II—Cluster cues and identify data gaps.

3. *Cluster significant cues*; look for patterns and relationships.
4. *Categorize clusters* according to your framework.
5. *Identify data gaps and inconsistencies.*

Level III—Draw conclusions about present health status.

6. *Think of as many explanations as possible for each cue cluster. Then decide which hypothesis best explains it.* (Note: You can sometimes identify both the problem and the etiology in this step.)
7. *Identify problem* (wellness diagnoses; actual, potential, and possible nursing diagnoses; collaborative problems; and medical problems).
8. *Identify patient and family strengths.*

Level IV—Determine etiologies and categorize problems.

9. *Determine the etiologies of the problems.*
10. *Categorize problems according to your framework.*

Verify the Diagnoses

11. *Verify diagnoses and strengths* with the patient, family, other professionals and references.

Label the Diagnoses

12. *Choose standardized problem label.* Write the formal health status statements: nursing and wellness diagnoses, collaborative problems, and strengths.
13. *Prioritize the problems.*

Record the Data

14. *Record the problem statements* on the appropriate documents: patient care plan, chart, and so on.

Functional Health Patterns as a framework for data analysis, continuing the example of Luisa Sanchez from Chapter 3.

Interpreting Data

After you organize and record the assessment data, you must analyze and interpret it in order to determine what it means. This section presents data interpretation as a series of steps in order to help you understand the process. In reality, it is a complex process, not a rigid set of linear steps to be accomplished one at a time. You must, of course, take some steps before others, but you should use these steps as guidelines, realizing you will do some of them simultaneously, move back and forth among them, and perhaps even intuit portions of them, especially as you gain clinical experience.

Data interpretation occurs at four levels (see Box 4–3). In the first level, you identify significant cues; in the second level, you cluster cues and identify data gaps; in the third level, you identify the client's health status; and in the final level, you determine the probable causes of the problems.

Level I: Identify Significant Cues

In your initial analysis (level one), you will organize data and compare them with established norms to identify significant cues (Steps 1 and 2).

Step 1. Organize the data. If you have made an initial, comprehensive assessment, the data will already be grouped by your data collection form.

  a. *Rewrite all the database information according to your preferred framework* (Box 4–4). While you are learning, this will make data gaps and inconsistencies more obvious and help you to see relationships among the cues.

  b. *You do not have to use the same framework as the data collection form.* Luisa Sanchez's admission assessment (see Figure 3–2 in Chapter 3) was organized according to body systems and specific nursing concerns (e.g., screening for falls). In Box 4–4, those data are organized according to Gordon's Functional Health Patterns. As a rule, nurses use the assessment form categories to organize data. However, different models are used here to show differences in organizing frameworks and to demonstrate that you are not limited to the framework of the data collection form.

Step 2. Compare individual data with standards and norms (Table 4–6). In this step you will use your knowledge of anatomy, physiology, psychology, developmental theory, and so on to *find significant cues.* Compare all data with such standards as norms for height and weight, lab values, nutritional requirements, social functioning, and coping skills. It may help you to *highlight, circle, or underline significant (abnormal) data,* as in Box 4–4.

Level II: Cluster Cues and Identify Data Gaps

The second level of analysis involves grouping the significant cues and identifying missing and inconsistent data (Steps 3–5).

Step 3. Cluster significant cues, looking for patterns and relationships among them.

  a. *To begin clustering, look for cues that are repeated in more than one category (or pattern).* For example, Mrs. Sanchez reports being "too tired to mess with hair and makeup" in the Self-Perception/Self-Concept pattern. She reports "weakness" in both the Cognitive/Perceptual and Activity/Exercise patterns as well. Therefore, weakness is probably an important diagnostic cue.

BOX 4–4

DATA FOR LUISA SANCHEZ, ORGANIZED ACCORDING TO GORDON'S FUNCTIONAL HEALTH PATTERNS

Luisa Sanchez, 28 years old, was admitted to the hospital with a productive cough and rapid, labored respirations. She stated that she has had a "chest cold" for 2 weeks and has been short of breath on exertion. Yesterday she began to experience a fever and "pain in my lungs." (See Figure 3–2 in Chapter 3.)

Health Perception/Health Management

Knows her medical diagnosis
Gives thorough medical history
Complying with thyroid hormone regimen
Relates progression of illness in detail
Realistic expectations (to have antibiotics
    and "go home in a day or two")
States usually eats "three meals a day"

Nutritional/Metabolic

5 ft 2 in (158 cm) tall; weight 125 lb (56 kg)
"No appetite" since having "cold"
Reports nausea
Oral temp 103°F (39°C)
Decreased skin turgor
Mucous membranes dry and pale
Skin hot and pale, cheeks flushed
Synthroid 0.1 mg per day
History of appendectomy and partial
    thyroidectomy
Old surgical scars: anterior neck,
    RLQ abdomen
Has not eaten today; last fluids at noon today

Eliminination

Last bowel movement yesterday: formed,
    "normal"
Urinary frequency and amount
    decreased X2 days
Abdomen soft, not distended
Diaphoretic

Activity/Exercise

No musculoskeletal impairment
States, "I feel weak."
Short of breath on exertion
Exercises daily
Respirations shallow; chest expansion < 3 cm
Blood pressure 122/80 mm Hg sitting
Radial pulse weak, regular, rate = 92
    beats/min
Cough productive of pale, pink sputum
Inspiratory crackles auscultated throughout
    right upper and lower chest
Diminished breath sounds on right side

Sleep/Rest

Difficulty sleeping because of cough
"Can't breathe lying down"

Cognitive/Perceptual

No sensory deficits
Pupils 3 mm, equal, brisk reaction
Oriented to time, place, and person
Responsive, but fatigued
Responds appropriately to verbal and
    physical stimuli
Recent and remote memory intact
"I can think OK. Just weak."
States "short of breath" on exertion
"Pain in lungs," especially when coughing
Experiencing chills
Reports nausea

BOX 4–4

DATA FOR LUISA SANCHEZ, ORGANIZED ACCORDING TO GORDON'S FUNCTIONAL HEALTH PATTERNS *continued*

Roles/Relationships

Lives with husband and 3-year-old daughter
Sexual relationship "satisfactory"
Husband out of town; will be back tomorrow
Child with neighbor until husband returns
States "good" relationships with friends and
  coworkers
Working mother, attorney
Husband helps "some" at home

Self-Perception/Self-Concept

Expresses "concern" and "worry" about
  leaving daughter with neighbors until
  tomorrow
Well-groomed; says, "Too tired to mess with
  hair and makeup"

Coping/Stress Tolerance

Anxious: "I can't breathe."
Facial muscles tense; trembling
"I can think OK. Just weak."
Expresses concerns about work: "I'll never
  get caught up."

Value/Belief

Catholic. No special practices desired
  except last rites
Middle-class, professional orientation
No wish to see chaplain or priest at present

---

b. *Next, group together (cluster) the cues that seem related.* Think about the relationships among facts.

- Does Mrs. Sanchez's report of decreased urinary frequency (Elimination pattern) have anything to do with her decreased skin turgor and elevated temperature (Nutritional/Metabolic pattern)?
- Why is she feeling weak? Is it related to her nausea (Nutritional/Metabolic), her cough (Activity/Exercise), or both? Or neither?

As you compare data across the categories of your framework, some seemingly normal data may take on new significance. In Box 4–4, in the Roles/Relationships pattern, the fact that Mrs. Sanchez's husband is out of town is, by itself, not a concern. However, taken with her expression of worry (Self-Perception/Self-Concept) and her anxiety (Coping/Stress), the information about her husband seems more significant. That is why it is underlined in Box 4–4 even though it seems normal when considered by itself.

c. *While you are learning, you should make another written list using only the significant (abnormal) clustered data.* The way you form cue clusters will depend on whether you reason deductively or inductively (refer to "Reasoning" in Chapter 2).

TABLE 4–6   Comparing Cues to Standards and Norms (Examples)

Type of Cue	Client Cues (Examples)	Standard/Norm
Deviation from population norms	Height is 158 cm (5 ft, 2 in). Woman with small frame. Weighs 109 kg (240 lb).	Height and weight tables indicate the "ideal" weight for a woman 158 cm tall with a small frame is 49–53 kg (108–121 lb).
Developmental delay	Child is 18 months old. Parents state child has not yet attempted to speak. Child laughs aloud and makes cooing sounds.	Children usually speak their first word by 10 to 12 months of age.
Changes in client's usual health status	States, "I'm just not hungry these days." Ate only 15% of food on breakfast tray. Has lost 13 kg (30 lb) in past 3 months.	Client usually eats three balanced meals per day. Adults typically maintain stable weight.
Dysfunctional behavior	Amy's mother reports that Amy has not left her room for 2 days. Amy is 16 years old.	Adolescents usually like to be with their peers; social group very important.
	Amy has stopped attending school and has withdrawn from social contact.	Functional behavior includes school attendance.
Changes in usual behavior	Mrs. Stuart reports that lately her husband angers easily. "Yesterday he even yelled at the dog." "He just seems too tense now."	Mr. Stuart is usually relaxed and easygoing. He is friendly and kind to animals.

Source: Adapted with permission from Kozier, B., Erb., G., Berman, A., et al. (2000). *Fundamentals of nursing* (6th ed.). Upper Saddle River, NJ: Prentice Hall Health, p. 296.

If you use *deductive reasoning*, you would list all the significant cues, underlined in Box 4–4, under the appropriate categories of your framework. For example, the abnormal cues from two categories in Box 4–4 would be listed as follows:

Self-Perception/Self-Concept

Expresses "concern" and "worry" about leaving daughter with neighbors until tomorrow
"Too tired to mess with hair and makeup"

Roles/Relationships

Husband out of town (back tomorrow)
Child with neighbor

Using inductive reasoning, as shown in Table 4–7, you would make your new list of cue clusters by grouping all significant cues (underlined in Box 4–4) that are related,

TABLE 4–7   Luisa Sanchez Data—Related Cues Suggesting Problem Responses (Clustered Inductively)

Related Cues (Clusters)	Functional Health Pattern	Tentative Problem Statement (Inference)
Cluster 1 No significant cues	Health Perception/Health Management	*Strength*: Healthy lifestyle; understanding and compliance with treatment regimens
Cluster 2 "No appetite" since having "cold" Reports nausea X2 days Has not eaten today; last fluids at noon today	Nutritional/Metabolic	*(Nursing diagnosis)* Imbalanced Nutrition: Less than Body Requirements
Cluster 3 "No appetite" since having "cold" Reports nausea X2 days Last fluids at noon today Oral temp 103°F (39.4°C) Skin hot and pale; cheeks flushed Mucous membranes dry Poor skin turgor Decreased urinary frequency and amount X2 days Diaphoresis	Nutritional/Metabolic (includes hydration) or ~~Elimination~~	*(Nursing diagnosis)* Deficient Fluid Volume. Cues include elimination data but are not an elimination problem. Decreased urine is a symptom of a fluid volume problem.
Cluster 4 Difficulty sleeping because of cough "Can't breathe lying down" States, "I feel weak." Short of breath on exertion	Sleep/Rest or ~~Activity Exercise~~	*(Nursing diagnosis)* Disturbed Sleep Pattern
Cluster 5 Taking Synthroid 0.1 mg/day Old surgical scar on anterior neck	Nutritional/Metabolic	*(Medical treatment)* Not a problem as long as patient follows regimen
Cluster 6 Difficulty sleeping because of cough "Can't breathe lying down" Short of breath on exertion States, "I feel weak." Responsive but fatigued "I can think OK, just weak." Radial pulse rate 92 beats/min, weak	~~Sleep/Rest~~ or Activity/Exercise or ~~Cognitive/Perceptual~~	*(Nursing diagnosis)* Activity Intolerance or Self-Care Deficit (needs help with hygiene and so on because of weakness) Cues from other patterns are contributing to the problem in the Activity/Exercise pattern.
Cluster 7 Reports chills Oral temp 103°F (39.4°C) Diaphoretic	Cognitive/Perceptual or ~~Nutritional/Metabolic~~	*(Nursing diagnosis)* Problem is altered comfort (chills); elevated temp is contributing to problem.

(continued)

TABLE 4–7 Luisa Sanchez Data—Related Cues Suggesting Problem Responses (Clustered Inductively) (*continued*)

Related Cues (Clusters)	Functional Health Pattern	Tentative Problem Statement (Inference)
Cluster 8		
Husband out of town; will be back tomorrow Child with neighbor until husband returns	Roles/Relationships or ~~Coping/Stress~~	*(Nursing diagnosis)* Interrupted Family Processes because parents temporarily unavailable to care for child
Cluster 9		
Husband out of town; will be back tomorrow Child with neighbor until husband returns Expresses "concern" and "worry" over leaving child with neighbors until husband returns Anxious: "I can't breathe." Facial muscles tense; trembling Concerns about work: "I'll never get caught up."	~~Roles/Relationships~~ or Self-Perception/ Self-Concept or ~~Coping/Stress~~	*(Nursing diagnosis)* Anxiety is a problem; the Roles/Relationships and Coping/Stress cues are contributing to (causing) the anxiety.
Cluster 10		
"Pain in lungs," especially when coughing Cough productive of pale, pink sputum	Cognitive/Perceptual	*(Nursing diagnosis)* Chest pain
Cluster 11		
Skin hot and pale Respirations shallow; chest expansion <3 cm (1 1/4 in) Cough productive of pale, pink sputum Inspiratory crackles auscultated throughout right upper and lower chest Diminished breath sounds on right side Mucous membranes pale	Activity/Exercise (pattern includes respiratory and cardiovascular status)	*(Medical problem)* Pneumonia *(Collaborative problems: respiratory insufficiency, septic shock)* *(Nursing diagnosis)* Ineffective Airway Clearance caused by disease process

regardless of the pattern in which individual cues are found. For each significant cue, look for all other data that seem related to it. You may find the same cue appearing in more than one cluster (e.g., in Table 4–7, "Can't breathe lying down" appears in Clusters 4 and 6). The remainder of this chapter illustrates an inductive approach to data interpretation.

4-3 THINK & REFLECT!

Think about each of the following cue clusters. Do the cues fit together? Explain your reasoning.

Cluster 1—Osteoarthritis, difficulty getting out of bed, stiff joints, walks with walker

Cluster 2—Long-standing diabetes, legally blind, states feels lonely, wears glasses

Cluster 3—Incontinent of urine, wears incontinence pants, drinks adequate fluids, reddened area over coccyx

Cluster 4—Has bowel movement only every 3–4 days, sedentary lifestyle, history of urinary tract infections

See suggested responses to #4-3 Think & Reflect! in Appendix A.

Step 4. Next, decide which framework category (pattern) is represented by each new cue cluster. Identifying the category in which the problem occurs helps to narrow your search for the specific problem. Clustering is messy because there are many ways to group cues, and they do not fall neatly into a single category.

- *You may have more than one cue cluster in a pattern* (e.g., in Table 4–7, Clusters 2 and 3 represent the Nutritional/Metabolic pattern).
- *A cue cluster may suggest more than one pattern.* If so, list them all—it may be that the cue cluster represents more than one problem. Cluster 3, for example, yields two problems: a fluid volume problem and a potential oral mucous membrane problem.
- *A cue cluster may fit only one pattern, but you may not be sure at first which one.* If this occurs, list all the patterns that seem to fit (as in Table 4–7). After you think more about the relationships among the cues and recognize specific problems, you may be better able to identify the pattern. For example, some Cluster 3 cues fit in both the Nutritional/Metabolic and the Elimination patterns. Only as you begin to determine cause and effect does it become clear that the problem response occurs in the Nutritional/Metabolic pattern and that the Elimination cues are merely symptoms of the problem.

Look for overlap in the clusters. If there is overlap, see if you can find a way to combine the clusters or the cues differently. The goal is to find a set of clusters that is thorough and efficient—that addresses all the patient's strengths and problems but does not include problems the nurse can do nothing about. Be sure to consider various ways to group the cues.

Step 5. Identify data gaps and inconsistencies. Ideally, data will have been completed and validated during the assessment phase. However, the need for certain data may not be apparent until you cluster and begin to look for meaning in the data.

- *Look for inconsistencies.* Does the information in one cue cluster contradict that in another? Do your objective findings conflict with what the patient has said? Has the client given you the same information about concerns and strengths as other team members?

- *See if you have enough data to support or rule out your hunches about the meaning of the clusters.* For example, if in Clusters 8 and 9 you did not know that Mrs. Sanchez's husband was "out of town and coming back tomorrow," you would probably look at the clusters and think, "I wonder where her husband has gone and when he'll return. How long will the child need to stay with the neighbors? Why is she worried about leaving the child with them?"

4-4 THINK & REFLECT!

Your patient complains of abdominal cramping. He states that even though he takes a laxative every day, he must strain to have a bowel movement. What is your first hunch about the meaning of these data? Is there a problem? What is it? What data do you still need to feel more confident about your diagnosis? (Hint: Look up "Constipation" and "Perceived Constipation" in a nursing diagnosis handbook.)

See suggested responses to #4-4 Think & Reflect! in Appendix A.

Level III. Draw Conclusions about Present Health Status

In Steps 6 through 8, you determine the meaning of the cue clusters. Begin by making initial judgments about the meaning of each cue cluster. Does the cluster represent a problem? Or is it the cause of a problem in another cluster? The following discussion continues to use an inductive process. It would vary slightly if you were using a deductive approach.

Step 6. Think of as many explanations as possible for each cue cluster. This helps keep you from drawing premature conclusions about the meaning of the data. Continue looking for data gaps. You may rule out some hypotheses because of insufficient data and confirm others based on your knowledge and experience. For Cluster 3 in Table 4–7, two possible explanations are:

1. Mrs. Sanchez's decreased urine output could represent a urinary tract problem. She also has chills and a fever, which are symptoms of a kidney infection. However, she has already been seen by a physician and has a medical diagnosis of pneumonia, and she shows no other signs of a urinary tract problem. So this explanation is unlikely.
2. Mrs. Sanchez's decreased urine output could be a result of a Nutrition/Metabolic problem. Inadequate fluid intake, combined with fluid loss from fever and diaphoresis, may mean there is scant fluid for her kidneys to eliminate. In this explanation, her fever is the cause, rather than a symptom, of a problem.

Step 7. Identify problems and wellness diagnoses. In this step, you choose the best explanation for each cue cluster, making a judgment about which of the following each cluster represents:

- *No problem:* No need for nursing intervention.
- *A wellness diagnosis:* Patient wishes to achieve a higher level of wellness.
- *A medical problem:* Possible need for referral.
- *A collaborative problem:* Patient's medical diagnosis indicates the need to monitor for development of predictable complications.

- *An actual nursing diagnosis:* Client data indicate a need for nursing assistance.
- *A potential (risk) nursing diagnosis:* There are no signs or symptoms of an actual problem, but risk factors exist; a problem may occur if you do not intervene.
- *A possible nursing diagnosis:* You have reason to suspect a problem but not enough data to confirm it.

Table 4–7 includes the inferences made about all eight cue clusters. For the explanations for Cluster 3 (proposed in Step 6, preceding), you would probably conclude the following:

1. There is no Elimination problem.
2. There is an actual nursing diagnosis, Deficient Fluid Volume, in the Nutritional/Metabolic category.

All but three of Luisa Sanchez's problems are nursing diagnoses. The nurse can order the definitive actions to prevent or treat all except these three problems. Cluster 5 is a medical problem: hypothyroidism as a result of having had a thyroidectomy. This problem is being controlled by the Synthroid, prescribed by a physician. Cluster 11 reflects the medical diagnosis of pneumonia, which had already been made by a physician. It will be managed medically and need not be written on a nursing plan of care (there may even be a critical pathway for pneumonia). Cluster 11 also contains some collaborative problems (Potential Complications of Pneumonia: Respiratory Insufficiency and Septic Shock) that are not apparent from the cue clusters in Table 4–7. They are identified from the fact that Mrs. Sanchez has pneumonia and would be included in the standardized plan of care or critical pathway for any patient with pneumonia.

Step 8. Identify patient and family strengths. Examine your original list of cues (see Box 4–4); you cannot use the clustered cues because they consist of abnormal data. Ask the client and family how they have coped successfully in the past and what they see as their strengths. The following are some of Mrs. Sanchez's strengths:

Pattern	Strength
Health Perception/Health Management	Shows healthy lifestyle, understanding of and compliance with treatment regimen
Nutritional/Metabolic	Normal weight for height
Roles/Relationships	Husband supportive; neighbors available and willing to help

Level IV. Determine Etiologies and Categorize Problems

This is the final level of the diagnostic reasoning process. Refer to Box 4–3.

Step 9. Determine the etiologies of nursing diagnoses. In this step, you determine the most likely causes of the nursing diagnoses you identified in Step 8. These are the problem **etiologies**—the physiological, psychological, sociological, spiritual, or environmental factors believed to be causing or contributing to the problem. The etiologies must be correctly identified in order for your nursing actions to be

SOURCES OF PROBLEM ETIOLOGIES (EXAMPLES)

Environmental	Congenital malformations
Socioeconomic	Hereditary or genetic
Personal loss	Role changes
Religious, ethical	Political
Physiological	Cultural
Psychological	Communication difficulties
	Lack of education or information

effective. See Box 4–5 for examples of some sources of etiologies. Ask yourself the following questions:

- What is causing this problem?
- Which is the problem, and which is the etiology?
- How likely is it that this etiology is contributing to the problem?
- What data, knowledge, or past clinical experience support the link between the etiology and this problem? Or do not support it?

You must make inferences in this step because you cannot actually *observe* the link between the problem and the cause. For example, in Cluster 3, you can observe that Mrs. Sanchez has dry mucous membranes, decreased urine output, hot skin, and poor skin turgor and conclude that she has a problem: Deficient Fluid Volume. However, you cannot observe that the elevated temperature, diaphoresis, and limited fluid intake are the *causes* of this problem. You must infer this link between the problem and cause based on your knowledge of the metabolic effects of a fever and the physiology of fluid balance in the body, as well as your experience with similar patients.

You will not always find the etiology within the same pattern as the problem. In the following example from Table 4–7, a problem in the Activity/ Exercise pattern is caused by stressors in the Nutritional/Metabolic, Activity/Exercise, and Cognitive/Perceptual patterns.

Problem	**Functional Health Pattern**
Ineffective airway clearance	Activity/Exercise

Etiology	
(1) Viscous secretions because of fluid volume deficit	Nutritional/Metabolic
(2) Shallow chest expansion because of pain, weakness, and fatigue	Cognitive/Perceptual Activity/Exercise

Although patients may have the same problem, the etiologies may be different.

EXAMPLE: All three of the following patients have "Noncompliance with prescribed medication regimen" as their problem.

Patient A, etiology: Denial of illness

Patient B, etiology: Forgetfulness

Patient C, etiology: Both forgetfulness and denial of illness

When writing a nursing diagnosis, focus on those etiologies that can be influenced by independent nursing interventions.

Take-away point: You cannot actually observe the link between problem and cause, so all etiologies must be inferred.

Step 10. For each problem, make the final decision about which framework pattern it represents. Relating problems to framework patterns (see Table 4–7, center column) can help you to choose a label when you begin to write your diagnostic statements. It may help you to look back at the discussion of nursing frameworks in Chapter 3.

Cluster 3 at first appears to involve both the Nutritional/Metabolic and Elimination patterns. However, the most reasonable explanation of the cues is that Mrs. Sanchez's fluid volume deficit (Nutritional/Metabolic) is causing her decreased urine output (Elimination). Her fluid volume deficit is the problem—the human response that needs to be changed. In this step, you are categorizing the problem, not the etiology, so Cluster 3 fits best in the Nutritional/Metabolic pattern. When you write your formal diagnoses (in a later step), you will look first at the diagnostic labels in the Nutritional/Metabolic pattern. Follow this same process for each group of cues until you have listed and identified the appropriate pattern for all the patient's problems (see the "Tentative Problem" column of Table 4–7).

4-4 WHAT DO YOU KNOW?

List the four main levels of data interpretation.

See answer to #4-4 What Do You Know? in Appendix A.

Verifying Diagnoses

After identifying the patient's health status, you should verify your conclusions with the patient. A diagnosis is your interpretation of the data, and interpretation is not the same as fact. You can never be absolutely certain that an interpretation is correct even after verifying it. Try not to think of diagnoses as right or wrong but as being on a continuum of more or less accurate. Make your diagnoses as accurate as possible but remain open to changing them as you obtain new data or insights. If the client is unable to participate in the decision making, you may be able to verify your diagnoses with significant others.

EXAMPLE: You might say to Mrs. Sanchez, "It seems to me that you are worried about getting behind in your work but that your main worry is about leaving your daughter with your neighbors. Does this seem accurate to you?"

If the patient confirms your hypothesis, you will include the problem on her plan of care. If the patient does not agree with the problems you have identified, you will clarify and re-state them until they accurately reflect her health status. You may occasionally include a problem in a plan of care even though the patient does not verify it. It may be a problem the patient is not aware of (as in the case of an unconscious patient) or one she is denying.

EXAMPLE: A client may not perceive that she has Low Self-Esteem. Yet because your data strongly suggest it, you may wish to continue to assess for this problem and use nursing interventions to promote self-esteem. If you want to ensure that other nurses will also do this, you must include the problem in the care plan as a possible problem.

You should further validate each diagnosis by comparing it with the criteria in Box 4–6. If the client verifies it and it meets the criteria, your diagnosis should be high on the accuracy continuum.

Labeling and Recording Diagnoses

After identifying and verifying the client's problems and strengths, the final step is to state them formally. To choose the labels for the nursing diagnoses, you simply compare the cue clusters with the definitions and defining characteristics of the NANDA-I diagnostic labels in a nursing diagnosis handbook (e.g., *Prentice Hall Nursing Diagnosis Handbook*). The process of selecting labels and writing diagnostic statements for nursing diagnoses and collaborative problems is covered in detail in Chapter 5.

Health Promotion: Diagnosing Wellness

Nurses engaged in health promotion may use a slightly different diagnostic process. Because clients are basically well, a health-promotion process considers them to be their own experts. Therefore, much of the power and responsibility for defining health needs

---

BOX 4-6

CRITERIA FOR VALIDATING DIAGNOSES

- The database is complete and accurate.
- The data analysis is based on a nursing framework.
- The cue clusters demonstrate the existence of a pattern.
- The cues are truly characteristic of the problems hypothesized.
- There are enough cues present to demonstrate the existence of the problem.
- The tentative cause-and-effect relationship is based on scientific nursing knowledge and clinical experience.

belongs to those experiencing them. The nurse merely facilitates the process. The nurse engages in a dialogue with the client, reflecting on the client's experiences and raising critical questions. Together the client and nurse begin to see behavioral patterns that facilitate or hinder the client's potential for healing. Health promotion focuses not on client problems but on client potential, positioning the client in a better position to manage his own health and healing. Statements of client potential may take the form of wellness diagnoses.

Critical Thinking and Diagnosis

When diagnosing, you will use critical thinking to analyze and synthesize data, apply knowledge, recognize patterns, and draw conclusions. To check the quality of your thinking in the diagnosis phase of the nursing process, ask yourself the questions in Table 4–8 (review "Standards of Reasoning" in Table 2–3, in Chapter 2, as needed).

Reflective Practice

Critical thinkers look for the best way to do things: the best interventions for a problem, the best technique for a procedure, and so on. In the diagnosis phase, you will look for the "best way" to describe the patient's health status. The core questions for reflection are:

- What is the most useful and accurate way to describe the patient's present health state?
- What is the central issue (theme) for this patient?

Finding the central issue will help you to prioritize your care and decide which problems should be the main focus for care. First reflect on the cue clusters to find a balance between omitting clusters and having too many overlapping clusters; then reflect on the diagnoses. Look for a theme. For example, Luisa Sanchez's problems (see Table 4–7) include Ineffective Airway Clearance, Anxiety, and Disturbed Sleep Pattern. Ineffective Airway Clearance is a part of the etiology of both Anxiety and Disturbed Sleep Pattern. As you reflect, you will notice Ineffective Airway Clearance (or its effects) in other diagnoses. It emerges as a theme—as the central issue. If Mrs. Sanchez's airway clearance improves, she will be less anxious and able to sleep better. As you can see, intervening effectively for a central problem also relieves some peripheral problems. Think about the total picture for the patient at the same time you examine each diagnosis. Truly, you need to think about everything at once during this part of the process—that is why reflection is needed.

Avoiding Diagnostic Errors

Although you can never be absolutely certain a diagnosis is correct, it is important for diagnoses to be as accurate as possible. The following suggestions may help you avoid diagnostic errors. Keep in mind that most sources of diagnostic error are also legitimate sources of hypotheses about the meaning of patient data. They cause errors only when you rely too heavily on them. See Box 4–7 for ways to avoid diagnostic errors.

Diagnosis: Think About Your Thinking

d of Reasoning	Questions to Ask Yourself
Clarity—A statement must be clear in order to know whether it is accurate, relevant, and so on.	■ Have I clustered the cues without too much overlap? ■ How have I clustered these cues in the past? ■ When I verified my diagnoses, did the patient understand my descriptions of his problems and strengths? ■ Have I expressed the problems and strengths clearly? ■ Do they give a clear picture of the patient's health status?
Accuracy—A statement can be clear but not accurate.	■ Is this the best explanation for the cue cluster? ■ Do I have enough data to support my diagnoses? Did I identify all the data gaps? ■ Did the patient verify my diagnoses?
Precision—A statement can be both clear and accurate but not precise.	■ Did I use the most specific description of the patient's health status (e.g., "severe headache" is more specific than "pain")?
Relevance—A statement can be clear, accurate, and precise but not relevant to the issue.	■ Have I focused on the significant cues? What data are outside normal ranges? Is it normal for this patient? ■ Have I omitted any relevant cues from the clusters? ■ Are the problems within the domain of nursing practice?
Significance—Related to relevance. What is most important?	■ Considering the whole situation, what are the most important problems right now? ■ What problems can I realistically deal with? ■ Do I need to refer or report any problems immediately?
Depth—A statement can be clear, accurate, precise, and relevant but superficial.	■ What are the different possibilities for clustering the cues? ■ Am I qualified to determine what the problem is, or do I need help? ■ Is my diagnosis within the domain of nursing practice? ■ Did I consider social, cultural, and spiritual factors? ■ For problems and etiologies, did I look beyond the medical diagnosis to consider human responses?
Breadth—A line of reasoning can meet all of the other standards but be one sided.	■ What other problems do the cue clusters suggest? ■ Did I verify the diagnoses with the client and family? ■ Do I have biases, stereotypes, or preconceived notions about the patient's health status? ■ Did I identify wellness diagnoses, strengths, and collaborative problems, as well as nursing diagnoses?
Logic—Reasoning brings various thoughts together in some kind of order. If the thoughts make sense in combination, then thinking is logical.	■ How are the cues related within each cluster? ■ How is the etiology related to the problem? Would it really produce that human response? ■ Did I jump to conclusions about the patient's health status? Or did I take the time to think carefully about the data analysis/synthesis?

Based on Paul, R. (1996). *Critical thinking workshop handbook*. Dillon Beach, CA: Foundation for Critical Thinking. See http://www.criticalthinking.org.

BOX 4–7

COMMON DIAGNOSTIC ERRORS

Researchers found the following diagnostic errors were commonly made by students.
- Using only the label definition without comparing patient data with defining characteristics for the diagnosis
- Missing etiological or related factors
- Inferring beyond the data; that is, drawing a conclusion not supported by the assessment data
- Misinterpreting a patient's realistic worry (e.g., identifying it as Anxiety or Ineffective Coping)
- Reading data or diagnostic criteria inaccurately
- Missing cues because of lack of knowledge and experience

Source: Adapted from O'Neil, J. A. (1997). The consequences of meeting "Mrs. Wisdom": Teaching the nursing diagnostic process with case studies. In M. J. Rantz & P. LeMone (Eds.), *Classification of nursing diagnoses: Proceedings of the Twelfth Conference, North American Nursing Diagnosis Association.* Philadelphia: NANDA, pp. 131–138.

Take-away point: Avoid diagnostic errors by:
- Being aware of sources of error
- Keeping an open mind
- Ensuring data are complete
- Supporting diagnostic conclusions with data
- Validating diagnoses with the patient

1. **Don't jump to conclusions based on just a few cues. Look for patterns in the data, and look at behavior over time rather than at isolated incidents**. For example, in Table 4–7, you would not diagnose Interrupted Family Processes on the basis of the two cues in Cluster 8. There are no data to show that the family was ever before disrupted or that it will ever be again. You would need to see if the situation persists or if other data were found to support such a hypothesis.

2. **Suspend judgment when data are incomplete.** In the following example, the nurse should have gathered more data before interpreting the cues to mean Pain.

   EXAMPLE: On entering the room for a scheduled postoperative observation, the nurse sees that Ms. Foley is crying. The nurse quickly leaves the room, saying, "I'll be right back with your pain medication." On checking the medication record, the nurse discovers that the patient has already received an analgesic. The patient actually was crying because she had just received bad news from the surgeon about the results of her operation.

3. **Build a good knowledge base and acquire clinical experience.** Principles from other disciplines (e.g., physiology) help you to understand patient data in different ways, thereby improving the accuracy of your diagnoses.

A good knowledge base helps you recognize significant cues and patterns. You need to know what is normal for most people, for such things as vital signs, lab tests, speech development, breath sounds, and so on. In addition, you must determine what is normal for a particular person, taking into account age, physical makeup, lifestyle, culture, and the person's own perception of normal. Compare findings with the patient's baseline data when possible. For example, normal blood pressure for adults ranges from 110/60 to 120/80 mm Hg. However, a blood pressure of 90/50 mm Hg may be perfectly normal for a particular individual. For a person with long-standing hypertension, blood pressure of 150/90 mm Hg may not be a significant cue.

A good knowledge base helps you to have faith in your own reasoning and keeps you from relying too much on authority figures. You should certainly consult experienced nurses for input about the meaning of patient data. But realize that even experienced nurses can make errors. Patient problems you identify with the help of an authority must be verified in the same manner as any other problem.

4. **Examine your beliefs and values.** Beliefs are not usually acquired rationally, and they can be misleading. We tend to believe what those around us believe, what we are rewarded for believing, what serves our own interests, and what makes us comfortable. Reflect on your beliefs, keeping the ones that are supported by good reasons and evidence, to help you avoid the errors of bias and stereotyping.

   Bias is the tendency to slant one's judgment in a particular way. We all have ideas about what people are like and what causes them to behave in certain ways and even why they become ill. Some people believe they will catch a cold if they get their feet wet; others believe that illness is punishment for wrongdoing. Such ideas are based on life experience, not evidence, and may or may not be accurate.

   EXAMPLE: A nurse feels strongly that people are responsible for their own health. This nurse makes biased judgments about a patient with lung cancer who has a 40-year smoking history and about a patient with emphysema who asks to have his ventilator shut off. The nurse's personal theory likewise affects his data interpretation for patients with AIDS and other sexually transmitted diseases.

   Stereotypes are expectations about a person based on beliefs about his group (e.g., physicians, elderly people, nurses, drug users). Two examples of stereotypes are that fat people are jolly and that women are emotional. A negative stereotype is a **prejudice**. Stereotypes are based more on hearsay than on fact or experience. If you rely on stereotypes instead of patient data, you will miss the uniqueness of each person. A common example of this is referring to patients as "the hysterectomy patient" or "the teenager in room 220."

5. **Keep your mind open to all possible explanations of the data clusters.** Remember that diagnoses are only tentative conclusions. Be ready to change your diagnoses as you reflect on and acquire more data. This will help you to avoid the following thinking errors:

   a. *Forming premature conclusions based on context.* Nurses sometimes make judgments before even meeting the client, based on the client's medical diagnosis, the setting they are in, the chart, or what others say about the client (e.g., "she's a complainer"). Such information can help you to think of possible meanings in the data, but be careful not to let it bias your thinking. For example, Nurse Thomas has read that grief is a response to loss of a body part. She also knows the theory that childbearing is an important aspect of a woman's identity. She therefore expects that patients having a hysterectomy will grieve over the loss of childbearing ability. This nurse fails to see each patient as an individual and is quick to develop a diagnosis of grieving at the first sign of crying, sadness, or other emotional upset—based on what she "knows." Patients become upset for many reasons, and Nurse Thomas's inference of grief is highly inaccurate for some of them.

b. *Relying too much on past experience.* This is different from stereotyping because stereotypes are formed on the basis of little or no experience. Basing conclusions on past experience with similar situations is a common and legitimate practice. Generalizing from experience can help you to formulate tentative diagnoses, but it can also lead to error unless you validate your assumptions.

EXAMPLE: In the past 6 months, Nurse Thomas has cared for several women who have undergone hysterectomies. All of her patients have experienced at least some level of grief after surgery. Unconsciously, she has used the specific cases in her experience to generalize a rule about all cases. She now expects to see a grief reaction after hysterectomy and frequently identifies cue clusters in that manner.

6. **Validate all diagnoses with data; don't rely on intuition alone.** Be able to back up your diagnosis with patient data (signs and symptoms) and verify your conclusions with the patient and family. You may have a feeling, but no evidence, that a problem exists. This should be a signal for you to watch the patient more closely than usual for signs and symptoms that the problem is developing. You may want to share your feeling with another nurse, the patient, or the physician—"I can't put my finger on it, but I just have a feeling that something is going on."

7. **Develop cultural sensitivity.** A situation may be considered a problem in one culture but not another. For example, in the mainstream United States culture, it is acceptable to bottle feed a baby. However, some cultures (e.g., Navajo) believe that breastfeeding promotes respect and obedience, while bottle feeding does not. From that cultural perspective, bottle feeding might be considered a problem or a symptom of a problem. The key is to understand that personal and cultural meanings are attached cue clusters. The following guidelines will improve the accuracy of your diagnoses:

- Learn about the cultural or ethnic groups in your area.
- Do not assume the meaning of a behavior (cue) without considering the patient's culture and ethnicity.
- Be aware of your own beliefs and attitudes about health; examine their logic and origins.

Take-away point: For a quick check of your diagnostic reasoning, ask these questions:
- Is the problem correctly identified?
- Does it describe the patient's health status?
- Is there anything I can do to help with it?

Ethical Considerations

Nursing process deals with persons rather than things or objects. Therefore, every act of nursing, including diagnosis, has a moral or value dimension. Your values, especially about nursing roles and responsibilities, determine your choices about what data are even worthy of collection, especially when you are pressed for time. For example, when a nurse values decreased length of stay, assessments for the medical diagnosis—which are required by the critical pathway—may be a higher priority for him than a more holistic nursing assessment (Gordon et al., 1994).

When analyzing assessment data, you may interpret some of that data to represent moral or ethical problems—for the patient and family, other healthcare professionals, or yourself. For example, if a cue cluster suggests Chronic Confusion as a nursing diagnosis, then ethical questions arise about the patient's ability to give informed consent for treatments. Identification of an actual or potential ethical problem signals the need to gather information about all involved parties, what they want to happen, and the moral basis for their claims. You would then formulate a problem statement, the same as for other aspects of health status.

Defining or describing ethical problems requires sensitivity to the needs of others and awareness of your own moral duties or obligations to others in a situation. You also need some general knowledge about ethical principles and problems. That, of course, is beyond the scope of this text. Refer to a fundamentals of nursing or an ethics text for that information.

SUMMARY

The diagnostic process is summarized in Box 4–3.

Diagnosis

- Is a pivotal step in the nursing process.
- Is the process of interpreting data, verifying hypotheses about the data (with the client or other professionals), labeling the problems, and recording the diagnoses.
- May identify nursing diagnoses, collaborative problems, other health problems, or wellness diagnoses.
- May identify actual risk, or possible problems, as well as patient strengths.
- Requires knowledge, critical thinking, not making premature judgments, and keeping an open mind.
- May identify ethical problems.

Nursing diagnoses

- Involve human responses to disease and other stressors in the area of health.
- Are problems that nurses can independently treat or prevent.
- Are culturally influenced.
- Can be used to individualize standardized plans of care such as critical pathways.

CRITICAL THINKING AND CLINICAL REASONING: A CASE STUDY

Discuss the following case with classmates. Look up unfamiliar terms (e.g., COPD) as needed.

Imagine that you are providing home care for a client who has chronic obstructive pulmonary disease (COPD). He has often been admitted to the hospital for acute respiratory distress and at times even requires mechanical ventilation. His activities are always limited because of his inadequate oxygenation; he requires assistance from home health aides for cooking and bathing. His home smells of stale cigarette smoke, and you see ashtrays full of ashes and cigarette stubs. The client begins smoking a cigarette during your visit.

1. What feelings would you have? (Just identify your feelings at this time.)
2. What thoughts, perhaps about past experiences, might be contributing to your feelings?
3. What values do you have that might influence the way you see this situation? (Examples of values are, "Mothers should take good care of their children" and "It is important to be honest.")
4. With items 1–3 in mind, what, if anything, would you say to this client when he lights the cigarette?

When you begin to discuss smoking with the client (in item #4), he becomes very angry. He bangs his fist on the table and shouts, "I wish you would mind your own business!"

5. What do you think the client is feeling?
6. What thoughts or past experiences may have contributed to his anger?
7. Would you make a nursing diagnosis of Noncompliance for this patient? If so, what is the etiology? If not, why not?
8. Would you make a nursing diagnosis of Deficient Knowledge (effects of smoking on COPD) for this patient? Why or why not?
9. Are there any other nursing diagnoses you would want to make, based on the available data?

See suggested responses to Critical Thinking and Clinical Reasoning: A Case Study in Appendix A

Pearson Nursing Student Resources

Find additional review materials at **www.nursing.pearsonhighered.com**
Prepare for success with additional NCLEX®-style practice questions, interactive assignments and activities, Web links, animations and videos, and more!

Diagnostic Language

5

Introduction

In Chapter 4, you learned to identify and verify nursing diagnoses, collaborative problems, and patient strengths. This chapter explains how to use the NANDA International (NANDA-I) standardized terminology to write nursing diagnoses, describes formats for collaborative problems, and presents frameworks for prioritizing patient problems. Figure 5–1 highlights the aspects of the diagnosis phase that are emphasized in this chapter.

Standardized Nursing Languages

Standardized languages are essential for structuring and communicating knowledge and practice, as well as for evaluating the cost and quality of nursing care. Examples of standardized languages include the musical scale, Arabic numerals, and symbols of chemical elements. As nursing knowledge has developed, nurse theorists and scientists have begun to develop vocabularies to describe and explain what nurses know and do and systems to organize that knowledge for practice, education, and research.

Classification Systems

A **classification system** (also called a **taxonomy**) identifies and classifies ideas or objects on the basis of their similarities. For example, in anatomy, parts of the body are named and then classified according to body systems—the radius and ulna are bones in the skeletal system. Classification systems are created and used

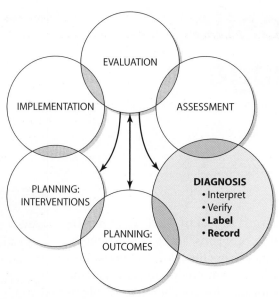

FIGURE 5–1

The diagnosis phase: writing the diagnostic statement

for various purposes. The following are examples of some non-nursing classification systems used in healthcare.

- The International Classification of Disease (ICD) names and classifies medical conditions, including mental disorders (World Health Organization, 2007).
- The Current Procedural Terminology (CPT) names and defines all services and procedures performed by physicians. It is used for reimbursement of physician services (American Medical Association, 2010).
- The *Diagnostic and Statistical Manual* (DSM) of the American Psychiatric Association (2000) is used by mental health professionals to name and describe psychiatric disorders.

Take-away point: Standardized languages are necessary for structuring and communicating knowledge and practice and for evaluating the cost and quality of nursing care.

The Need for Uniform Nursing Language

Well-developed classifications of standardized nursing languages are needed for the following reasons:

1. **Expanding nursing knowledge.** Taxonomies structure memory, thinking, and decision making. Their systematic organization structures a body of knowledge, making it possible to identify gaps and relationships in the knowledge. Existing nursing taxonomies have already collected and organized the major concepts needed to construct practice-level theories for nursing (Blegen & Tripp-Reimer, 1997).

2. **Supporting computerized records.** Computer information systems and computerized patient records require standardized languages that can be converted to numerical codes. A common nursing language is required in order for nursing data and documentation to be included in patient records and research databases.

3. **Defining and communicating unique nursing knowledge.** Nurses are the largest group of healthcare professionals in the United States. Nevertheless, there is confusion, even among nurses, about what nurses do. A common language could be used by all nurses to communicate with each other and with those outside of nursing, enabling nurses to describe what they do for patients and to show the difference it makes in patient outcomes.

   In an effort to reduce costs, most healthcare institutions are reorganizing and questioning traditional roles, especially those of nurses. If nursing is to survive as a discipline, we need to answer two questions: (a) What do nurses do? and (b) Do nurses' actions make a difference in patient outcomes? This requires research-based findings, which depend on standardized nursing languages to reflect nursing contributions.

4. **Improving nursing care quality.** Each discipline should delineate the data elements needed to define and evaluate a clinical encounter. For nursing, the data elements are diagnoses, interventions, and outcomes. When standardized nursing vocabularies are included in clinical documentation systems, data can be generated to evaluate the effectiveness of nursing interventions.

5. **Influencing health policy decisions.** Standardized terms would generate data that more accurately represent nursing practice than outcomes-related measures currently used (Rutherford, 2008). Such data would make it possible to compare the effectiveness and cost of nursing treatments, not just in an institution but across locations. Results from such studies could be used to influence health policy decisions locally, regionally, and nationally.

Existing Nursing Taxonomies

Table 5–1 contains a list of some of the standardized nursing languages currently recognized by the American Nurses Association (ANA) and used in the United States. Each system will be discussed in more detail throughout this and subsequent chapters. NANDA-I, Nursing Interventions Classification (NIC), and Nursing Outcomes Classification (NOC) each focus on only one element of nursing. The Clinical Care Classification (CCC) and the Omaha System contain all three elements: diagnoses, outcomes, and interventions. Because this chapter focuses on nursing diagnoses, the NANDA-I taxonomy is discussed in more detail than the other classification systems.

In addition to the U.S. taxonomies, the International Council of Nurses (ICN) has developed an International Classification for Nursing Practice (ICNP) that classifies nursing phenomena (diagnoses), nursing outcomes, and nursing actions (ICN, 2009). This classification intends to provide a common language for nurses throughout the world.

TABLE 5–1   Some Nursing Taxonomies Recognized by the American Nurses Association

Taxonomy	Elements Classified	Comments
NANDA International	Diagnoses	The first nursing language taxonomy in the United States. Development of standardized language systems for nursing-sensitive outcomes and nursing interventions followed. Comprehensive across specialty and practice areas.
NIC (Nursing Interventions Classification)	Interventions	The first comprehensive standardized classification of nursing interventions. Developed by a research team at the University of Iowa, it describes both direct and indirect care activities performed by nurses (McCloskey & Bulechek, 1992). Comprehensive across specialty and practice areas.
NOC (Nursing Outcomes Classification)	Outcomes	The first standardized classification of nursing-sensitive patient outcomes. Developed by a research team at the University of Iowa, it describes outcomes that can be influenced by independent nursing actions (Johnson & Maas, 1997). Comprehensive across specialty and practice areas.
Clinical Care Classification	Diagnoses, Outcomes (expected and actual), Interventions	Designed for home health or ambulatory care. Specifically designed for computer-based documentation systems. Developed from research conducted at Georgetown University School of Nursing (Saba, 1995, 1997).
Omaha System	Diagnoses, Interventions, Outcomes	A system for classifying and coding problems, outcomes, and nursing interventions for patients receiving care in the community. Developed by the Visiting Nurses Association of Omaha, Nebraska (Martin & Scheet, 1992).

Source: Nursing Information and Data Set Evaluation Center (last updated 2006). Available at http://www.nursingworld.org/npii/terminologies.htm.

5-1 WHAT DO YOU KNOW?

1. List four reasons standardized nursing languages are needed.
2. (True or false) Taxonomies classify ideas and objects on the basis of their similarities.

See answer to #5-1 What Do You Know? in Appendix A.

NANDA International

In the 1950s and 1960s, nursing leaders recognized the need to describe nursing work and nursing knowledge. Several studies were done to identify patient problems requiring nursing intervention. These evolved into lists of *nursing problems* (Abdellah, 1957) and *client needs* that might require basic nursing care (Henderson, 1964). Although neither of these was actually a list of patient problems as we now define them, they did demonstrate that nursing care focuses on something other than disease processes. In 1973, the ANA identified nursing diagnosis as an important function of the professional nurse.

Before 1973, there was no language to describe the conclusions that nurses reached through assessment. Although NANDA-I is a volunteer organization and mostly unfunded, it pioneered the work in nursing language and classification with its classification of nursing diagnoses. It began in 1973, when nursing faculty at St. Louis University, led by Kristine Gebbie and Mary Ann Lavin, called the first conference on classification. A national task force was formed, and 100 nurses attended the First Conference on Nursing Diagnosis (Gebbie, 1976). This group continued to meet every 2 years and, at the Fifth Conference in 1982 (Kim et al, 1984), formally became the North American Nursing Diagnosis Association. Membership consists of nurses from education, practice, research, and administration, as well as from all nursing specialty areas (e.g., intensive care, maternal-child, home health). This diversity ensures input from a variety of perspectives. The major functions of the early groups were to generate, name, and implement diagnostic categories. Emphasis then shifted to clarifying existing labels, developing etiologies, and defining characteristics. These priorities still exist, along with others, such as revising the taxonomy, promoting research to validate the diagnostic labels, and encouraging nurses to use standardized language in their practice.

In 1994, The **Nursing Diagnosis Extension Classification** (**NDEC**) research team at the University of Iowa reached a collaborative agreement with NANDA-I to extend and refine the NANDA-I work by addressing some of the issues about comprehensiveness, specificity, clinical usefulness, and clinical testing of the NANDA-I taxonomy. Many of the diagnoses on the official NANDA-I list have been tested only minimally.

The NANDA-I Taxonomy

Any number of ordering principles can be used to classify things (e.g., size, weight, color). The first NANDA taxonomy was alphabetical and nonhierarchical (as in the list inside the front cover of this text). A framework known as NANDA Taxonomy II (shown in Table 3–12), is used to organize the NANDA-I diagnostic labels. Taxonomy development is ongoing, and changes are published in a biannual publication, *Nursing Diagnoses: Definitions & Classification.*

NANDA-I works with the ANA and other organizations to include the NANDA-I labels in other classification systems—for example, the World Health Organization ICD. NANDA-I diagnosis-related articles are currently indexed in the Cumulative Index of Nursing and Allied Health (CINAHL) and in the National Library of Medicine Medical Metathesaurus for a Unified Medical Language.

NANDA-I Review Process

Review and refinement of diagnostic labels is ongoing. New and modified labels are discussed at each biannual conference. All individual nurses can submit diagnoses to NANDA-I. Diagnoses are also submitted by NDEC and nursing specialty organizations (e.g., the Association of Operating Room Nurses). The elected Diagnostic Review Committee stages each diagnosis according to how well it is developed and supported (e.g., by concept analysis or research). Diagnoses on the official NANDA-I list are not finished products but are approved for clinical use and further study. NANDA-I reports ongoing work in its official journal, *International Journal of Nursing Terminologies and Classifications.*

Choosing a Problem Label

The NANDA-I diagnostic labels provide a common language for nurses to use in describing health problems for any type of client and in all healthcare settings. You must understand the meaning of the NANDA-I labels if your written statements are to accurately reflect your clinical judgments.

Components of a NANDA-I Diagnosis

Take-away point: Each NANDA-I diagnosis has four components: label, definition, defining characteristics, and either related factors or risk factors.

Label

Also referred to as the *title* or *name,* the **label** is a concise word or phrase describing the client's health. Labels can be used as either the problem or the etiology in a diagnostic statement. Most labels include qualifying terms such as *Actual, Risk, Ineffective, Impaired,* or *Increased.*

Taxonomy II includes seven "axes" that are used to describe a diagnosis. Table 5–2 shows the axes to use when writing diagnostic statements. The diagnoses on the NANDA-I-approved list are worded using these axes. Not all of the axes are needed for every diagnosis. For example, for an adolescent who has risk factors for a parenting problem, you might write: *Risk for Impaired Parenting (by an individual adolescent).* Notice that "Risk for Impaired Parenting" is on the NANDA-I-approved list. You would add words from other axes (e.g., "individual, adolescent") only as needed to clarify the diagnosis.

From Axis 1: Parenting

From Axis 2: Individual

From Axis 3: Impaired

From Axis 7: Risk

Notice that many of the NANDA-I labels are very general; you cannot know what a diagnostic concept includes by looking at the label alone. For example, do you think "Activity Intolerance" means that the patient tires easily when playing football or that he has chest pain when he walks up the stairs? What is the difference between the labels "Activity Intolerance" and "Fatigue"? The other components of a NANDA-I diagnosis help to clarify these questions.

TABLE 5–2 Qualifiers for Nursing Diagnoses (from NANDA International Taxonomy II)

Axis 1: Diagnostic Concept

This is the essential, fundamental part of the diagnosis. It consists of one or more nouns. Examples include activity intolerance, adjustment, and parenting. Each diagnostic label has a root concept.

Axis 2: Subject of the Diagnosis

This is the person for whom the diagnosis is made.

Individual	A single human being distinct from others, a person
Family	Two or more people having continuous or sustained relationships, perceiving reciprocal obligations, sensing common meaning, and sharing certain obligations toward others; related by blood or choice
Group	A number of people with shared characteristics
Community	A group of people living in the same locale under the same governance. Examples include neighborhoods and cities.

Axis 3: Judgment

A descriptor or modifier that limits or specifies the meaning of the diagnostic concept. Together with the concept, it forms the diagnostic label.

Descriptor	Definition
Compromised	To make vulnerable to threat
Complicated	Intricately involved, complex
Decreased	Lessened (in size, amount, or degree)
Defensive	Used or intended to defend or protect
Deficient	Insufficient, inadequate
Delayed	Late, slow, or postponed
Disabled	Limited, handicapped
Disorganized	Not properly arranged or controlled
Disproportionate	Too large or too small in comparison with norm
Disturbed	Not operating normally
Dysfunctional	Abnormal, incomplete functioning
Effective	Producing the intended or desired effect
Enhanced	Improved in quality, value, or extent
Excessive	Greater than necessary or desirable
Imbalanced	Out of proportion or balance
Impaired	Damaged, weakened
Ineffective	Not producing the intended or desired effect
Interrupted	Having its continuity broken
Low	Below the norm
Organized	Properly arranged or controlled
Perceived	Observed through the senses
Readiness for	In a suitable state for an activity or situation
Situational	Related to particular circumstance(s)

(Continued)

TABLE 5–2 Qualifiers for Nursing Diagnoses (from NANDA International Taxonomy II) (*continued*)

Axis 4. Location	
The parts or regions of their body or their related functions	
Auditory	Olfactory
Bladder	Oral
Bowel	Peripheral
Cardiac	Peripheral vascular
Cardiopulmonary	Renal
Cerebral	Skin
Gastrointestinal	Tactile
Gustatory	Tissue
Intracranial	Vascular
Kinesthetic	Verbal
Mucous membranes	Visual
Neurovascular	Urinary

Axis 5: Age
Fetus, neonate, infant, toddler, preschool child, school-age child, adolescent, adult, older adult

Axis 6: Time	
Acute	Lasting less than 6 months
Chronic	Lasting more than 6 months
Intermittent	Stopping or starting again at intervals, periodic, cyclic
Continuous	Uninterrupted, going on without stop

Axis 7: Status of the Diagnosis	
Actual	Existing in fact or reality, existing at the present time
Health Promotion	Behavior motivated by the desire to increase well-being and actualize human health potential
Risk	Vulnerability, especially as a result of exposure to factors that increase the chance of injury or loss
Wellness	The quality or state of being healthy; may be stated as "actual" (although it is understood to exist if not specifically stated)

Source: NANDA International. (2009). *NANDA International nursing diagnoses: Definitions and classification 2009–2011.* Ames, IA. Wiley-Blackwell.

5-1 THINK & REFLECT!

Use the Taxonomy II (Table 5–2) axes to write a problem statement for the following data: An elderly client with left-sided paralysis has a red area of abraded ("broken") skin over his sacrum. (The concept, Axis 1, is Skin Integrity.)

See suggested responses to #5-1 Think & Reflect! in Appendix A.

Definition

The **definition** expresses clearly and precisely the essential nature of the diagnostic label; it differentiates the label from all others. For example, Activity Intolerance and Fatigue both involve decreased energy and abilities; however, whereas the Activity Intolerance definition focuses on the inability to "complete . . . daily activities," the Fatigue definition requires the presence of "an overwhelming sustained sense of exhaustion."

Defining Characteristics

Defining characteristics are the *cues* (subjective and objective data) that indicate the presence of the diagnostic label. For actual diagnoses, the defining characteristics are the patient's *signs and symptoms*; for risk diagnoses, they are *risk factors*. It is not necessary for all of the defining characteristics to be present in order to use a label; usually, the presence of two or three confirms a diagnosis.

> **EXAMPLE:** You could diagnose Constipation if only one or two of the following defining characteristics were present:

  a. Indigestion
  b. Hard, dry, formed stool
  c. Straining with defecation
  d. Pain with defecation
  e. Abdominal distention
  f. Palpable abdominal mass

It is easy to see that a client with a diagnosis of Constipation might experience one or more of these symptoms in various combinations. A palpable mass is present in most clients who have Constipation, but some clients may not have a palpable mass. Furthermore, you would probably diagnose Constipation for a client who had only symptoms *b* and *c*, but you would not make that diagnosis for a client who had only symptoms *a* and *e*.

Related or Risk Factors

Related or **risk factors** are the conditions or situations that are associated with the problem in some way. They are conditions that precede, influence, cause, or contribute to the problem. They can be biological, psychological, social, developmental, treatment related, situational, and so on. Each diagnosis lists the related factors seen most often; however, do not interpret this as a complete list of factors that *could* be associated with the label. Imagine, for example, the variety of situations or factors that could contribute in some way to Anxiety; it would be impossible to list them all.

Related factors are often, but not always, used as the etiologies of a diagnostic statement. A related factor may be a part of the etiology for several problems, or a single problem may have several related factors as its etiology (cause).

EXAMPLE

Problem   *Etiology*

Altered Sexuality Patterns
Constipation ——————————————————— Lack of privacy
Disturbed Sleep Pattern

                                                    ——— Lack of privacy
Constipation ————————————— Inadequate fiber intake
                                                    ——— Inadequate fluid intake

For potential nursing diagnoses, such as Risk for Deficient Fluid Volume, risk factors are similar to defining characteristics: They are the cues that must be present in order to make the diagnosis. Risk factors are nearly always at least a part of the etiology of the risk diagnostic statement.

EXAMPLE: Using the factors below, you might write the following diagnosis for a patient: "Risk for Deficient Fluid Volume related to increased urinary output secondary to diuretic medications."

Risk factors for the label Risk for Deficient Fluid Volume are excessive fluid losses through both normal and abnormal routes, medications (e.g., diuretics), factors influencing fluid needs (e.g., hypermetabolic state), deviations affecting access to or intake or absorption of fluids (e.g., physical immobility), extremes of weight, and knowledge deficiency related to fluid volume.

The related factors listed in handbooks are written in general terms and are used only as suggestions. Related factors are unique to each person, so you will usually need to individualize them. For example, one of the related factors for Impaired Physical Mobility is "prescribed movement restrictions." For a given patient, it is important to know exactly what the restrictions are, so you would need to write the diagnostic statement as, "Impaired Physical Mobility related to prescribed bed rest" or ". . . related to medical order for no weight-bearing on right leg," for example.

5-2 WHAT DO YOU KNOW?

1. What are the four components of a NANDA-I diagnosis?
2. Define the term *NANDA-I label.*
3. What is the difference between related factors and risk factors?

See answer to #5-2 What Do You Know? in Appendix A.

How to Choose a Label

To choose the correct label, you simply match patient symptoms (cues) with the definitions and defining characteristics of one of the NANDA-I labels. Remember, though, that there are around 200 different labels, so random searching is not practical. By the time you are ready to choose a label, you should already have narrowed the possibilities. Recall that during data interpretation you identified the most likely explanation (problem and etiology) for each cluster of cues and decided which of your framework patterns fit it best. Finding labels on the list that appear to have the same meaning as your hypothesized explanation should then be a simple matter. Refer again to Table 4–7, the clustered abnormal cues for Luisa Sanchez. Cluster 11 is shown as follows:

Cluster 11 from Table 4–7	Functional Health Pattern
1. Cough productive of pale, pink sputum	Activity/Exercise (pattern includes respiratory status)
2. Respirations shallow	
3. Chest expansion < 3 cm	
4. Inspiratory crackles through right chest	
5. Mucous membranes pale	
6. Diminished breath sounds on right side	
7. Skin hot and pale	

The nurse hypothesized the following explanation for Cluster 11:

Cues 1 through 4 are defining characteristics for Ineffective Airway Clearance. This problem may be causing inadequate oxygenation, resulting in Cue 5. Cues 1, 6, and 7 are indicators of pneumonia, the medical problem that is creating the Ineffective Airway Clearance. Other problems are contributing as well: Deficient Fluid Volume is probably causing the patient's mucus to be thick and hard to bring up (Cues 4 and 6); Pain and weakness are contributing to Cues 2 and 3.

The nurse concluded that this explanation represented an actual problem and that the problem is a nursing diagnosis, not a collaborative or medical problem. Her informal problem statement was "ineffective airway clearance."

To find the appropriate NANDA-I label for this problem, you could simply look at an alphabetized list (e.g., the one inside the front cover of this text) for labels that seem related in some way to the explanation. You would, in this case, look for labels with words such as *airway, breathing,* or *respiration* and then find the labels in a nursing diagnosis handbook (e.g., *NANDA International Nursing Diagnoses: Definitions & Classification 2009–2011;* Wilkinson & Ahern, 2009) and compare them with your cluster of cues.

Use a Theoretical Framework to Organize the Labels

It is more efficient, however, to organize your list of diagnostic labels according to a theoretical framework (the same one you used to organize your data) so that related diagnoses are listed together. Because Luisa Sanchez's data analysis used the Gordon Functional Health Patterns, you would look for your labels under the Activity/Exercise pattern in that table (see inside back cover). There are quite a few titles under this pattern but certainly fewer than the roughly 200 listed in the alphabetical table on the inside front cover. Of the labels under Activity/Exercise, the only ones with possible connections (and some are remote, indeed) to Cluster 11 are the following:

Ineffective Airway Clearance

Impaired Gas Exchange

Ineffective Breathing Pattern

Choose the Label that Best Matches the Cue Cluster

Next, look up the most likely sounding label. Does the definition for Ineffective Airway Clearance match the nurse's explanation of the cues (Cluster 11)? Do the cues match the defining characteristics of that label? How about Ineffective Breathing Pattern? Does that fit better?

For Mrs. Sanchez, Ineffective Airway Clearance is the best-fitting label for Cluster 11. She does not have enough of the defining characteristics for Impaired Gas Exchange or Ineffective Breathing Pattern. Notice, too, that one of Mrs. Sanchez's cues is found in the related factors listed for Ineffective Airway Clearance: infection. The complete nursing diagnosis for Mrs. Sanchez would be Ineffective Airway Clearance related to thick secretions and shallow chest expansion secondary to pain, deficient fluid volume, and fatigue.

Other Diagnostic Statements for Mrs. Sanchez

The diagnostic statements for Mrs. Sanchez's other cue clusters are given as follows. Compare the cue clusters in Table 4–7 to the definitions and defining characteristics in a nursing diagnosis handbook (e.g., *NANDA-I*, 2009; Wilkinson & Ahern, 2009). Notice that NANDA-I labels can be used for both problems and etiologies. Review information on human responses in Chapters 1 and 4 as needed. Recall that responses occur on many levels and that a response can function as a stimulus that produces another response.

Cluster 1	No problem. Strengths are healthy lifestyle and understanding of and compliance with treatment regimens.
Cluster 2	Imbalanced Nutrition: Less than Body Requirements related to decreased appetite and nausea and increased metabolism secondary to disease process. (Note that this is a short-term problem that will be corrected primarily by medical treatment of her pneumonia. Meanwhile, though, she will need nutritional assessment and support.)
Cluster 3	Deficient Fluid Volume related to intake insufficient to replace fluid loss secondary to fever, diaphoresis, and nausea.
Cluster 4	Disturbed Sleep Pattern related to cough, pain, orthopnea, fever, and diaphoresis.
Cluster 5	No problem as long as medical regimen is followed.
Cluster 6	Self-Care Deficit (Level 2) related to Activity Intolerance secondary to Ineffective Airway Clearance and Disturbed Sleep Pattern.

Cluster 7   [Altered Comfort: Chills] related to fever and diaphoresis.

Cluster 8   Risk for Interrupted Family Processes related to mother's illness and temporary unavailability of father to provide child care. (Note that the defining characteristics for this diagnosis are not present in Cluster 8; however, there are risk factors.)

Cluster 9   Anxiety related to difficulty breathing and concerns over work and parenting roles.

Cluster 10   Chest Pain (Acute) related to cough secondary to pneumonia.

Cluster 11   (See the preceding discussion about this cluster.)

The following collaborative problems (potential complications) complete the list of problems for Mrs. Sanchez:

Potential complications of pneumonia: (a) Respiratory insufficiency, (b) septic shock

Potential complications of intravenous therapy: (a) Inflammation, (b) phlebitis, (c) infiltration

Potential complications of antibiotic therapy: (a) Allergic reactions, (b) gastrointestinal upset, (c) other side effects, depending on specific medication

Mrs. Sanchez's potential complications do not require collaboration unless they develop into actual problems. The nurse independently monitors for all three and can take independent action to prevent the potential complications of intravenous therapy. Because Mrs. Sanchez is not at higher risk than the normal population of pneumonia patients, individualized nursing diagnoses (e.g., Risk for Infection) are not written for these problems. They are prevented by agency routines and standards of care and require no special interventions. This will be explained further in Chapter 10, "Creating a Plan of Care."

Learning to Recognize the NANDA-I Labels

As you become familiar with the NANDA-I problem labels, it will be easier to recognize cue clusters in your patients—it is always easier to see something if you know what you are looking for. The best way to learn the labels is by using them; however, like most clinical skills, you need a certain degree of familiarity in order to use them. Refer to a nursing diagnosis handbook frequently for definitions, defining characteristics, and related/risk factors. To further help you learn what the labels mean, see "What Do You Know About Diagnostic Language," in Chapter 5, at Pearson Nursing Student Resources.

Format for Writing Diagnostic Statements

As shown in Box 5–1, ANA Standards of Practice specifically address the format and content of diagnostic statements. As you have already learned, a diagnostic statement describes the patient's problem and the related or risk factors. This basic *Problem + Etiology*

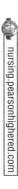

nursing.pearsonhighered.com

BOX 5–1

STANDARDS OF PRACTICE

American Nurses Association Standard 2: Diagnosis

The registered nurse analyzes the assessment data to determine the diagnoses or issues.

Competencies

The registered nurse:

1. Derives the diagnoses or issues based on assessment data.
2. Validates the diagnoses or issues with the patient, family, and other healthcare providers when possible and appropriate.
3. Documents diagnoses or issues in a manner that facilitates the determination of the expected outcomes and plan.
4. Identifies actual or potential risks to the patient's health and safety or barriers to health which may include but are not limited to interpersonal, systematic, or environmental circumstances.
5. Uses standardized classification systems, when available, in naming 1068 diagnoses.

(NOTE: There are additional measurement criteria for advanced practice registered nurses.)

Note: This material is from the draft for public comment (ANA, 2010, in press); its wording may be somewhat changed in the final published version (August 2010). For that version of the ANA standards, visit http://www.nursingworld.org.

Source: Reprinted with permission from American Nurses Association (2010, in press). In *Nursing: Scope and standards of practice* (2nd ed.). (Public Comment draft, January). Silver Spring, MD. Available at http:/nursebooks.org.

format varies slightly, depending on whether you are writing a nursing diagnosis, wellness diagnosis, or a collaborative problem and depending on nursing diagnosis status (actual, risk, or possible). Briefly, the basic components of a diagnostic statement are as follows and as shown in Table 5–3.

1. **Problem.** The problem describes the client's health status clearly and concisely. Remember that it identifies what should be changed about the client's health status, so it should suggest client goals or outcomes. Use a NANDA-I label for this part of your statement when possible.

TABLE 5–3   NANDA International Components in Diagnostic Statements

	Diagnostic Statement Components		
	Problem	**Etiology**	**A.M.B.**
Actual Diagnoses	Label	Related factors, other diagnosis labels	Defining characteristics
Potential Diagnoses	Label	Risk factors	None

2. **Etiology.** The etiology describes factors causing or contributing to actual problems. For potential problems, it describes the risk factors that are present. The etiology may include a NANDA-I label, some of the defining characteristics, a NANDA-I risk factor or related factor, or something entirely outside the NANDA-I standardized language. The etiology enables you to individualize nursing care for a client. For example, even though the problem is the same, Impaired Verbal Communication *related to inability to speak English* would suggest different interventions than Impaired Verbal Communication *secondary to tracheostomy*.

3. **Related to (r/t).** This phrase connects the two parts of the statement. The phrase *due to* is not used because it implies a direct cause-and-effect relationship, which is hard to prove in a nursing diagnosis. Human beings and human responses are complex. Usually, there are multiple factors that interact to "cause" a problem, and it is possible that even if those factors were eliminated, the problem response might still exist. At best, you can say that it is highly likely that the factors are influencing, creating, or contributing to the problem.

5-3 WHAT DO YOU KNOW?

Why do nurses use "r/t" instead of "due to" to join the problem and etiology of a nursing diagnosis?

See answer to #5-3 What Do You Know? in Appendix A.

Actual Nursing Diagnoses

When a client's signs and symptoms match the defining characteristics of a label, an actual diagnosis is present. Note that the word *actual* is assumed, so you should not write it in the diagnostic statement. This section presents the basic format and several variations for actual diagnoses.

Take-away point: Actual nursing diagnoses may be written as a one-, two-, three-, or four-part statement.

Basic Format: Two-Part Statement

The basic format for an actual nursing diagnosis consists of two parts: the problem and the etiology.

Problem	r/t	*Etiology*
↓		↓
(NANDA-I label)	r/t	(Related factors)
↓		↓
Constipation	r/t	Inadequate dietary fiber

Some NANDA-I labels contain the word *Specify*. For these, you need to add words to indicate more specifically what the problem is.

EXAMPLE: Noncompliance (*specify*)

Noncompliance (*diabetic diet*) r/t unresolved anger about having diabetes

The NANDA-I labels in most listings are arranged with the qualifiers after the main word (Infection, Risk for) for ease of alphabetizing. Do not write your diagnoses in that manner; instead, write them as you would say them in normal conversation.

EXAMPLE: *Incorrect:* Airway Clearance, Ineffective r/t weak cough reflex

Correct: Ineffective Airway Clearance r/t weak cough reflex

P.E.S. Format

Besides *Problem + Etiology*, you may wish to include the defining characteristics as a part of your diagnostic statement. This is called the **P.E.S. format**, for "problem, etiology, and symptom." The P.E.S. format is especially recommended when you are first learning to write nursing diagnoses. If you use this method, simply add *as manifested by (A.M.B.)* followed by the patient's signs and symptoms that led you to make the diagnosis. Use the following format:

Problem	(r/t)	Etiology	(A.M.B.)	Symptoms
↓	↓	↓	↓	↓
(NANDA-I label)	(r/t)	(Related factors)	(A.M.B.)	(Defining characteristics)
↓	↓	↓	↓	↓
Self-Esteem Disturbance	r/t	Being rejected by husband	A.M.B.	Hypersensitive to criticism; states, "I don't know if I can manage by myself." Rejects positive feedback.

Another example of the P.E.S. format follows. Notice that this method creates a very long statement.

EXAMPLE: Noncompliance (low-salt diet) r/t unresolved anger about diagnosis A.M.B. elevated blood pressure, 10-lb weight gain, and statements: "forget to take my pills," and "can't live without salt on my food."

Patient symptoms are helpful in planning interventions, so it is important that they be easily accessible. If they result in a statement that is too long, you can record them in the nursing progress notes when you first make the diagnosis. Another possibility, recommended for students, is to record the signs and symptoms *below* the nursing diagnosis, grouping the subjective (S) and objective (O) data.

    EXAMPLE: Noncompliance (low-salt diet) r/t unresolved anger about diagnosis.

        S—"I forget to take my pills."

          "I can't live without salt on my food."

        O—Weight 215 (gain of 10 lb)

          BP 190/100

A common error among beginning diagnosticians who use the P.E.S. format is to write a vague, nonspecific problem and etiology, hoping that the client's health status will be explained by listing the signs and symptoms. Guard against this tendency by making the Problem + Etiology as specific and descriptive as possible before adding the signs and symptoms. Your diagnostic statement should present a clear picture of your client's health status even without the listing of symptoms.

"Secondary to"

Sometimes the diagnostic statement is clearer if the etiology is divided into two parts with the words *secondary to* (2°). The part following secondary to is often a pathophysiology or a disease process, as in "Risk for impaired skin integrity r/t decreased peripheral circulation 2° diabetes." Use "2°" only if it is the only way to make your statement precise.

"Unknown Etiology"

You can make a diagnosis when the defining characteristics are present even if you do not know the cause or contributing factors. For instance, you might write, "Noncompliance (medication regimen) r/t unknown etiology." If you think you know an etiology, but still need more data to confirm it, use the phrase *possibly related to*. When you have confirming data you can rewrite the diagnosis more positively. You might say, for example, "Noncompliance (medication regimen) *possibly r/t* unresolved anger about diagnosis."

"Complex Etiology"

Occasionally, there are too many etiological factors or they are too complex to be stated in a brief phrase. The actual causes of Decisional Conflict or Chronic Low Self-Esteem, for instance, might be long term and complex. In such unusual cases, you can omit the etiology and replace it with the phrase *complex factors* (e.g., Chronic Low Self-Esteem *r/t complex factors*).

5-2 THINK & REFLECT!

Think of a problem, other than Decisional Conflict and Chronic Low Self-Esteem, that could be caused by a complex etiology.

See suggested responses to #5-2 Think & Reflect! in Appendix A.

Three-Part and Four-Part Statements

Some diagnostic labels consist of two parts: The first indicates a general response, and the second makes it more specific. Adding an etiology to these labels creates a three-part diagnosis; adding *secondary to* makes it four parts.

EXAMPLE:

Labels: Dysfunctional Family Processes: Alcoholism
Imbalanced Nutrition: Less than Body Requirements
Feeding Self-Care Deficit (Level 3)
Nursing Diagnosis: Imbalanced Nutrition: Less than Body Requirements r/t nausea
2° chemotherapy

You may need to add a third part to other NANDA-I labels as well. Diagnostic statements must precisely describe the client's health concern because general concepts and categorizations are ineffective for planning nursing care. Not all NANDA-I labels provide this level of precision. You can sometimes make them more descriptive by using the P.E.S. format or by using a two-part etiology with *secondary to*, as in the preceding example. Sometimes, however, you may need to add a colon and third part using your own words. Notice that the following example does not indicate the specific difficulty with mobility even though the etiology is very descriptive. Can the patient use her hands at all? Or is her mobility only partially limited? Can she pick up silverware and feed herself, for example, or brush her hair? In some cases, the label definition makes the problem more specific, but in this instance, it does not offer much help.

EXAMPLE: Impaired Physical Mobility r/t stiffness and pain in hands secondary to arthritic joint changes

Label Definition: Limitation in independent, purposeful physical movement of the body or of one or more extremities.

To make the nursing diagnosis more specific, you should add a third part (descriptor):

Problem	*Descriptor* +	*Etiology*
↓	↓	↓
(NANDA-I label)	(Specific problem description)	r/t (related factors)
↓	↓	↓
Impaired Physical Mobility	(*Decreased fine motor skills*)	r/t pain and stiffness in the hands 2° arthritic joint changes

In this example, using the P.E.S. format does not help because the signs and symptoms are the same as the etiology: pain and stiffness in the hands. The statement is improved by adding *secondary to*. Nevertheless, pain and stiffness in the hands are really *symptoms* of the problem rather than a *cause* of the impaired mobility; therefore, you should not use them on the right side of the statement in the etiology phrase. The most logical way to write the diagnosis is to add a colon and a more specific description to the general problem of Impaired Physical Mobility.

EXAMPLE: Impaired Physical Mobility r/t stiffness and pain in hands

> *P.E.S.:* Impaired Physical Mobility r/t stiffness and pain in hands A.M.B. stiffness and pain in the hands
>
> *Better:* Impaired Physical Mobility r/t stiffness and pain in hands 2° arthritic joint changes
>
> *Best:* Impaired Physical Mobility: decreased fine motor skills r/t stiffness and pain in hands 2° arthritic joint changes
>
> *Format:* *General Problem: (Specific descriptor) r/t etiology*

Pain is another label that often needs an added third-part descriptor. Even when considered with its etiology and definition, it does not always fully specify the client's problem. In the following example, you cannot tell how severe the pain is or where it is located. In the *Better* example, words are added to make the diagnosis thoroughly descriptive and specific to the client. Notice that in the *Better* example, the NANDA-I label describes the general area of the problem, and the descriptor describes the specific type of problem in that area.

EXAMPLE: Acute Pain related to fear of addiction to narcotics

> *Better:* Acute Pain: Severe headache r/t fear of addiction to narcotics

You may see this diagnosis written as "Pain r/t severe headache." However, headache is a *type* of pain, not the *cause* of pain; the second part of the statement is supposed to consist of etiological factors, not problems. Furthermore, although this statement clarifies the location and severity of the pain, it does not indicate the cause.

Risk for Infection and Interrupted Family Processes are other labels that may need a third part added to make them more specific. Risk for Infection can often be made more specific by adding *secondary to*. However, in the following example, the first statement does not indicate whether the client is at risk for systemic infection or a localized infection of a wound or incision.

EXAMPLE: Risk for Infection r/t susceptibility to pathogens 2° compromised immune system

> *Better:* Risk for Infection: Systemic r/t susceptibility to pathogens 2° compromised immune system, or
>
> Risk for Infection: Abdominal Incision r/t susceptibility to pathogens 2° compromised immune system

Remember that the diagnostic statement must thoroughly and specifically describe the problem and its causes (or risk factors). This is what dictates your format. In order to be fully descriptive, you will use secondary to, the P.E.S. format, qualifying words, a third-part descriptor, or a combination of these as needed.

One-Part Statements

A few NANDA-I labels are so specific that you do not need an etiology in the diagnostic statement. Most nurses write *wellness diagnoses* (e.g., Effective Breastfeeding, Readiness for Enhanced Spiritual Well-Being) without etiologies. The following NANDA-I syndrome diagnoses are also written without an etiology (a syndrome diagnosis is actually a collection of several nursing diagnoses grouped under one label):

Disuse Syndrome

Impaired Environmental
   Interpretation Syndrome

Post-Trauma Syndrome

Rape-Trauma Syndrome

Relocation Stress Syndrome

In addition, for the following labels it is difficult to think of an etiology other than a medical diagnosis, or if an etiology is written, it is somewhat redundant:

Death Anxiety

Decreased Cardiac Output

Defensive Coping

Latex Allergy Response

Unilateral Neglect

Death Anxiety, for instance is fully described by its definition, which states that it is fear related to dying. In a statement such as "Death Anxiety r/t fear of dying," the etiology adds nothing to the understanding of the problem.

See Table 5–4 for a summary of formats used for actual nursing diagnoses.

Potential (Risk) Nursing Diagnoses

A *potential (risk)* nursing diagnosis is one that is likely to develop if you do not intervene to prevent it. It is diagnosed by the presence of risk factors rather than defining characteristics.

TABLE 5–4 Formats for Actual Nursing Diagnoses

Basic Two-Part Statement	Problem r/t etiology
Two-Part Statement with P.E.S. Format	Problem r/t etiology A.M.B. symptoms
Three-Part Statement ("Secondary to")	Problem r/t etiology 2° pathophysiology
Four-Part Statement	General problem: Specific description r/t etiology 2° pathophysiology
Unknown Etiology	Problem r/t unknown etiology
Complex Etiology	Problem r/t complex factors

Risk nursing diagnoses have the same *Problem + Etiology* format as actual diagnoses—the client's risk factors form the etiology.

> **EXAMPLE:** Risk for Impaired Skin Integrity (pressure sores) *r/t immobility 2° casts and traction*

Risk diagnoses may have most of the previously mentioned variations in format (e.g., one-part statement, three-part statement, multiple etiology). Of course, the P.E.S. format cannot be used because the patient does not have any defining characteristics of the diagnosis—if signs and symptoms are present, the diagnosis is actual, not risk.

Possible Nursing Diagnoses

When you do not have enough data to confirm a diagnosis that you suspect is present or when you can confirm the problem but not the etiology, write a *possible* nursing diagnosis. The word *possible* can be used in either the problem or the etiology. As in other kinds of diagnoses, the etiology may be multiple, complex, or unknown.

> **EXAMPLES:** *Possible Situational Low Self-Esteem* related to loss of job and rejection by family.
>
> Disturbed Thought Processes *possibly related to unfamiliar surroundings*
> *Possible Low Self-Esteem* related to unknown etiology

Use *r/t unknown etiology* if you do not know the etiology; use *possibly r/t* if you suspect but cannot confirm the etiology. Remember, though, that etiologies are inferred, so you can never be *absolutely* certain an etiology is correct.

Wellness Diagnoses (Format)

New NANDA-I wellness labels (Box 5–2) are preceded by the phrase *Readiness for Enhanced* and will be one-part statements (e.g., *Readiness for Enhanced* Parenting). However, some wellness labels still have different one-part formats (e.g., *Effective* Breastfeeding and *Health-seeking Behaviors*).

Collaborative Problems

As a rule, you will not write an etiology for a collaborative problem. Collaborative problems are complications of a disease, test, or treatment that nurses cannot treat independently. Nurses focus mainly on monitoring and preventing such problems. The etiologies of collaborative problems are likely to be diseases, treatments, or pathologies. Notice in the following example that if you use the usual *Problem + Etiology* format, the etiology suggests the need for medical interventions.

> **EXAMPLE:** (Incorrect) Potential for Increased Intracranial Pressure r/t head injury.

The problem statement should include both the possible complication for which you are monitoring and the disease, treatment, or other factors that produce it. In the

BOX 5–2

WELLNESS DIAGNOSES, NANDA INTERNATIONAL

Effective Breastfeeding

Effective Therapeutic Regimen
   Management

Readiness for Enhanced
   Communication

Readiness for Enhanced Community
   Coping

Readiness for Enhanced Coping

Readiness for Enhanced Family Coping

Readiness for Enhanced Family
   Processes

Readiness for Enhanced Fluid Balance

Readiness for Enhanced Knowledge
   (specify)

Readiness for Enhanced Nutrition

Readiness for Enhanced Organized
   Infant Behavior

Readiness for Enhanced Parenting

Readiness for Enhanced Religiosity

Readiness for Enhanced Self-Concept

Readiness for Enhanced Sleep

Readiness for Enhanced Spiritual
   Well-Being

Effective Therapeutic Regimen
   Management

Readiness for Enhanced Urinary
   Elimination

Source: NANDA International. (2009). *NANDA International nursing diagnoses definitions and classification 2009–2011.* Ames, IA: Wiley-Blackwell

following example, you would monitor for signs and symptoms of increased intracranial pressure that might result from the patient's head injury.

EXAMPLE: Potential Complication of Head Injury: Increased Intracranial Pressure.

Sometimes you will be monitoring for a group of complications associated with a disease or pathology. In that case, state the disease and follow it with a list of the complications.

EXAMPLE: Potential Complications of Pregnancy-Induced Hypertension:

Seizures	Premature labor
Fetal distress	Central nervous system (CNS) hemorrhage
Pulmonary edema	Hepatic or renal failure

You cannot use the P.E.S. format for collaborative diagnoses because they are usually potential problems. The patient does not have the signs and symptoms—you are monitoring to see if they occur. However, for some collaborative problems, an etiology can be helpful in planning interventions; for example, the complication may be caused by something more specific than a disease process. While you are a student, you should write the etiology, as in the following examples, (a) when it clarifies your statement, (b) when it can be concisely stated, or (c) when it helps to suggest nursing actions.

EXAMPLE:

Disease/Situation	*Complication*	*r/t*	*Etiology*

↓   ↓   ↓

Potential complication of *childbirth:*	Hemorrhage	r/t	1. uterine atony 2. retained placental fragments 3. bladder distention

↓   ↓   ↓

Potential complication of *diuretic therapy*	Arrhythmias	r/t	low serum potassium

See Table 5–5 for a summary of formats to use for actual, potential, possible, and wellness diagnoses, as well as for collaborative problems.

Relationship of Nursing Diagnoses to Outcomes and Nursing Orders

The first part of the diagnostic statement (the problem) states what needs to change; thus, it determines the patient outcomes needed to measure this change. In the following example, the goal would be to relieve the anxiety. This suggests a need to observe for symptoms such as rapid speech and shakiness.

EXAMPLE: Anxiety r/t lack of knowledge of scheduled venogram

↓

Goals (Outcomes)

The second part of the diagnostic statement (the etiology) identifies factors contributing to the actual problem or the risk factors for a risk problem. In many cases, the etiology directs the choice of nursing interventions. In the preceding example, the

TABLE 5–5   Formats for Various Problem Statuses

Actual Nursing Diagnosis	Problem r/t etiology
Potential Nursing Diagnosis	Risk for problem r/t risk factors
Possible Nursing Diagnosis	Possible problem r/t actual (or possible) etiology
Wellness Nursing Diagnosis	■ Readiness for enhanced (NANDA label) ■ Effective (label)
Collaborative Problem	Potential complication of disease or treatment: (Specify complication)

etiology suggests a nursing order for patient teaching. In addition to teaching the patient about the venogram, however, the nurse would probably intervene more directly to relieve the anxiety—for instance, by helping the patient to recognize and express his anxiety. As you can see, nursing interventions can be suggested by either part of the diagnostic statement.

EXAMPLE: Anxiety r/t lack of knowledge of scheduled venogram

$$\downarrow \qquad \downarrow$$

**Nursing   Nursing
Orders   Orders**

A few other problem labels also suggest particular nursing interventions regardless of the cause of the problem, for example: Decisional Conflict, Fear, Hopelessness, Ineffective Denial, and Risk for Self-Directed, or Other-Directed, Violence.

As the NANDA-I labels become more specific, you will probably discover more instances in which the etiology cannot be treated by independent nursing actions, so the nursing orders will flow from the problem rather than from the etiology. In the following example, the nurse cannot treat a spinal cord lesion. Both the outcome and nursing orders are suggested by "Reflex Incontinence."

EXAMPLE: Reflex Incontinence   r/t   spinal cord lesion

Outcomes and Nursing Orders

When possible, though, you should rewrite the etiology so that it will provide direction for nursing intervention. Usually this means replacing a disease or medical condition with a principle or pathophysiology. This is not necessary for experienced nurses.

EXAMPLE: Risk for Infection r/t *surgical incision*

Rewritten: Risk for Infection r/t portal of entry for pathogens 2° surgical incision

In every case, the nurse should be able to prescribe definitive prevention and treatment for at least one side of the nursing diagnosis.

?

5-4 WHAT DO YOU KNOW?

1. Which part of the diagnostic statement determines the patient outcomes needed to measure change in the problem status?
2. (True or false) Interventions are sometimes suggested by the problem label instead of the etiology.

See answer to #5-4 What Do You Know? in Appendix A.

Thinking Critically about the Content of Diagnostic Statements

In addition to using the correct format for your diagnostic statements, you must consider the quality of their content—reflect on their meaning. After writing your diagnoses, judge them against the following criteria, which are based on the "standards of reasoning" set forth in preceding chapters. If you need to review these standards, refer to Chapter 2 and Table 4–8.

1. *(Standard: Clarity)* **The statement is stated clearly and gives a clear picture of the patient's situation.** It uses terminology generally understood by other professionals and limits jargon and abbreviations.

    EXAMPLE:

    Incorrect: Toileting *SCD* r/t inability to get *OOB w/o help*
    Correct: Toileting *Self-Care Deficit* r/t inability to get *out of bed without help*

2. *(Standard: Clarity)* **The statement is concise**. Wordy statements are often unclear. Using NANDA-I labels helps to keep the problem statement brief.
    a. If etiological factors are long and complicated, use "r/t complex etiology."
    b. If P.E.S. format produces a long statement, list the signs and symptoms under the diagnostic statement.

    EXAMPLE: Chronic Low Self-Esteem related to long-standing feelings of failure aggravated by recently being rejected by her husband as manifested by being hypersensitive to criticism, stating, "I don't know if I can manage by myself," rejecting positive feedback, and not making eye contact.

    Better: Chronic Low Self-Esteem r/t complex factors, A.M.B.
    S—"I don't know if I can manage by myself."
    O—Hypersensitive to criticism, rejects positive feedback, no eye contact

3. *(Standard: Accuracy)* **The statement is accurate and valid**. Diagnostic statements should meet the following criteria:
    - Patient signs and symptoms match NANDA-I defining characteristics.
    - For potential problems, patient risk factors match NANDA-I risk factors.
    - The cue cluster fits the NANDA-I label definition.
    - The patient has validated the diagnosis.

4. *(Standard: Precision)* **The statement is descriptive and specific.** The statement should fully describe the client's problem. Meet this criterion even if it makes the statement longer than you would like. The NANDA-I labels are always made more specific by:
    a. Knowledge of the label definition (If you know the definition, you may realize the label is more precise than you thought.)
    b. Adding the etiology to make the complete problem statement
    c. Adding the patient's defining characteristics (P.E.S. format)

If the statement still is not descriptive enough, make it more specific by:

d. Adding qualifying words (e.g., *mild, moderate, intermittent*)

e. Adding "secondary to" in the etiology

f. Adding a third part (a colon and more specific problem)

EXAMPLE: Acute Pain r/t fear of addiction to narcotics

Better: Acute Pain: *Severe Headache* r/t fear of addiction to narcotics

5. **(Standard: Depth) The statement uses legally advisable language.** Ask yourself, "What are some of the complexities of this diagnosis" (e.g., legal implications)? The statement should not affix blame or refer negatively to aspects of patient care.

   EXAMPLE:

   Incorrect: Impaired Skin Integrity: Pressure Sores *r/t not being turned frequently enough*
   Correct: Impaired Skin Integrity: Pressure Sores r/*t inability to turn self*

6. **(Standards: Depth, Breadth) The complete list of nursing diagnoses and collaborative problems reflects the client's overall health status.** Although collaborative problems are not always written on the plan of care, the master problem list for the patient should include all the patient's collaborative problems, as well as the actual, risk, and possible nursing diagnoses and client strengths. A complete list will enable you to plan all the nursing care the patient requires.

7. **(Standard: Breadth) The statement uses nonjudgmental language.** Remember to ask, "Do I have preconceived notions or values that affect how I see the problem?"

   EXAMPLE:

   Incorrect: Risk for Injury: Falls *r/t poor housekeeping*
   Better: Risk for Injury: Falls *r/t cluttered floors*

8. **(Standard: Logic) Cause and effect are correctly stated.** That is, the etiology "causes" the problem, or puts the client at risk for the problem.

   EXAMPLE:

   Correct: Impaired Oral Mucous Membrane r/t fluid volume deficit A.M.B. xerostomia and oral lesions

   Incorrect: Deficient Fluid Volume r/t altered oral mucous membrane A.M.B. xerostomia and oral lesions

   To check this logic, insert the parts of your statement in this sentence format (you are reading your diagnosis backward, actually):

   "*(Etiology)* causes *(Problem)*"

   EXAMPLE: Dysfunctional Grieving r/t inability to accept death of spouse.

   Read backward:

Inability to accept death of spouse *causes* Dysfunctional Grieving

   ↑ ↑ ↑

(Etiology)	*causes*	*(Problem)*

EXAMPLE: Risk for infection r/t interruption of body's first line of defense 2° abdominal incision.

Read backward:

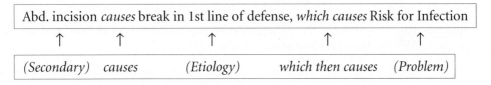

9. *(Standard: Logic)* **The problem side of the statement contains only one diagnostic label.**

   EXAMPLE:

Incorrect	*Correct*
Risk for Deficient Fluid Volume and Constipation r/t inadequate fluid intake	Constipation r/t inadequate fluid intake Risk for Deficient Fluid Volume r/t inadequate intake of fluid

10. *(Standard: Logic)* **The etiology is not merely a rewording of the problem.**

    EXAMPLE:

Incorrect	*Correct*
Chronic Pain r/t headache	Chronic Pain (Headache) r/t unknown etiology

11. *(Standard: Logic)* **At least one side of the statement provides direction for nursing actions.** If you cannot prescribe the interventions to change either the problem or the etiology, then you should reevaluate the statement. Perhaps what you have identified as the problem is actually the stimulus for other problem responses. In the following example, the nurse cannot change what was first identified as a "hearing problem." However, the hearing problem produced a social interaction problem, which the nurse can address.

    EXAMPLE:

    Incorrect: Disturbed Sensory/Perceptual (Auditory) r/t progressive hearing loss 2° nerve degeneration

    Correct: Impaired Social Interaction r/t embarrassment at being unable to follow conversations because of progressive hearing loss 2° nerve degeneration

    a. Nursing diagnoses suggest independent nursing actions to treat or prevent.
    b. Collaborative problems suggest independent nursing actions to detect and prevent.

12. **The statement does not include any of the errors described in Table 4–2 (i.e., stating a patient need; a nursing goal or action; or medical test, equipment, or treatment rather than a problematic human response).**

Wellness Diagnoses

Wellness diagnoses are especially useful for healthy clients, such as schoolchildren or new parents, who require teaching for health promotion, disease prevention, and personal growth. Following is the NANDA-I definition of wellness diagnoses.

> **Wellness diagnoses** "describe human responses to levels of wellness in an individual, family, or community that have a readiness for enhancement" (2009 p. 26).

All new wellness diagnoses are preceded by the phrase *Readiness for Enhanced* and are one-part statements. Box 5–2 contains the wellness labels that are included in the NANDA-I taxonomy. Others may be created by preceding the diagnostic concept with "Readiness for Enhanced."

The Omaha System for classification in community health nursing (see Table 5–1) deals with wellness diagnoses by using modifiers. For each diagnosis used, the nurse must describe the status as "health promotion, potential, or actual." When no signs, symptoms, or risk factors are present, the nurse identifies a health promotion status (e.g., Emotional stability: Health promotion).

Wellness diagnoses provide a clear focus for planning interventions without indicating that a problem exists. For some nurses, health promotion is their primary role. However, even patients with many health problems may have health promotion needs or areas of wellness. For example, you might use a wellness diagnosis for the following:

- Chronically ill clients in long-term care settings for whom you wish to improve functioning and quality of life by providing physical exercise to improve strength and flexibility
- Acute-care patients in ambulatory care settings, such as clinics and emergency departments, for whom your secondary role would be to prevent further problems and enhance well-being, perhaps by referring patients to preventive or health promotion services

Situations where you might use a wellness diagnosis include patients who are gaining new information, learning new skills, improving physical functional status, weaning from ventilators, acquiring new roles, achieving maturational or developmental tasks, or experiencing wound healing.

Describing healthy states for acutely ill hospitalized patients presents some difficulties. Hospitalized patients often have many nursing diagnoses and collaborative problems. From a practical standpoint, you can address only a limited number of problems during a workday, so you will usually address the high-priority diagnoses first. Because wellness diagnoses are usually lower in priority, the acute-care nurse may never find the time to carry out the health-promotion interventions that a wellness diagnosis suggests. For hospitalized patients, it may be better to describe healthy responses by identifying strengths to use in planning interventions for the problems you identify. Concluding that a set of cues represents "no problem" does not necessarily mean you need to write a wellness diagnosis for that set. It is quite acceptable to identify health responses as strengths rather than writing them as wellness diagnoses, especially in short-term situations. Some examples of strengths include communicates adequately in dominant language, stable family situation, and adequate financial support. For a discussion of patient strengths, see "Step 8: Identify Patient and Family Strengths" in Chapter 4.

Spiritual Diagnoses

Spirituality both affects and is affected by a person's health status. Thus, from a holistic perspective, nurses need to be able to describe problems of spirituality. Six NANDA-I labels that directly relate to spiritual status are Spiritual Distress, Readiness for Enhanced Spiritual Well-being, Risk for Spiritual Distress, Impaired Religiosity, Risk for Impaired Religiosity, and Readiness for Enhanced Religiosity. The following NANDA-I diagnoses may also be related to a client's spiritual status, either as symptoms or causes of a spiritual problem:

Complicated Grieving	Ineffective Denial
Death Anxiety	Ineffective Individual or Family Coping
Decisional Conflict	Powerlessness
Fear	Chronic Low Self-Esteem
Hopelessness	Disturbed Sleep Pattern

If the patient does not have the defining characteristics for these diagnoses, you may be able to use one of the following terms to describe the patient's spiritual status. O'Brien (1982, p. 81) further categorizes spiritual distress as follows:

- *Spiritual pain*: Difficulty accepting the loss of a loved one or intense physical or emotional suffering
- *Spiritual alienation*: Separation from religious or faith community
- *Spiritual anxiety*: Challenge to beliefs and value systems (e.g., by moral implications of therapy, such as abortion or blood transfusion)
- *Spiritual guilt*: Failure to abide by religious rules
- *Spiritual anger*: Difficulty accepting illness, loss, or suffering
- *Spiritual loss*: Difficulty finding comfort in religion
- *Spiritual despair*: Feeling that no one cares

Others describe spiritual problems on a continuum from mild to severe:

- *Spiritual concerns*—In which the patient shows mild anxiety and discouragement and expresses concerns about relationships with God
- *Spiritual distress*—In which anxiety is more severe; the patient cries, expresses guilt; feels anger toward staff, family, or higher power; and experiences loss of meaning or purpose in life
- *Spiritual despair*—In which patient loses hope and spiritual belief, is severely depressed, refuses to participate in treatment, does not communicate with family, and wishes to die (Sumner, 1998)

Spiritual Distress may be the etiology of the preceding problems, and others as well. For example:

Chronic Low Self-Esteem r/t *Spiritual Distress* 2° failure to live according to the principles of one's religion

Disturbed Sleep-Pattern r/t *Spiritual Distress*

Family and Home Health Diagnoses

Efforts are being made to incorporate family diagnoses into the NANDA-I classification system. The labels in Box 5–3 could be used to describe family health status, and others could be adapted by adding "family" (e.g., Family Decisional Conflict, Family Social Isolation). Home health nurses use both individual and family diagnoses. Box 5–4 shows the labels used most often by home healthcare nurses in a 1997 study. Because Medicare and other insurers consider client education to be a reimbursable skill, it is especially important to include a Deficient Knowledge diagnosis in a home health plan of care.

Take-away point: The nursing diagnoses in the CCC system (See Table 5–1) are appropriate for individuals, families, or communities.

The CCC uses the NANDA-I definition of nursing diagnosis and many of its diagnoses were adapted from NANDA-I labels (Saba, 2006).

BOX 5–3

NANDA INTERNATIONAL FAMILY DIAGNOSES

Effective Breastfeeding
Interrupted Breastfeeding
Ineffective Breastfeeding
Caregiver Role Strain (Actual and Risk for)
Compromised Family Coping
Disabled Family Coping
Readiness for Enhanced Family Coping
Dysfunctional Family Processes
Interrupted Family Processes

Readiness for Enhanced Family Processes
Impaired Home Maintenance
Impaired Parenting (Actual and Risk for)
Readiness for Enhanced Parenting
Risk for Impaired Attachment
Parental Role Conflict
Impaired Social Interaction
Ineffective Therapeutic Regimen Management

Source: NANDA International. (2009). *NANDA International nursing diagnoses definitions and classification 2009–2011.* Ames, IA: Wiley-Blackwell

FREQUENTLY USED HOME HEALTH DIAGNOSES

A survey of 96 home healthcare nurses found the following diagnoses were rated as high frequency, high treatment priority. They represent four diagnostic areas: health management, activity, nutrition, and cognitive/perceptual patterns. The highest-ranked label was Knowledge Deficit (now called Deficient Knowledge).

Knowledge Deficit	Pain
Self-Care Deficit: Bathing/Hygiene	Nutritional Deficit (Specify)
Self-Care Deficit: Dressing/Grooming	Risk for Injury
Risk for Infection	Impaired Mobility
Risk for Impaired Skin Integrity	Activity Intolerance
Impaired Skin Integrity	Decreased Cardiac Output

Source: From Gordon, M., & Butler-Schmidt, B. (1997). High frequency–high treatment priority nursing diagnoses in home health care nursing. In M. J. Rantz & P. LeMone (Eds.), *Classification of nursing diagnoses: Proceedings of the Twelfth Conference, North American Nursing Diagnosis Association*. Glendale, CA: CINAHL Information Systems.

Community Health Diagnoses

Community health nurses need labels to describe the health status of individuals, families, groups (e.g., all pregnant adolescents in the community), and entire communities. For example, a community may have high levels of air pollution or widespread unemployment, both of which have implications for the health of its citizens. Efforts are being made to incorporate community diagnoses into the NANDA-I classification system. Currently, the following are the only NANDA-I labels to describe the health status of communities:

Ineffective Community Coping

Readiness for Enhanced Community Coping

Ineffective Community Management of Therapeutic Regimen

Lesh (1997) reported that public health nurses most frequently used the following 10 nursing diagnoses:

Inadequate Income

Knowledge Deficit

Health Management Deficit

Altered Parenting

Altered Health Maintenance

Potential for Altered Parenting

Potential Noncompliance

TABLE 5–6 The Omaha System Domains and Problems

Domains	Problem Labels
Environmental	Income, neighborhood or workplace safety, residence, sanitation
Psychosocial	Abuse, caretaking or parenting, communication with community resources, grief, growth and development, interpersonal relationship, mental health, neglect, role change, sexuality, social contact, spirituality
Physiological	Bowel function, circulation, cognition, communicable or infectious condition, consciousness, digestion or hydration, hearing, neuromusculoskeletal function, oral health, pain, pregnancy, postpartum, reproductive function, respiration, skin, speech and language, urinary function, vision
Health-Related Behaviors	Family planning, healthcare supervision, medication regimen, nutrition, personal care, physical activity, sleep and rest patterns, substance use

Source: The Omaha System (2009, updated). Problem classification scheme. Domains and problems of the problem classification system. Available at http://www.omahasystem.org/problemclassificationscheme.html and Martin, K. S. (2005). *The Omaha System: A key to practice, documentation, and management*, (2nd ed.). New York: Elsevier.

Impaired Home Maintenance Management

Support System Deficit

Compliance with Immunization Regulations

Take-away point: The Omaha System was developed by community health nurses (see Table 5–1) for use in settings such as home care, public health, school health, and prisons.

See Table 5–6 for domains and problem labels. There are two sets of modifiers that the nurse must use with each diagnosis:

1. Health promotion, Potential deficit, Deficit
2. Family, Individual

So, for example, a family diagnosis might read "*Deficit* in *Family* Income." Even with this system, there are no terms to describe the health status of communities or groups. It has been suggested that the term *Group* should be added to the modifiers (Martin, 2005). A example of a group diagnosis, then, might be "*Deficit* in *Group* (shelter for the homeless) Income."

Issues Associated with the NANDA-I Classification

There are various criticisms of the NANDA-I taxonomy and of individual labels: They are unclear, too abstract (e.g., Impaired Parenting), too medical (e.g., Decreased Cardiac Output), not understood by others, and so on. These problems probably will be corrected as the system evolves and diagnoses are refined. Meanwhile, if you disagree with a diagnostic label, you do not have to use it, or you can add words to make it more specific and clear. You should not reject the idea of standardized diagnostic language just because of a few awkward diagnoses. The system is evolving, as do all classification systems. In the medical diagnosis taxonomy, only in recent years was *toxemia of pregnancy* changed to *preeclampsia/eclampsia*, and only recently has *AIDS* become a medical diagnosis. Both NANDA-I and NDEC continue working to test, refine, and clarify the diagnoses and the classification structure.

Unrealistic Expectations

The more serious issues involve the whole system rather than individual diagnoses. We may be expecting too much from nursing diagnosis in terms of what it can do for the profession and for patients. Does it truly define nursing? If so, will that make any difference in the long run? Nursing is changing rapidly and being shaped by events outside the profession (e.g., technology, the economy, demographic changes). We must remember that nursing diagnosis is simply an important part of nursing. Do not expect it to singlehandedly remedy such problems as lack of autonomy and third-party payment; other (political) measures will be necessary.

Effect on Holistic Perspective

Some believe that using a list of ready-made labels causes nurses to miss creative inferences they would otherwise make. Others believe that a step-by-step, scientific approach inhibits intuitive problem solving and prevents a holistic perspective. Certainly, we have all seen examples of the dehumanizing effects of science and technology. However, we can use our science in a humanistic manner. According to Kritek, "Naming our phenomena of concern does not narrow our perception of clients, but broadens it. . . . When a child weeps, you work hard to discover why. You try to solve the problem. But of course, you always comfort the entire child, not just the problem. Nursing will retain its fidelity to holism if it chooses to do so" (1985, p. 396). Using a common language and logical thinking should actually help nurses to identify and communicate unique aspects of patients that they might otherwise miss.

Ethical Considerations

Neither the diagnostic process nor diagnostic statements are value free. A nurse's values may lead him to emphasize or ignore certain data during assessment, resulting in inaccurate or missed diagnoses. Because nursing diagnoses direct the way others view and relate to the patient, as well as the nursing care that is given, inaccurate diagnoses mean that the most effective interventions may not be selected.

EXAMPLE: A nurse's highest patient-care value is safety. Autonomy has never been a big issue in his life. When he cares for an elderly client, he diagnoses Risk for Injury r/t Disturbed Thought Processes 2° aging A.M.B. confusion and disorientation. He does not take into account that confusion is a side effect of one of the client's medications. Seeing this diagnosis, other nurses begin to perceive the client as needing more supervision than he actually does. Gradually, the client loses his autonomy and becomes more dependent.

Even if it were possible for the *diagnostic process* to be value neutral, the *phrasing* of a diagnostic statement can have ethical implications. A diagnosis stated in value-laden terms may influence how other caregivers treat the patient. The etiology is the part of the diagnosis most likely to harbor negative or judgmental terms because it is often complex and not stated in standardized language.

EXAMPLE: Compromised Family Coping r/t *sexual promiscuity of the mother*

Anxiety r/t *unrealistic expectations of others*

The problem side of the statement can also create difficulty because the NANDA-I diagnostic labels are not entirely value free. For example, *Noncompliance* may imply that the patient is not cooperating as he "should"; this can negatively affect nurses' attitudes toward the patient (Keeling et al, 1993). You may be able to remove some of the stigma from such problem labels by writing the etiology carefully, as in the following: "Noncompliance with clinic appointments r/t inability to find reliable transportation for long trip." Geissler (1991) suggests *Nonadherence* as a less negative term than *Noncompliance.*

Some NANDA-I labels are not negative in and of themselves but can be perceived as negative by nurses because of their own values. *Anxiety* carries a negative connotation for those who value strength and self-control; they may see an "anxious" patient as weak or unworthy of attention. *Deficient Knowledge* may imply lack of ability or lack of motivation to learn, either of which could evoke a negative reaction from caregivers who place a high value on learning.

Remember that it is the nurse, not the diagnostic statement, who determines the quality and the morality of a patient's care. Some nurses were surely making value judgments about their patients long before nursing diagnoses existed. As a part of their role, nurses interpret patient experiences, regardless of whether these interpretations are named as nursing diagnoses, and like all interpretations, nursing judgments are influenced by values. Many judgments go unstated as assumptions and are never examined. By writing a diagnostic statement, the nurse's judgment at least becomes open and explicit and is available for examination by the nurse and by others.

Even though it is impossible to be value neutral, diagnosing does not need to be unethical. To diagnose in an ethical manner, you must be aware of your values and their influence on the diagnostic process. You must realize the effect of your nursing diagnoses on other caregivers and try to phrase them in neutral, nonjudgmental language. And finally, you should validate your nursing diagnoses with the patient, to be sure that in the *patient's* judgment, the cue cluster represents a *problem* (dysfunction, impairment) and not just a difference in perspectives and values. The ill person is vulnerable and in a position of inequality with healthcare providers, so you need to promote a relationship in which the patient feels free to voice disagreement.

Cultural Considerations

Many nurses (e.g., Geissler, 1992; Leininger, 1990) believe that NANDA-I nursing diagnoses are not culturally sensitive. This characteristic can lead to misdiagnosis of problems and etiologies. Remember that diagnoses represent responses that clients and families find problematic from *their* perspective, cultural or otherwise. Undoubtedly, all problems and etiologies are influenced by cultural factors. However, it is especially easy to see how the following labels would be interpreted differently from different cultural perspectives:

Impaired Health Maintenance	Imbalanced Nutrition
Ineffective Role Performance	Anxiety
Decisional Conflict	Effective/Ineffective Breastfeeding
Impaired Social Interaction	Impaired Verbal Communication
Ineffective Denial	Disabled Family Coping
Ineffective Coping	Pain

5-3 THINK & REFLECT!

In Culture A, pain is considered a punishment for sins, so the person is expected to tolerate pain without complaint in order to make atonement. In Culture B, expressions of pain elicit attention and sympathy. Suppose you are caring for a client with a fractured arm. He is holding his arm, pacing the floor, cursing, and complaining loudly of unbearable pain.

- If you are from Culture A, what would be your most likely interpretation of these cues?
- If you are from Culture B, what would be your most likely interpretation?
- If you and the client are both from Culture A, would your interpretation be accurate?
- If you are from Culture A and the client is from Culture B, would your interpretation be accurate?

See suggested responses to #5-3 Think & Reflect! in Appendix A.

Recording Nursing Diagnoses

After validating and labeling the nursing diagnoses, you will write them in priority order in the appropriate documents (or computer): either the client's chart or the care plan. Some documentation systems include a multidisciplinary problem list at the front of the client record (chart). In many agencies, the care plan becomes a part of the client's permanent record on dismissal, so diagnoses should be written in ink. When a diagnosis is resolved or changed, you can draw a single line through it or mark over it with a highlighter pen. Some care plans include a space beside the diagnosis to write the date the diagnosis is resolved or discontinued. Refer to Box 5–1 for ANA standards for documenting nursing diagnoses.

Prioritizing Diagnoses

Prioritizing is sometimes considered a part of the planning phase of the nursing process, but if the diagnoses are to be recorded in priority order, then prioritizing must occur in the diagnosis phase. Priorities are assigned on the basis of the nurse's judgment and the client's preferences. You can rank the diagnoses from highest to lowest priority (1, 2, 3, etc.), or you can assign each problem a high, medium, or low priority. Prioritizing problems helps to ensure that care is given first for the more important problems. This does not necessarily mean that one problem must be resolved before you address another.

> **EXAMPLE:** Bathing Self-Care Deficit might be a long-term problem for a patient. This does not mean you should wait until the patient can bathe himself before addressing the next highest priority, Risk for Constipation.

You should also consider risk problems when setting priorities. It is often as important to prevent a problem as it is to treat an actual one.

> **EXAMPLE:** For a poorly nourished, immobile patient, Risk for Impaired Skin Integrity is of higher priority than actual Deficient Diversional Activity.

Preservation of Life

If you use preservation of life as a criterion, you would rate the client's diagnoses based on the amount of threat they pose to the client's life. Life-threatening problems would take priority over those that cause pain or discomfort. A **high-priority problem** is one that is life threatening, such as severe fluid and electrolyte loss or respiratory obstruction. A **medium-priority problem** does not directly threaten life, but it may produce destructive physical or emotional changes (e.g., Rape-Trauma Syndrome). A **low-priority problem** is one that arises from normal developmental needs or requires only minimal supportive nursing intervention (e.g., Ineffective Sexuality Patterns related to deficient knowledge). After assigning high, medium, and low priorities, you can rank the diagnoses from most to least important.

EXAMPLE:

Rank	Diagnosis	Priority
1	Deficient Fluid Volume related to vomiting	Medium
2	Disturbed Sleep Pattern . . .	Low
3	Deficient Diversional Activity . . .	Low

Maslow's Hierarchy

Maslow's Hierarchy of Human Needs also provides a good framework for prioritizing nursing diagnoses. Recall from Chapter 3 that in Maslow's model, there are five levels of human needs. Starting with the most basic (highest priority) need, they are physiologic, safety and security, social, esteem, and self-actualization. As a rule, the more basic needs must be met before the client can deal with the higher needs.

Kalish (1983) has made Maslow's system even more useful by dividing the physiological needs into survival and stimulation needs. Survival needs are the most basic; only when they are satisfied can the client be concerned about higher level needs. When survival needs are met, the client tries to meet stimulation needs before moving up the hierarchy to safety, social, and other higher-level needs. Kalish's division of physiological needs includes the following:

Survival needs: Food, air, water, temperature, elimination, rest, pain avoidance

Stimulation needs: Sex, activity, exploration, manipulation, novelty

In this framework, diagnoses involving survival needs have priority over those involving stimulation needs.

EXAMPLE: The following diagnoses are ranked from highest to lowest priority:

Need	*Nursing Diagnosis*
Survival	Imbalanced Nutrition: Less than Body Requirements related to fatigue
Stimulation	Deficient Diversional Activity related to infectious disease isolation
Esteem	Chronic Low Self-Esteem related to inability to perform role functions

---

5-5 WHAT DO YOU KNOW?

1. Using preservation of life as a criterion, state whether the following are high, medium, or low priority diagnoses. Those that:
   a. Are life threatening
   b. Are concerned with developmental needs and need minimal nurse support
   c. Would bring about destructive physical or emotional changes
2. List the Maslow/Kalish needs in order from lowest (survival) to highest.

See answer to #5-5 What Do You Know? in Appendix A.

Patient Preference

Consider patient preference as much as possible when setting priorities. Give high priority to the problems the patient feels are important as long as this does not interfere with survival needs or medical treatments. Because she is exhausted after delivery, a new mother's first priority may be to sleep. However, you must observe her closely for signs of postpartum hemorrhage, so you cannot safely follow her priorities in this situation. If you explain your priorities, you may be able to persuade the patient to agree with them.

Attending to problems that are high priorities for the patient increases the likelihood that they will be successfully resolved: patients will cooperate most enthusiastically to solve problems they consider important. As in the following example, patients may not be motivated to address other problems until their main concerns are dealt with.

EXAMPLE: Pat Sams is an 18-year-old woman who has just given birth to her first baby. The nurse knows she must teach Ms. Sams how to bathe her infant before she is dismissed—within 24 hours after delivery. The nurse has given highest priority to Ms. Sams's Deficient Knowledge diagnosis. However, Ms. Sams finds it difficult to concentrate on the bath demonstration because she has a different priority. She is hoping the baby's father will come to visit and has been washing her hair and putting on makeup. She has not heard from him since coming to the hospital, and she is worried he will not want to see her and the baby.

Take-away point: Balance patient preferences with therapeutic and safety needs.

SUMMARY

- Standardized nursing languages are essential for developing and communicating nursing knowledge and practice and for evaluating the cost and quality of nursing care.
- Five standardized nursing languages recognized by the ANA are NANDA-I, NIC, NOC, the CCC, and the Omaha System.

Nursing diagnosis statements:
- Use NANDA-I labels.
- Use the format of Problem related to (r/t) Etiology (or the P.E.S. variation).
- Are varied by one-part statements, use of secondary to, unknown and complex etiologies, and three- and four-part statements.
- Should be descriptive, accurate, and specific using nonjudgmental, legally advisable language.
- Can be used to describe the health responses of individuals, families, or communities.
- Are not value free and require nurses to be aware of their own values and the perceptions of others.
- Have ethical, cultural, and spiritual dimensions.
- May describe wellness states as well as health problems.
- Should be recorded on the care plan in priority order.

Collaborative problems:
- Use the format of Potential Complication of (disease, test, or treatment): (complication).

CRITICAL THINKING AND CLINICAL REASONING: A CASE STUDY

Discuss the case with your peers. Look up unfamiliar terms, medical diagnoses, and treatments as needed. Refer to a nursing diagnosis handbook for information about specific nursing diagnoses.

Situation: Mr. Gomez, a 55-year-old man, visits his primary care provider because of fatigue and a 7-lb weight gain. He has a history of anterior myocardial infarction 1 year ago. Since then, he has not changed his lifestyle. He continues to work at least 60 hours a week, consumes a high-fat diet, and has been unable to stop smoking.

Physical examination reveals labored respirations at 34 breaths/min; crackles (auscultated) in all lung fields; heart rate 130 bpm, with occasional irregularity and an S3 sound noted; blood pressure 184/110 mm Hg; and 3+ pitting edema in lower extremities. He tells his provider, "I'm just working too hard. I just need some more of those water pills you gave me a while back."

Referral is made for home health nursing visits. In preparing a report to the home health agency, the nurse is considering the following nursing diagnoses:

- Ineffective Denial r/t unknown etiology
- Noncompliance r/t lack of knowledge about treatment regimen
- Ineffective Management of Therapeutic Regimen r/t failure to change lifestyle

1. Assume that the defining characteristics for Ineffective Denial are present. Evaluate the etiology of that diagnosis. Based on these data, is it correct? Why or why not?
2. Assume that the defining characteristics for Noncompliance are present. Evaluate the etiology of that diagnosis. Based on these data, is it correct? Why or why not?
3. Assume that the defining characteristics for Ineffective Management of Therapeutic Regimen are present. Evaluate the etiology of that diagnosis. Based on these data, is it correct? Why or why not?
4. Now, make *no* assumptions about the defining characteristics of the problem. Choose the NANDA-I label based on the data presented in the situation. Which of the three best fits Mr. Gomez?
5. Using *only* the problems and etiologies shown in the nurse's three nursing diagnoses, recombine them to make *one* nursing diagnosis for Mr. Gomez. Use this format: *NANDA-I label (specific description of problem) r/t etiology A.M.B. signs and symptoms.*
6. In addition to the psychosocial nursing diagnosis you developed in Item 5, the nurse also diagnoses (a) Fatigue and (b) Potential Complications of Congestive Heart Failure: Fluid Overload and Cardiac Decompensation. Which of these three problems would you give highest priority? Why?
7. Which of these three problems do you think is Mr. Gomez's highest priority? Explain your reasoning.
8. What biases do you have (about anything in this situation) that might affect how you interpret these data?

See suggested responses to Critical Thinking and Clinical Reasoning: A Case Study in Appendix A

Planning: Overview and Outcomes

Introduction

Planning patient care is a responsibility of professional nurses (Box 6–1). This chapter discusses planning as a step of the nursing process, compares various types of planning, and explains how to write individualized patient outcomes. Figure 6–1 presents an overview of the planning phase.

Overview of Planning: Third and Fourth Phases of Nursing Process

In the planning phases (planning outcomes, planning interventions), the nurse, with patient and family input, derives desired outcomes from the diagnostic statements and identifies nursing interventions to achieve those goals. The purpose and end product of the two planning phases is a holistic plan of care tailored to the patient's problems and strengths. The planning steps end when this plan has been made. A *plan* is not always a written, individualized nursing care plan. It may be a mental plan the nurse has for achieving an outcome, or it may be a standardized set of routines (e.g., take vital signs every 4 hours) that meets the needs that certain patients have in common (e.g., all postoperative patients on a unit).

In the planning phases, the nurse engages in the following activities:

1. Deciding which problems need individually developed plans and which can be addressed by critical pathways, standards of care, policies and procedures, and other forms of preplanned, standardized care.

After completing this chapter, you should be able to do the following:

- Describe the nursing activities that occur in the planning phase of the nursing process.
- Explain the relationship between planning and the other phases of the nursing process.
- Discuss the importance of initial, ongoing, and discharge planning.
- Explain how to derive measurable, observable, individualized client goals/outcomes from nursing diagnoses.
- Develop outcomes to address special needs (e.g., wellness, teaching, spiritual).
- Give examples of family and community outcomes.
- Describe three standardized languages for patient outcomes.
- Explain how to use the Nursing Outcomes Classification (NOC).
- Discuss the use of computers in choosing outcomes.
- Use guidelines and critical thinking standards to evaluate the quality of your outcomes and the thinking you used.
- Discuss the ethical, cultural, and legal considerations involved in developing client goals.

BOX 6–1

PROFESSIONAL STANDARDS OF PRACTICE

American Nurses Association Standard 3. Outcomes Identification

The registered nurse identifies expected outcomes for a plan individualized to the patient or the situation.

Competencies

The registered nurse:

1. Involves the patient, family, significant others, and other healthcare providers in formulating expected outcomes when possible and appropriate.
2. Derives culturally appropriate expected outcomes from the diagnoses.
3. Considers associated risks, benefits, costs, current scientific evidence, expected trajectory of the condition, and clinical expertise when formulating expected outcomes.
4. Defines expected outcomes in terms of the patient, patient values, ethical considerations, environment or situation with such consideration as associated risks, benefits and costs, and current scientific evidence.
5. Includes a time estimate for the attainment of expected outcomes.
6. Develops expected outcomes that provide direction for continuity of care.
7. Modifies expected outcomes based on changes in the status of the patient or evaluation of the situation.
8. Documents expected outcomes as measurable goals.

(*NOTE:* There are additional measurement criteria for advanced practice RNs.)

Note: This material is from the draft for public comment (ANA, 2010, in press); its wording may be somewhat changed in the final published version (August 2010). For that version of the ANA standards, visit http://www.nursingworld.org.

Source: Reprinted with permission from American Nurses Association (2010, in press). In *Nursing: Scope and standards of practice* (2nd ed.). (Public Comment draft, January). Silver Spring, MD. Available at http:/nursebooks.org.

---

2. Choosing and adapting standardized, preprinted interventions and plans of care where appropriate. (This activity is explained in detail in Chapter 10, "Creating a Plan of Care.")
3. Choosing and writing individualized outcomes and nursing orders for problems that require nursing attention beyond preplanned, routine care.

Remember that the nursing process phases are interdependent and overlapping. Planning outcomes and planning interventions are no exception. Their effectiveness depends directly on the assessment and diagnosis phases. If assessment data (assessment) are complete and accurate and the diagnostic statements are correct (diagnosis), then the goals and nursing interventions flow logically (planning) and are likely to be effective. In the same way, implementation and evaluation depend on the planning phases. The outcomes and nursing orders written during planning serve to guide the nurse's actions during implementation. Furthermore, the outcomes developed during planning are the criteria used in evaluating whether patient care has had the desired effects (more about this in Chapter 9).

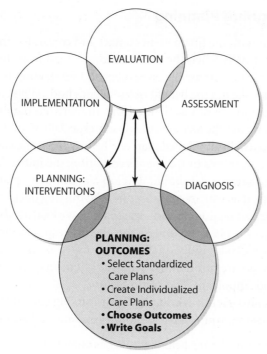

FIGURE 6–1
The planning phase: outcomes and goals

Informal and Formal Planning

The nursing process phases overlap when nurses do *informal planning* while carrying out the activities of the other steps. For example, while listening to a patient's lung sounds (assessment), the nurse may be making a mental note (planning) to notify the primary care provider of her findings. This chapter emphasizes **formal planning**, which is a conscious, deliberate activity involving decision making, critical thinking, and creativity.

Time-Sequenced Planning

In addition to the planning involved in creating a nursing plan of care, nurses often use **time-sequenced planning** when they plan a patient's care for a shift or for a 24-hour period:

- The timing and order of nursing activities for a patient must often be planned (e.g., giving pain medication before a painful dressing change).
- Nurses must coordinate the timing of nursing care with the actions of other healthcare team members, visits from family and friends, and the patient's circadian rhythms.
- Nurses must plan a daily work schedule. In addition to planning care for *each* patient, nurses must structure their own time so they can give care to all the patients assigned for that shift.

Initial versus Ongoing Planning

Initial planning begins with the first patient contact and continues until the nurse–patient relationship is ended, usually when the patient is discharged from the healthcare agency. The nurse who performs the admission assessment should develop the initial comprehensive plan of care because she has the benefit of the client's body language and some intuitive kinds of information that are not available from the written database alone. Planning should be initiated soon after the assessment is done, especially with the trend toward short hospital stays. Even a partially developed plan can be helpful in the early nurse–client contacts. Because of time constraints or the client's condition, the initial database is sometimes incomplete. In such situations, you should develop a preliminary plan using the information available and refine it as you are able to gather the missing data.

Ongoing planning can be done by any nurse who works with the client. It is carried out as new information is obtained and as the client's responses to care are evaluated. The initial plan of care can be individualized even more as the nurses get to know the client better. Nurses who are not familiar with the client may not recognize the significance of new data, and important data could be lost.

Ongoing planning also occurs as you plan your nursing care at the beginning of each day. In your daily planning, you will use ongoing assessment data to do the following:

1. Determine whether the client's health status has changed.
2. Set the day's priorities for the client's care.
3. Decide which problems to focus on during this shift.
4. Coordinate your activities so you can address more than one problem at each client contact.

6-1 WHAT DO YOU KNOW?

Give an example of each of the following: informal planning, formal planning, time-sequenced planning, initial planning, ongoing planning.

See answer to #6-1 What Do You Know? in Appendix A.

A Practice Example

THINK ABOUT THIS CLINICAL SCENARIO

You receive the following messages almost simultaneously.

2:49 P.M.	Mr. C. has requested pain medication: "I'm hurting real bad. Please come now."
2:50 P.M.	Mrs. A., who is confined to bed, asks for a drink of water.
2:51 P.M.	Mrs. B., who needs help to ambulate, says she needs to go to the bathroom right now: "Hurry, please!"
2:52 P.M.	The nursing assistant says. "Come quick. Mr. D's dressing is all wet with blood, and it's trickling out from under it."

How will you structure your time so you can meet all of these patients' needs? Which patient would you help first? Think about it for a minute before reading ahead.

What was your plan for this situation? Certainly you must have looked at the needs of each individual as well as the needs of the whole group. You would, of course, try to meet the most urgent needs first. In this situation, you might have decided to check Mr. D's dressing first to evaluate whether the bleeding needed immediate attention. When needs are of equal priority (perhaps Mr. C. and Mrs. B.), you have to sequence your care on the basis of good time management. You might deal with a simple problem first in order to free some uninterrupted time for more complex actions. For example, you might quickly administer Mr. C.'s pain medication on your way to help Mrs. B. Ambulate. All of those solutions assume you must deal with these patients alone. However, there may be assistive personnel to whom you can delegate some activities.

Discharge Planning

Discharge planning is the process of preparing the patient to leave the healthcare agency. It includes preparing the person for self-care as well as providing for continuity of care among present caregivers and those who will care for the person after discharge. Because most patients are in the hospital for only a short time, it is essential to begin discharge planning on admission and continue it until the patient leaves the agency. As a rule, discharge is not the end of the illness episode for the patient but is the transition to another phase of it. Research shows that discharge planning can reduce complications and readmissions (Dedhia, 2009). Schneider et al, 1993). Tuazon (1992) has suggested using the word *MODEL* as a mnemonic device to help you concentrate on discharge planning basics:

M   Make a written plan.

O   Offer resources (e.g., social worker).

D   Devise ways to increase compliance.

E   Evaluate your teaching with immediate feedback.

L   Legal implications: Document.

Take-away point: Discharge planning should begin on admission and continue until the patient leaves the agency.

Collaborative Discharge Planning

All patients need some degree of discharge planning, but you may not always need a separate, written discharge plan. You can sometimes include discharge assessments and teaching as nursing orders on the comprehensive plan of care. For example, one nursing order for Mrs. Sanchez (in Chapters 3, 4, and 5) is to teach her to continue taking her antibiotics after discharge until they are all gone, even if she feels better. Most institutions have a standardized, preprinted discharge plan such as Figure 6–2.

FOLLOW UP CARE	When to call the doctor; symptom management (pain, nausea); plan for meeting outcomes not met during hospitalization::
	Call Your primary physician to find out if an insurance referral form is needed for follow up appointments. After discharge, you need to call for an appointment to see physician Clinic/Physician Phone # Date Time _____ _____ _____ _____ or ____days ____weeks ____months _____ _____ _____ _____ or ____days ____weeks ____months _____ _____ _____ _____ or ____days ____weeks ____months Plans for follow up Labs/Tests/Treatments Date Time Test/Treatment Location Ordered by
PERSONAL CARE	**Bathing**: ☐ No restrictions ☐ Other: **Treatment/Therapy/Wound or Skin Care/ Supplies Needed** 2-Day Supply Sent Home ? ☐Yes
ACTIVITY/ REHAB	☐ No restrictions ☐ Do not climb stairs ☐ Drive_____ ☐ Return to Work _____ ☐ Do not lift ☐ May lift up to _____lbs ☐ Weight Bearing _____# ☐ Other
DIET	☐ No restrictions ☐ Other: Food/Drug Interactions: ☐ Coumadin ☐ MAO Inhibitors ☐ Other:
MEDICAL EQUIPMENT	☐ 2nd pair of TED hose given
COMMUNITY RESOURCES	**Referral Resource** **Agency** **Phone #** Transportation Arrangements for discharge:___ Home IV Therapy _____ _____ _____ Home Health _____ _____ Home Oxygen _____ _____ Education/Community Resources:_____ Home PT/OT/Speech _____ _____ _____ Ask-A-Nurse 816-932-6220

Preprinted Discharge Instruction Sheet given to patient ☐ NA ☐Yes
 List Instruction Sheets:

I understand these instructions and agree with this plan of care _____
Patient/SO Signature

MULTIDISCIPLINARY DISCHARGE INSTRUCTIONS
Shawnee Mission Medical Center
9100 W. 74th Street
Shawnee Mission, Kansas 66204

FIGURE 6–2

Discharge plan record (*Source:* Courtesy of Shawnee Mission Medical Center, Shawnee Mission, KS. Used with permission.)

A written discharge plan is required for patients with special needs (e.g., complex self-care needs, newly diagnosed chronic diseases such as diabetes). Patients are often discharged from the hospital still in need of skilled nursing care. They may be placed in a long-term care setting or sent home to continue complicated treatments and therapies (e.g., apnea monitors, intravenous [IV] therapies, mechanical ventilators). Post-hospital needs are often met by members of a multidisciplinary team, which may include private-duty nurses; home care services; social services; physical therapists; housing departments; speech, occupational, and hearing therapists; physicians; and the client's family. Discharge planning must include all involved disciplines.

Discharge to Home Care

With the decreased length of hospital stays, transition to home and self-care has become very important. Home health nurses, too, must emphasize discharge planning as a part of their role. Box 6–2 contains priorities to consider when discharging

---

BOX 6–2

DISCHARGE PLANNING PRIORITIES

1. To what extent does the patient wish to be involved in the planning?
2. How will the following affect the patient's self-care ability?
   - Age
   - Medical condition
   - Financial resources
   - Disabilities or limitations (e.g., secondary conditions such as poor vision)
   - Nutritional status (e.g., special dietary needs)
   - Primary caregiver (e.g., feelings about patient, abilities)
   - Home environment (e.g., hazards, stairs, wheelchair access)
3. Is there a need for:
   - Referral to community agencies (e.g., home-delivered meals)?
   - Someone to coordinate with the insurance company?
4. Home care teaching:
   - Determine what information the client believes he needs.
   - Begin teaching when the patient is receptive.
   - Include family members.
   - Notify home care agency of teaching done or needed.
5. At discharge, see that all plans are in place. For example, have arrangements been made for:
   - Transportation home (medically equipped or other)?
   - Medical supplies at home?
   - A nurse or home health aide?

Source: Adapted from Anthony & Hudson-Barr (2004), Berman et al (2008), Nazarko (1998), Tirk (1992), Tuazon (1992), Weissman & Jasovsky (1998), and Wilkinson & Treas (2011).

a client to home care. The following example illustrates the need for discharge planning:

> **EXAMPLE:** Anna was hospitalized for bacteremia and renal failure. After 2 months, she went home, severely debilitated, to a one-room apartment. The diet that her nurse and dieticians had so carefully taught her in the hospital was impossible for her to follow with her low energy level and minimal cooking facilities. She could not afford to fill the prescription the nurse practitioner had given her. Within 3 weeks, she was readmitted to the hospital, again with renal failure and bacteremia (adapted from Carr, 1990).

Patient Plans of Care

There are two kinds of care plans: comprehensive nursing plans of care and multidisciplinary (collaborative) plans of care. Both types may contain sections that are (a) standardized, preplanned, and preprinted or (b) individualized to fit the unique needs of individual patients. The most obvious benefit of a written care plan is that it *provides continuity of care*. It is important—sometimes essential—that all caregivers use the same approach with a patient.

> **EXAMPLE:** Jed Goldstein is being treated on an adolescent mental health unit. The staff has been trying to modify his manipulative behavior. Val Benitez, RN, has been floated to the mental health unit from the critical care unit. She does not know Jed, but she reads an order on the nursing plan: "Do not respond to negative talk about staff on other shifts." Later, Jed begins to complain about the night nurse. Val's usual response to patients in the critical care unit is to remain neutral but encourage them to express their feelings. Instead, she remembers the nursing order and changes the subject. Val is not an experienced psychiatric nurse; without the plan of care, her nurturing instincts and past experience might have prompted her to respond differently. This would not have been therapeutic for Jed and would have undermined the work of the nurses on the other shifts.

A written plan of care *promotes efficient functioning of the nursing team* by assuring that time is not wasted on ineffective approaches (as in the preceding Jed Goldstein example) and that efforts are not duplicated. By specifically outlining nursing interventions and expected client responses, written plans provide a convenient reference for organizing the nursing progress notes. They also help to ensure adequate discharge planning, provide documentation for third-party reimbursement and serve as a guide for making staff assignments.

Electronic Care Planning

Computer literacy has become an essential nursing skill. Computers are used to create both standardized and individualized plans of care. The nurse can access the patient's stored plan of care from a centrally located terminal at the nurses' station or from terminals in patient rooms. Computerized plans of care are easy to review and update, and because they do not rely on human memory, they are likely to be thorough and accurate. Figure 6–3 is a recreation of a computer screen showing an overview of the plan of care for a patient with the medical condition "respiratory disorder."

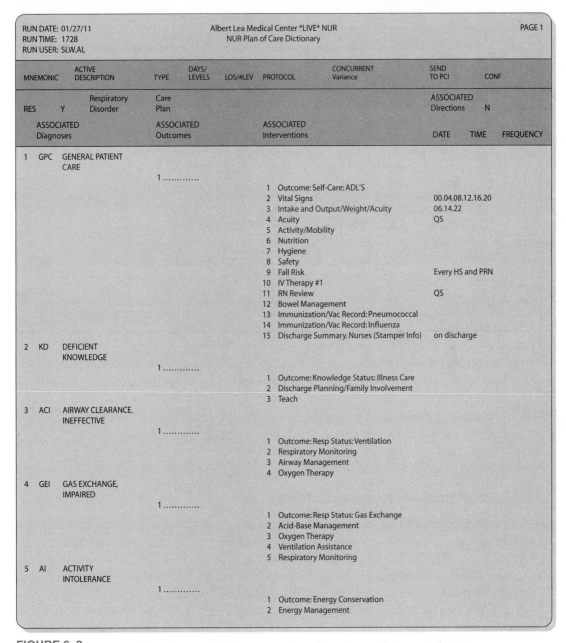

FIGURE 6–3

Computer screen for respiratory disorder plan of care (*Source:* By permission of Albert Lea Medical Center, Mayo Health System, Albert Lea, MN.)

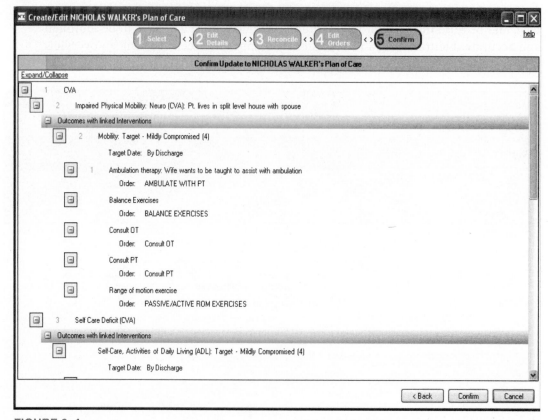

FIGURE 6–4

Computer plan of care for a single nursing diagnosis (*Source:* Copyright 2007–2009 McKesson Corporation and/or one of its affiliates. Used with permission. All rights reserved.)

It includes several nursing diagnoses, as well as a section for "general patient care." Figure 6–4 is an example of a computer plan of care for a single nursing diagnosis, using standardized nursing languages.

Comprehensive Nursing Plans of Care

A **comprehensive nursing plan of care** is made up of several different documents that integrate dependent, interdependent, and independent nursing functions. It provides a central source of patient information to guide care. The **nursing diagnosis care plan** is the section of the comprehensive plan that prescribes the outcomes and interventions for the patient's nursing diagnoses and collaborative problems. This chapter focuses on nursing diagnosis care plans; comprehensive plans are discussed more fully in Chapter 10.

Care plan forms differ from agency to agency. However, the format usually consists of at least three columns: nursing diagnoses, patient outcomes, and nursing orders. Some agencies add a column for evaluating patient responses to the nursing interventions.

Date	Nursing Diagnosis	Predicted Outcomes	Nursing Orders	Rationale	Evaluation
7/15/11	Decisional Conflict r/t value conflicts regarding termination of treatment A.M.B. tearfulness. Statements of inability to decide.	1. By 7/16 will discuss feelings about the situation with nurse and significant other. 2. etc.	1. Spend at least 15 minutes sitting with client during each visit. 2. Listen without making judgements. 3. etc.	1. Demonstrates support and caring. 2. Demonstrates acceptance of client's value and worth unconditionally. 3. etc.	7/16 Goal #1 Goal met. Discussed feelings of guilt with wife.

FIGURE 6–5
Sample format for nursing care plans

Planning usually progresses horizontally across the page: Nursing Diagnoses → Patient Outcomes → Nursing Orders → Evaluation. Figure 6–5 shows a typical format. In this format, you could write the assessment data in the same column as the nursing diagnosis if you use the *as manifested by (A.M.B.)* format for diagnoses (see Chapter 5). A few agencies add a column for **rationale**, which consists of principles or scientific reasons for selecting a specific nursing action. It may also explain why the action is expected to achieve the outcome. Professional functioning requires an understanding of the rationale underlying the nursing orders even when the rationale is not written on the plan of care.

To be useful in the clinical setting, plans of care must be concise and easy to use. Still, the format chosen should include adequate space to write individualized nursing orders even when preprinted plans are used.

Student Plans of Care

Care plans in practice settings are designed for nurses to use in delivering care. Student plans of care are designed, in addition, for these purposes:

- To help the student learn and apply the nursing process
- To provide a guide for giving nursing care to meet the client's needs while in the clinical setting
- To help the student learn about the client's pathophysiology or psychopathology and the associated nursing care

Therefore, you may be required to write your student plans of care without incorporating any preprinted plans. You may be expected to develop a list of all of your patient's actual and risk (potential) nursing diagnoses and collaborative problems, not just the unusual ones, and to develop detailed nursing interventions for them. Your instructors may also ask you to provide an in-depth rationale for your nursing interventions and perhaps to cite literature to support your rationale.

Mind-Mapped Plans of Care

Mind mapping uses pictures to show the relationships among concepts. It is an alternative method of writing a plan of care. Mind mapping can stimulate critical thinking as you brainstorm about how to illustrate the relationships among data, nursing diagnoses, and other elements of a plan of care. The mind-mapped plan is complete when you have related all elements of the nursing process (i.e., data, nursing diagnoses, outcomes, interventions, evaluation) in whatever order you think of them. To learn more about mind mapping a plan of care, see Chapter 10.

Multidisciplinary Plans of Care (Critical Pathways)

A **critical pathway** (also called *interdisciplinary plan, multidisciplinary plan, collaborative plan, critical path,* and *action plan*) is a standardized, multidisciplinary plan of care that sequences patient care based on diagnosis or case type. It outlines, by time (a) the crucial assessments and interventions that must be performed by nurses, physicians, and other health team members and (b) the daily, or even hourly, patient outcomes necessary in order to achieve discharge goals within the defined length of stay. For example, for a patient undergoing an abdominal hysterectomy, part of the critical pathway might be as follows:

	Postoperative Day 1	**Postoperative Day 2**
Outcomes	Will verbalize pain appropriately to nurse; will state pain is < 5 on a 1–10 scale.	Will verbalize pain appropriately to RN; will state pain is < 2 on a 1–10 scale.
Interventions	Self-controlled administration of morphine per IV pump	Tylenol #3, tabs 1, p.o. as needed

Most critical pathways are developed for medical or surgical diagnoses, conditions, or procedures (e.g., tests, treatments) and tend to emphasize biomedical problems and interventions. They work best for cases that occur frequently in an agency or that have relatively predictable outcomes. A different critical pathway is created for each case type (e.g., myocardial infarction, cardiac catheterization, pneumonia, total hip replacement). A critical pathway addresses the needs that *all* patients with a certain condition have in common. It does not take into account a patient's unique needs; those must be addressed by an individualized nursing diagnosis plan of care—sometimes through variances (refer to "Using Nursing Diagnoses with Critical Pathways" in Chapter 4). A **variance** occurs when (a) an outcome is not met in the specified time or (b) an intervention is not performed at the specified time. See Figure 10–7 for an example of a critical pathway.

Planning Outcomes

Powerful political and market forces demand decreased healthcare costs, preferably without decreased quality. Therefore, healthcare institutions must compete for their "customers," who are not individuals but employers and businesses. This has led to outcomes-based care delivery—the use of outcomes to drive treatment planning, evaluation of care, and reimbursement by third-party payers (e.g., Medicare, private insurers). The preceding discussion of critical pathways is one example of outcomes-based care. Critical pathways describe outcomes for multidisciplinary (including medical) interventions but do not provide a way to judge *nursing* effectiveness and therefore do not provide a mechanism for nursing accountability. The remainder of this chapter focuses on individualized care planning and patient outcomes that are influenced by nursing care.

After determining the patient's present health status (nursing diagnosis), the next step is to set goals for changing or maintaining health status. A **goal**, or **desired outcome**, describes the patient responses you expect to achieve as a result of interventions. A **nursing-sensitive outcome** is one that can be achieved or influenced by nursing interventions. Many nurses use the terms *goal* and *outcome* interchangeably. This text will usually use the Nursing Outcomes Classification (NOC) terminology, in which the word *outcome*, when used alone, is defined as any patient response (good or bad) to interventions. *Goals* and *desired outcomes* are used as in the two introductory sentences of this paragraph (other terms with the same meaning are *predicted outcomes, expected outcomes,* and *outcome criteria*).

EXAMPLE:

Outcome:	Ambulation: walking
Goal (expected outcome, desired outcome, predicted outcome):	Walks to end of hall without assistance

You should be aware that some literature uses a slightly different scheme, defining *goals* as broad statements about the desired effects of the nursing activities and *outcomes* (and other outcome terms) as the more specific, observable criteria used to evaluate whether the broad goal has been met.

EXAMPLE:

Broad Statements (Goals)	*Specific Outcomes (Criteria)*
Improve nutritional status ⟶	Will gain 5 lb by April 25.
Decrease pain ⟶	Will rate pain as < 3 on a 1–10 scale.
Increase self-care abilities ⟶	Will be able to feed self by end of the week.

When goals are defined broadly, as in the above examples, the patient plan of care must include *both* goals and outcomes. In fact, they are sometimes combined into one statement; the broad goal is stated first, followed by *as evidenced by*, followed by a list of the observable responses that demonstrate achievement of the goal. Do not confuse *as evidenced by* with the phrase *as manifested by*, used in writing nursing diagnoses.

EXAMPLE:

Correct	*Incorrect*
Nutritional status will improve *as evidenced by* weight gain of 5 lb by 4/25.	Nutritional status will improve *as manifested by* weight gain of 5 lb by 4/25.

While you are learning, writing the broad, general goal first may help you to think of the specific outcomes that are needed. Remember, however, that although broad goals can be a starting point for planning, the specific, measurable outcomes *must* be written on the plan of care.

Purpose of the Outcome Statement

Outcome statements guide the planning of care and the evaluation of changes in patient health status. When the outcomes state precisely and clearly what you wish to achieve, ideas for nursing actions flow logically from the desired outcomes, and it is relatively easy to select nursing orders to achieve the desired changes.

Outcome statements also provide a sense of achievement for both the client and the nurse and motivate them in their efforts to improve health status.

EXAMPLE: Kay Stein has essential hypertension. She has a demanding career and family life, and she needs to lose 50 lb. Even though she takes her antihypertensive medication faithfully, follows her low-calorie diet, and tries to decrease her stress, she still does not feel any better. In fact, she feels worse because the medication gives her a headache. However, she and her nurse have set measurable, achievable outcomes, such as "Loses 2 lb this week" and "B/P will be 124/80 by end of the week." When Kay's blood pressure reading is 120/80 mm Hg and the scale shows she has lost 4 lb, she has proof that her efforts are really accomplishing something. This helps motivate her to continue making lifestyle changes that she finds very difficult.

Writing Outcome Statements

Whether you use standardized language or your own wording, outcome statements must be specific and descriptive in order to be useful for planning and evaluating care. Figure 6–6 is an example of a computer screen that suggests outcomes for the nursing diagnosis entered by the nurse.

Deriving Desired Outcomes from Nursing Diagnoses

Except for wellness diagnoses, diagnostic statements describe human responses that are problems for the patient, family, or community. Stating a problem response suggests that the opposite response is preferred and is what you will try to achieve. The nursing diagnosis "Constipation r/t inactivity and inadequate fluid intake" indicates that the client's elimination status needs to change. An improvement in elimination status would be evidenced by an opposite (normal) response—that is, a regular, formed, soft bowel movement.

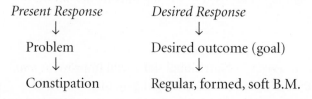

Present Response	Desired Response
↓	↓
Problem	Desired outcome (goal)
↓	↓
Constipation	Regular, formed, soft B.M.

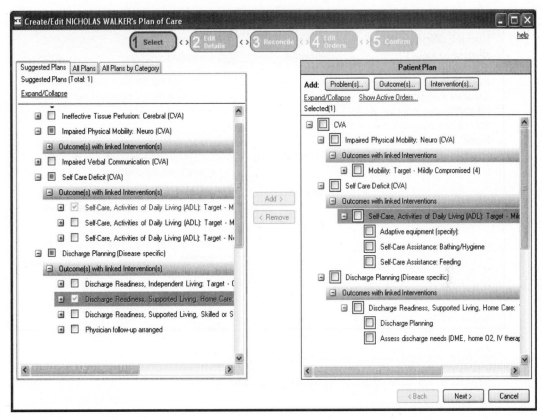

FIGURE 6–6

After the nurse enters a nursing diagnosis, a computer screen lists suggested outcomes
(*Source:* Copyright 2007–2009 McKesson Corporation and/or one of its affiliates. Used with
permission. All rights reserved.)

When developing goal statements, look at the problem and think: What would the alternative healthy response be? To describe the response in terms of specific behaviors, ask yourself the following:

1. If the problem is solved (or prevented), how will the client look or behave? What will I be able to see, hear, palpate, smell, or otherwise observe with my senses?
2. What must the client do to show that the goal is achieved? How well must he do it?

EXAMPLE: The nursing diagnosis is "*Deficient Fluid Volume* r/t insufficient fluid intake." The unhealthy response is deficient fluid volume; the alternative healthy response would be *adequate fluid volume.*

1. If the problem is solved (fluid volume is adequate), how will the client look or behave? One observable response you could see and palpate is *elastic skin turgor.*
2. What must the client do to demonstrate goal achievement? A possible answer to this is that he must *drink more fluids than he excretes.* Also, you might specify that he would *drink a minimum amount of fluids, perhaps 100 mL/h.*

TABLE 6–1   Examples of Alternative Healthy Responses

Nursing Diagnosis (Present Status)	Human Response	Desired Outcome
Ineffective Airway Clearance r/t poor cough effort 2° incisional pain & fear of "breaking stitches loose"	Appearance	Within 24 hours after surgery, will have no skin pallor or cyanosis during post-op period.
	Body functioning	Lungs clear to auscultation during entire post-op period.
	Symptoms	Within 48 hours after surgery, states having no shortness of breath when ambulating to chair.
	Knowledge	After reteaching, states rationale for turning, deep breathing, and coughing after surgery.
	Emotions	Within 48 hours after surgery, states he is no longer afraid to cough.

Therefore, your goal/outcome statement might be:

Will have adequate fluid volume, as evidenced by

a. elastic skin turgor
b. Intake = Output
c. drinks at least 100 mL/h

Outcomes, similar to nursing diagnoses, involve a variety of human responses, including appearance, body functions, symptoms, knowledge, interpersonal functioning, and emotions (Table 6–1). Because outcomes are derived directly from the nursing diagnoses, they will be appropriate only if you have stated the nursing diagnosis correctly.

EXAMPLE: Vincent Aarusa is highly anxious about the surgery he is about to undergo. He does not have a good understanding of the procedure or of its risks and benefits. Worse, his father died after having a similar surgery 20 years ago. His admitting nurse did not perceive the severity of his anxiety and wrote a nursing diagnosis of "Deficient Knowledge (Surgical Procedure) r/t no prior experience or teaching." The goal for this problem was stated as follows: "Will describe surgical procedure in general terms and discuss risks and benefits prior to surgery." When Mr. Aarusa was able to perform these behaviors, the nurse on the next shift discontinued the deficient knowledge problem, and the nursing staff attempted no further discussion of his surgery. Mr. Aarusa was sent to surgery with adequate information but with no relief of his anxiety.

Essential versus Nonessential Goals The essential patient goals are derived from the problem (first) clause. The second clause sometimes suggests some goals as well.

Problem + Etiology
↓

Goals/outcomes

Goals derived from the etiology are different from those derived from the problem. Their achievement may help to resolve the problem, but they could also be achieved *without* resolving the problem. In that case, the plan of care might be discontinued because the goals had been met, but the client would still have the problem.

EXAMPLE:

	Problem	*Etiology*
Nursing Diagnosis:	Imbalanced Nutrition: Less than Body Requirements for Calories	r/t Lack of appetite 2° depression
	—	↓
Goals/Desired Outcomes:	**1.** Will gain 5 lb by 12/14.	**3.** Will state his appetite is better within 3 days.
	2. Will consume at least 2,000 calories per day.	**4.** Will be hungry at mealtimes by 12/1.
		5. By 12/1, will be less depressed, as evidenced by **a.** no more than one crying spell per day. **b.** participation in unit activities.

Achieving goals 1 and 2 would actually show problem resolution. If the client gains 5 lb and consumes 2,000 calories per day, then he cannot have "less than body requirements for calories." This is not true for goals 3, 4, and 5. The client's depression might lift, and he might regain his appetite, but still continue to lose weight. If you discontinued the nutritional problem after measuring only objectives 3, 4, and 5, you would do the client a disservice. Therefore, for every nursing diagnosis, you must write at least one goal that, when achieved, shows direct resolution of the problem.

Goals for Actual, Risk, and Possible Nursing Diagnoses Outcome statements may reflect promotion, maintenance, or restoration of health, depending on the type of nursing diagnosis (Table 6–2). For an *actual nursing diagnosis*, goals focus on restoring healthy responses and preventing further complications. They specify patient behaviors that demonstrate resolution or reduction of the problem and that patients should be able to achieve with the aid of independent nursing activities.

TABLE 6–2 Goals or Desired Outcomes for Different Problem Types

Type of Problem	Patient Response Demonstrates:	Nursing Focuses on:
Actual nursing diagnosis	Resolution or reduction of problem	Resolution or reduction of problem Prevention of complication
Risk nursing diagnosis	Problem has not developed	Prevention and detection of problem
Possible nursing diagnosis	No patient responses	Confirmation or exclusion of problem
Collaborative problem	Problem has not developed	Detection and prevention of problem
Wellness diagnoses		
Health maintenance	Continuation of healthy functioning	Health maintenance
Health promotion	Achievement of a higher level of wellness	Health promotion

EXAMPLE:

Actual Nursing Diagnosis

Impaired Skin Integrity: Dermal Ulcer over coccyx r/t inability to move self in bed

Goal/Outcome Statement

Ulcer will not extend to deeper tissues.

Ulcer will not become infected, as evidenced by absence of purulent exudate.

By 12/1, healing will be evidenced by decreased redness and appearance of granulation tissue in wound bed.

Take-away point: Every nursing diagnosis must have at least one expected outcome that demonstrates resolution of the problem response.

Goals for *risk nursing diagnoses* focus on preventing the problem; the client responses should demonstrate a problem-free level of functioning or, if that is not possible, maintenance of the present level of functioning. Achievement of these goals should mean that the problem is not present at the time the assessment is made.

EXAMPLE:

Risk Nursing Diagnosis

Risk for Ineffective Breastfeeding r/t breast engorgement

Goal/Outcome Statements

Infant will be observed to "latch on," suck, and swallow at each feeding.

Mother will state satisfaction with breastfeeding.

Infant will regain birth weight within 14 days after birth.

Possible nursing diagnoses present an exception to the rule; they are *not* written in terms of desired patient response. You use a possible diagnosis when you do not have enough data to determine whether the patient has the problem. The goal for a possible nursing diagnosis is really a *nursing* goal: that the presence of the diagnosis will be confirmed or ruled out. You do not need to write goals for possible diagnoses. However, to help ensure that follow-up assessments will be done, you may wish to set a target time for confirming or ruling out the problem. If so, you could write a nursing goal. Nursing goals should not be written on the plan of care for actual or potential problems.

EXAMPLE:

Possible Problem: Possible Hopelessness r/t abandonment by significant other after onset of chronic illness

Nursing Goal: Confirm or rule out Hopelessness by 6/12.

Goals for Collaborative Problems Unlike collaborative problems, outcomes for nursing diagnoses are *nurse sensitive.* That is, they can be brought about primarily by nursing interventions. Nurses and physicians share accountability for achieving outcomes for *collaborative problems.* Therefore, outcomes for these problems are usually found in the agency's standardized care plans or critical pathways. Furthermore, it may not be legally advisable to write goals that imply nursing accountability, when accountability for the problem actually is shared with other professions.

Take-away point: Nursing care plans do not need goal statements for collaborative problems because they contain only nursing orders, and it is understood that the broad goal is prevention or early detection of the problem.

As a student, however, it may enhance your learning to write goals for collaborative problems. This will ensure that you know precisely what symptoms you are looking for and can recognize whether or not the problem is developing. When writing such outcomes, remember that a collaborative problem is a potential problem, not an actual problem. Nursing care focuses on prevention and early detection of the complication. Expected outcomes for collaborative problems should describe the patient responses you will observe as long as the problem has not developed. The goals may describe normal functioning or problem symptoms that you *do not* want to occur.

EXAMPLE:

Collaborative Problem	*Goal/Outcome Statements*
Potential Complication of Childbirth: Postpartum Hemorrhage	Postpartum hemorrhage will not occur, as evidenced by 1. saturating less than 1 vag. pad per hour during first 24 hours. 2. fundus firm and below umbilicus during first 24 hours. 3. pulse and B/P in normal range for patient.

Short-Term and Long-Term Goals

Short-term goals can be achieved within a few days or a few hours. Goals dealing with survival needs may even be stated in terms of minutes. For this reason, short-term goals are useful in acute-care settings, such as hospitals, where nurses often focus on the client's more immediate needs. The client may be discharged before the nurse can evaluate progress toward long-term goals. Some examples of short-term goals follow:

EXAMPLES:

> Voids within 6 hours after delivery of infant
> States relief of pain within 1 hour after receiving p.o. oxycodone
> Walks to end of hall and back, unassisted, by day 2 post-op

Short-term goals can be used to measure progress toward long-term goals. Achieving several short-term goals also provides reinforcement for the client, encouraging him to keep working on the problem.

EXAMPLES:

Long-Term Goal	Will have daily B.M. without use of laxatives *within 2 months.*
Short-Term Goals	After administration of enema will have B.M. *within 4 hours.*
	Will have next B.M. *within 36 hours* without aid of p.o. laxatives.
	Immediately, diet changes include prune juice and oatmeal (or other high-fiber cereal) for breakfast and substituting whole grain for white bread.
	Within 1 week, reports he is eating at least one good source of fiber at every meal.

As a student, you will probably care for a patient for only a few hours at a time. You should write short-term goals to measure what you can realistically accomplish while you are with the client so you can evaluate the results of the care you have given. In a comprehensive plan of care, you should also include longer-range goals that other nurses can use to evaluate patient progress when you are not there.

Long-term goals describe changes in client outcomes over a longer period—usually a week or more. The ideal long-term goal aims at restoring normal functioning in the problem area. When normal functioning cannot be restored, the long-term goal describes the maximum level of functioning that can be achieved given the client's health status and resources. Long-term goals are especially useful for clients with chronic health problems and those in home health care, rehabilitation centers, and other extended-care facilities. Some examples of long-term goals follow:

EXAMPLE: After attending six weekly childbirth-education classes, will correctly demonstrate abdominal and shallow chest breathing.

> By 12 weeks post-op, will have full range of motion of right shoulder.
> Within 3 months (12/24), will feed self using fork or spoon.

TABLE 6–3 Components of Goal or Expected Outcome Statements

Subject	Verb	Special Conditions	Performance Criteria	Target Time
Patient	will list	(after attending nutrition class)	two low-fat foods from each of the MyPyramid groups	before discharge.
Patient's lungs	will be	—	clear to auscultation	within 24 hours.
Client	will walk	(using walker)	to bathroom and back without shortness of breath	within 3 days.

Components of Goal Statements

As a rule, every goal statement (expected outcome) should contain a subject, an action verb, performance criteria, and a target time. It may sometimes be necessary to state special conditions as well. See Table 6–3 for examples of goal statement components.

Subject The subject of the goal is a noun. It is the client, any part of the client, or a property or characteristic of the client.

EXAMPLE:

Client   Mucous membranes
Ms. Atwell   Anxiety
Lung sounds

The subject is the client unless otherwise stated. Think, "Client will . . ." as you begin the goal statement but do not write "Client will."

EXAMPLE:

Incorrect: *Client will* describe pain as <3 on a scale of 1–10.
Correct: *Will* describe pain as <3 on a scale of 1–10.
               Describes pain as <3 on a scale of 1–10.

Action Verb The verb describes the desired client action (e.g., what the client is to learn or do). Using actions that can be seen, heard, smelled, felt, or measured will help make your outcomes specific and observable. Action verbs create a picture of the desired client condition or performance. Each goal should describe only one desired client condition; therefore, each should contain only one action verb.

EXAMPLE:

Incorrect: Will *describe* the food groups in MyPyramid and *choose* a balanced diet . . .
Correct: Will *describe* the food groups in MyPyramid.

Performance Criteria Performance criteria are the standards used to evaluate the quality of the client's performance. They describe the *extent* to which the client is expected to perform the behavior. The performance criteria indicate what should be measured in evaluating outcomes. Performance criteria may specify amount, quality, speed, distance, accuracy, and so forth—they tell *how, what, when,* or *where.*

EXAMPLE:

		What	**When**
Amount	Will lose	5 lb	during the first week.

		How	**What**
Accuracy	Will draw up	correct amount	of insulin.

		What	**How**
Quality	Will inject	insulin	using sterile technique.

		Where	**When**
Distance and Amount	Will walk	to the end of the hall	three times per day.

Target Time Each goal/outcome statement should specify the time by which you realistically expect a change in patient response (e.g., by discharge, by April 2, at all times). The target time helps to pace the patient's care, provides motivation by focusing on the future, and provides a deadline for evaluating patient progress.

EXAMPLE: Will name the food groups in MyPyramid *within 24 hours* after receiving pamphlet.

The target time is a type of performance criterion because it specifies the speed with which a goal is to be accomplished. In the preceding example, the client's progress would not be satisfactory if he took longer than 24 hours to learn the food groups.

Nursing knowledge and experience are needed for setting realistic target times. You will need to know the usual rate of progress for clients with the identified medical and nursing diagnoses and consider the client's particular capabilities and resources.

EXAMPLE: Esther Brady has just had an abdominal hysterectomy. Review of usual progress after this surgery indicates that most patients require IV or intramuscular narcotic analgesics for 24 hours and are then able to obtain relief from milder, oral analgesics. However, Ms. Brady is very anxious and has a history of poor pain tolerance. It would not be realistic to set a target time of 24 hours for resolution of her

Pain diagnosis. A more achievable goal might be: "Will obtain adequate pain relief from p.o. analgesics within 48 hours post-op, as evidenced by patient's statement that pain is <3 on a 1–10 scale."

Note that desired outcomes for risk problems do not need target times. The broad goal is to prevent the problem from occurring, so in a sense the target time is *at all times.*

EXAMPLE:

Nursing Diagnosis: Risk for Impaired Skin Integrity r/t immobility . . .
Predicted Outcome: Skin will remain intact with no redness over bony
                       prominences.
                       (Target time: At all times)
                       (Evaluate plan: Daily)

In the preceding example, the target time is assumed, so you would not need to write it in the plan of care. However, you may wish to schedule times for evaluating the outcomes and the accompanying plan of care.

Special Conditions If it is important to describe the conditions under which a client is to perform a behavior, you may need to add modifiers to the performance criteria. **Modifiers** describe the amount of assistance the client will need, the available resources, environmental conditions, or experiences the client should have before being expected to perform the behavior. As do performance criteria, modifiers describe *how, when, where,* and *how much.*

EXAMPLE:

                                              Type of assistance

How   Will walk to the end of the hall three times per day using a walker
           by April 8.

                                              Prior experience

When   Will list foods high in cholesterol after consulting with dietician.

           Environmental conditions

Where In one-to-one session, will express fear of abandonment by Friday.

Not all goals need special conditions; they are included only if they are important. If the performance criteria clearly specify the expected performance, then special conditions are not necessary.

6-2 WHAT DO YOU KNOW?

1. List the components of a goal statement.
2. (True or false) Special conditions should be a component of all goals.

See answer to #6-2 What Do You Know? in Appendix A.

The Nursing Outcomes Classification

The NOC is a standardized vocabulary used for describing patient outcomes. In this system, an **outcome** is "an individual, family, or community state, behavior, or perception, that is measured along a continuum in response to nursing interventions" (Moorhead et al, 2008, p. 30). The 2008 edition of the taxonomy has 385 outcomes organized in a taxonomy with seven domains: Functional Health, Physiologic Health, Psychosocial Health, Health Knowledge and Behavior, Family Health, Perceived Health, and Community Health. Each NOC outcome has a label (e.g., Mobility Level), a definition, a list of indicators, and a measurement scale (Table 6–4).

In the NOC taxonomy, the **outcome label** (also referred to as the *outcome*) is the broadly stated, one- to three-word, standardized name (e.g., coping, mobility level, knowledge: diet). The outcome is worded as a neutral state to allow for the identification of positive, negative, or no change in a patient's status. The nurse chooses outcomes based on the nursing diagnoses that have been identified. For example, for a patient with a diagnosis of Impaired Physical Mobility, the nurse might choose mobility level, transfer performance, and balance.

Indicators are concrete, observable, behaviors and states (e.g., balance performance, joint movement) that can be used to evaluate patient status. In Table 6–4, you would

TABLE 6–4 Example of a Nursing Outcomes Classification Outcome

Mobility Definition: Ability to move purposefully in own environment independently with or without assistive device					
Mobility Overall Rating	Severely compromised	Substantially compromised	Moderately compromised	Mildly compromised	Not compromised
	1	2	3	4	5
Balance	1	2	3	4	5
Coordination	1	2	3	4	5
Gait	1	2	3	4	5
Muscle movement	1	2	3	4	5
Joint movement	1	2	3	4	5
Body positioning performance	1	2	3	4	5
Transfer performance	1	2	3	4	5
Running	1	2	3	4	5
Jumping	1	2	3	4	5
Crawling	1	2	3	4	5
Walking	1	2	3	4	5
Moves with ease	1	2	3	4	5

Source: Reprinted from Moorhead, S., Johnson, M., & Maas, M., (Eds.) (2008). *Nursing Outcomes Classification (NOC)* (4th ed.). St. Louis: Mosby, p. 502. Used with permission from Elsevier Science.

TABLE 6–5 Examples of Nursing Outcomes Classification Measurement Scales

1	2	3	4	5
Severely Compromised	Substantially compromised	Moderately compromised	Mildly compromised	Not compromised
≥10 (number of occurrences)	7–9	4–6	1–3	None
Not adequate	Slightly adequate	Moderately adequate	Substantially adequate	Totally adequate

Source: Moorhead, S., Johnson, M., Maas, M., & Swanson, E. (Eds.) (2008). *Nursing Outcomes Classification (NOC)* (4th ed.). St. Louis: Mosby, pp. 44–45.

observe and rate the patient's balance performance and joint movement, for example, in evaluating his mobility level. Each outcome includes a list of indicators; the nurse selects the indicators that are appropriate for the patient and may add to the list. A five-point **measurement scale** is used to evaluate patient status on each indicator. Usually 1 is the least desirable and 5 is the most desirable patient condition along a continuum. Table 6–5 provides some examples of scales.

It is not necessary to state desired outcomes (or goals) when using this system. You merely rate the patient's status on each indicator (giving it a number) before and after interventions. You can, however, use the NOC outcomes to write goals (e.g., on a plan of care). You simply write the label, the indicators that apply to the patient, and the location on the measuring scale that is desired for each indicator. For example, using the outcome in Table 6–4, you might individualize goals for a patient as follows:

Mobility Level:

Transfer performance (5: completely independent)

Ambulation: walking (4: independent with assistive device)

Written traditionally as a goal statement, that goal would read:

"Mobility will improve, as evidenced by the ability to transfer independently (5) and walk with assistive device (walker) (4)."

Figure 6–3 illustrates the use of NOC outcomes in computerized care planning.

Family and Home Health Outcomes

Home health nurses use both individual and family outcomes. The NOC taxonomy includes nine outcomes specific to the family as a group (Moorhead et al, 2008):

Family Coping

Family Functioning

Family Health Status

Family Integrity

Family Normalization

Family Participation in
    Professional Care

Family Resiliency

Family Social Climate

Family Support During Treatment.

Other (individual) outcomes may be used with NANDA International (NANDA-I) family diagnoses. For a diagnosis of Ineffective Family Coping, for example, an outcome of Compliance Behavior might be used. Indicators of compliance behavior might be that the family seeks current information about illness and treatment and keeps appointments with a health professional.

The Clinical Care Classification (CCC) system (2006) provides three modifiers for creating outcomes: *improved, stabilized,* and *deteriorated.* The nurse attaches these to the diagnosis label to create an outcome goal for each nursing diagnosis, as in the following example:

EXAMPLE:

Nursing Diagnosis:	Disturbed sleep pattern
Goal/Expected Outcome:	Disturbed sleep pattern, improved
Actual Status at Discharge:	Disturbed sleep pattern, stabilized

Because the resulting goals are not clearly defined and measurable, they are not useful for testing the effects of nursing interventions (Parlocha & Henry, 1998). The CCC system is designed for home health care. However, none of the CCC nursing diagnoses is specific to families, so there are no family-specific outcomes. It seems reasonable to expect that future revisions, as NANDA-I has done, will include family diagnoses and outcomes.

The Omaha System can also be used to describe family outcomes. Refer to Chapter 4 and the next section.

Community Outcomes

Community health nurses need outcomes for individuals, families, and **aggregates** (groups of people or entire communities). NOC currently includes 10 outcomes specifically for use with aggregates (Moorhead et al, 2008).

Community Competence	Community Risk Control: Chronic
Community Health Status	Disease
Community Health: Immunity	Community Risk Control: Communicable Disease
Community Violence Level	Community Risk Control: Lead Exposure
Community Disaster Readiness	Community Risk Control: Violence
Community Disaster Response	

Using the Omaha System, the nurse creates desired outcomes by applying a "problem rating scale" to each nursing diagnosis. The rating scale measures what the client knows

TABLE 6–6   Omaha Problem Rating Scale for Outcomes

CONCEPT	1	2	3	4	5
Knowledge Ability of the client to remember and interpret information	No knowledge	Minimal knowledge	Basic knowledge	Adequate knowledge	Superior knowledge
Behavior Observable responses, actions, or activities of the client fitting the occasion or purpose	Never appropriate	Rarely appropriate	Inconsistently appropriate	Usually appropriate	Consistently appropriate
Status Condition of the client in relation to objective and subjective defining characteristics	Extreme signs/ symptoms	Severe signs/ symptoms	Moderate signs/ symptoms	Minimal signs/ symptoms	No signs/ symptoms

Source: The Omaha System. Problem rating scale for outcomes. Available at http://www.omahasystem.org/problemratingscaleforoutcomes.html.

(*knowledge*), does (*behavior*), and is (*status*) with regard to the nursing diagnosis (Table 6–6). An example of an expected outcome using this scale follows:

EXAMPLE:

Nursing Diagnosis: Deficit in family sanitation

Rating Scale	*Present Status*	*Expected Outcome*
Knowledge:	(2) Minimal knowledge	(3) Basic knowledge
Behavior:	(3) Inconsistently appropriate	(4) Usually appropriate
Status:	(3) Moderate signs/symptoms	(4) Minimal signs/symptoms

Because there are currently no aggregate nursing diagnoses in the Omaha System, there are no outcomes specific to groups.

The following are the four overarching goals recommended by the U.S. Public Health Service for improving the health of the nation (USDHHS, 2010). These are examples of group, or aggregate, goals.

1. Attain high-quality, longer lives free of preventable disease, disability, injury, and premature death.
2. Achieve health equity, eliminate disparities, and improve the health of all groups.
3. Create social and physical environments that promote good health for all.
4. Promote quality of life, healthy development, and healthy behaviors across all life stages.

For more information about public health objectives, visit www.healthypeople.gov.

Goals/Outcomes for Wellness Diagnoses

Recall that wellness diagnoses describe essentially healthy responses that the client wishes to maintain or improve. Desired outcomes for these diagnoses describe client responses that demonstrate health maintenance or achievement of a higher level of healthy functioning (e.g., "Over the next year, Mrs. Jacobs will continue participating in religious activities that provide spiritual support."). The national public health goals listed in the preceding section are examples of wellness outcomes for groups.

By using the highest number on the rating scale (5), both the NOC and the Omaha System can be used to write wellness outcomes.

EXAMPLE:

NOC: *Nursing Diagnosis*: Health-Seeking Behaviors
Expected Outcomes: (5) Very strong health orientation

Omaha: *Nursing Diagnosis*: Health Promotion: Physical Activity
Expected Behavior: (5) Superior knowledge, (5) consistently appropriate behavior with regard to physical activity

Nurses who use a wellness framework focus on the client potentials rather than on client problems. They lead clients to envisioning change and action rather than prescribing for the client. Nevertheless, goals are important. If the client commits to a plan of action (i.e., sets a goal), that is a good predictor of actual behavior change. Research suggests that nurses set goals with clients to begin their intended behaviors within a 2-month time frame (Frenn & Malin, 1998).

Patient Teaching Goals/Outcomes

Some patients need a special teaching plan to address their learning needs (see Chapter 10). **Teaching objectives** are patient outcomes that describe what the patient is to learn or how he will demonstrate learning. Objectives should reflect whether the learning is to take place in the cognitive, psychomotor, or affective domain. **Cognitive learning** involves perception, understanding, and the storing and recall of new information. **Psychomotor learning** involves physical skills. **Affective learning** involves changes in feelings, attitudes, and values.

EXAMPLE:

Cognitive domain Learner will *explain* the effect of weight on B/P.

Psychomotor domain Learner will *apply* B/P cuff correctly.

Affective domain Learner will state that he *feels* confident with his ability to obtain correct B/P readings.

As with all goals, choose active verbs for learning objectives; they will help you to think of teaching strategies and make it easier to evaluate whether learning takes place. Table 6–7 provides a few suggestions for active verbs in each of the learning domains.

TABLE 6–7   Active Verbs for Learning Objectives

Cognitive Domain	Psychomotor Domain	Affective Domain
Compare	Arrange	Choose
Define	Assemble	Defend
Describe	Construct	Discuss
Differentiate	Manipulate	Express
Explain	Organize	Help
Identify	Show	Justify
List	Start	Select
Name	Take	Share
State		

When writing objectives for the affective domain, keep in mind that you cannot directly observe a feeling or an attitude. Therefore, you could not write a goal such as: "Learner will feel happier by May 2." You can, however, observe behaviors that *indicate* the client's feelings or moods. The following examples allow you to infer that the client is happy:

EXAMPLE: By May 2, will state that he feels happier than before.
By May 2, will be observed smiling at least twice a day.
By May 2, will resume past habit of singing in the shower.

Critical Thinking: Reflecting on Planning

You will use critical thinking to decide which of the patient's problems can be addressed by standards of care, critical pathways, or other standardized approaches and to develop goals/outcomes for the nursing diagnoses that require an individualized approach. Outcome projection is an aspect of therapeutic judgment in which the nurse predicts what is possible to achieve based on available human, material, and economic resources (Gordon et al, 1994). Core questions for reflecting on the planning phase are:

- Is this a useful and usable plan of care?
- Do these outcomes provide a good picture of the changes desired in the patient's health status?
- Are these goals/outcomes stated in a way that makes them useful for planning and evaluating care?

Table 6–8 provides a summary of questions to help you think about your thinking in the planning phase. The remainder of this chapter discusses guidelines to help you think critically about your outcome statements and about the legal, ethical, spiritual, and cultural implications of outcome statements.

Guidelines for Judging the Quality of Outcome Statements

1. *(Standards: Accuracy, Logic)* **The outcome is appropriate to and derived from the nursing diagnosis.** For each diagnosis, at least one desired outcome demonstrates resolution of the problem clause. Outcomes b and c in Figure 6–7 demonstrate this guideline.

TABLE 6–8   Planning Outcomes: Think About Your Thinking

Standard of Reasoning	Questions for Reflection
Clarity	■ Are the goals or expected outcomes stated clearly so that any nurse could use them to measure patient progress? ■ Are the outcomes stated concisely?
Accuracy	■ Would goal achievement indicate problem resolution? ■ Is the outcome appropriate to and derived from the nursing diagnosis? ■ Are outcomes revised to reflect changes in patient status?
Precision	■ Are the goals or outcomes stated precisely and in detail rather than vaguely? ■ Are the outcomes observable or measurable?
Relevance, Significance, Depth	■ What are the most important goals to accomplish? ■ Overall, what is the primary focus of the care for this patient? ■ Am I qualified to make this plan, or do I need help? ■ Are there enough outcomes to completely address each nursing diagnosis? ■ Does each goal statement have the necessary components?
Breadth	■ Does the standardized plan or critical pathway address all the important patient needs, or do I need an individualized plan? ■ Did I make sure the patient and family agree with the goals? ■ Are the goals congruent with the total treatment plan? ■ Are the goals realistic and achievable?
Logic	■ Are the goals or outcomes derived from the patient problem? ■ Is each outcome derived from only one nursing diagnosis? ■ Is the outcome stated as a patient response, not a nurse activity?

Note: Refer to Chapter 2 for a review of standards of reasoning, as needed.

2. *(Standard: Logic)* **Each outcome is derived from only one nursing diagnosis.** An outcome should have only one patient behavior; otherwise, evaluation is difficult. In Outcome a, Figure 6–7, suppose the patient had no urge incontinence but was still having pain when voiding. Would you conclude that the goal was met or not met?

3. *(Standard: Logic)* **The outcome is stated in terms of patient responses rather than nurse activities.** Thinking "Patient will . . ." at the beginning of each goal can help you focus on patient behaviors rather than on your own actions, but do not write, "Patient will."

EXAMPLE:

Nurse Activity (Incorrect)   Prevent infection of incision.

Patient Response (Correct)   Incision will not become infected, as evidenced by:
1. absence of redness.
2. no drainage.
3. edges approximated.

4. *(Standard: Accuracy)* **The desired outcomes are revised to reflect changes in patient status.** As you work with a patient, you will gain a clearer idea of her health status and

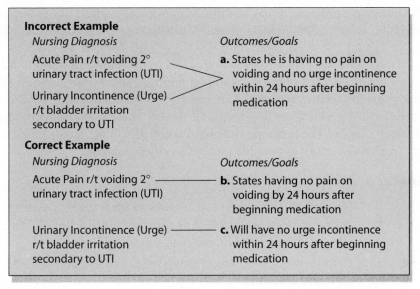

Incorrect Example

Nursing Diagnosis   *Outcomes/Goals*

Acute Pain r/t voiding 2°   **a.** States he is having no pain on
urinary tract infection (UTI)   voiding and no urge incontinence
                                             within 24 hours after beginning
Urinary Incontinence (Urge)   medication
r/t bladder irritation
secondary to UTI

Correct Example

Nursing Diagnosis   *Outcomes/Goals*

Acute Pain r/t voiding 2°   **b.** States having no pain on
urinary tract infection (UTI)   voiding by 24 hours after
                                             beginning medication

Urinary Incontinence (Urge)   **c.** Will have no urge incontinence
r/t bladder irritation   within 24 hours after beginning
secondary to UTI   medication

FIGURE 6–7
Example for guidelines 1 and 3

abilities. You will then be able to write more accurate, individualized outcomes. The following example shows how outcomes can be individualized and revised for a patient with a nursing diagnosis of Activity Intolerance r/t prolonged immobility.

EXAMPLE:

Initial Goal/Outcome: Ability to tolerate activity will improve, as evidenced by:
(General)   1. walking progressively farther each day.
                                 2. increased ability to perform self-care (e.g., hygiene).

Revised Goal/Outcome: Ability to tolerate activity will improve, as evidenced by:
(More specific)   1. by 5/12, walks to chair (8 ft) without shortness of
                                    breath.
                                 2. by 5/12, assists with bath by washing own hands,
                                    face, and torso.

Revised Goal/Outcome: Ability to tolerate activity will improve, as evidenced by:
(After condition   1. by 5/18, sits on side of bed with no change in vital
deteriorates)   signs.
                                 2. by 5/18, assists with bath by washing own face.

5. *(Standard: Clarity)* **Desired outcomes are phrased in positive terms.** In other words, they will be stated in terms of what you hope will occur rather than what you hope will *not* occur.

EXAMPLE:

Negative wording: Skin will not become broken or ulcerated.

Positive wording: Skill will remain intact.

For potential problems, it may be difficult to think of positive terms. It is easier, for example, to write, "No redness" than to describe exactly the color of normal skin. You cannot just write, "Skin color will be normal" because *normal* is too vague. In such instances, you may use negative terms. A measurable, negatively worded outcome is actually a list of the signs and symptoms you are trying to prevent. In Item 3, preceding, outcomes 1 and 2 are negatively worded; outcome 3 is positively worded. The nurse would try to prevent outcomes 1 and 2, and achieve outcome 3.

6. *(Standard: Clarity)* **The outcome statement is concise.** Outcome statements should be stated in as few words as possible without sacrificing clarity.

EXAMPLE:

Wordy: By April 15, the patient will demonstrate adequate knowledge of an appropriate low-calorie diet by listing foods to avoid and foods allowed in each of MyPyramid groups.

More Concise: By 4/15, lists for each food group foods to avoid and foods allowed on low-calorie diet.

As a rule, do not write "patient will." Specify who is to perform the behavior only when it is *not* the patient. You might write, for example, "By dismissal, *Ms. Rauh* will demonstrate ability to change Mr. Rauh's dressing according to printed guidelines she received."

7. *(Standard: Precision)* **The goal/outcome is directly observable or measurable.** Use action verbs to describe what the client will be able to do and to what extent. This ensures that others can make observations to determine whether the goal has been met and the problem has been resolved. In the following example, you cannot observe what the patient knows. However, you could observe whether she can name the high-sodium foods.

EXAMPLE:

Incorrect: By 11/30 will *know* which foods to avoid.

Correct: By 11/30 will *name* the high-sodium foods to avoid in each food group.

You cannot observe actions such as *understands, knows, feels,* or *appreciates.* If you cannot avoid using such verbs, make them more precise by adding the phrase "as evidenced by," followed by the responses you wish to see.

8. *(Standard: Precision)* **The goal/outcome is specific and concrete.** Other nurses should have no doubt about the focus for nursing care when reading an outcome. Vague, general words can be interpreted in several ways and lead to disagreement about whether the outcome has been met. Avoid performance criteria such as *normal, adequate, sufficient, more, less,* and *increased.* Does "increased activity tolerance" mean that the patient can run a mile, or does it mean that he can walk from the chair to the bed with no shortness of breath?

When possible, individualize outcomes to describe the patient's normal baseline measurements. The upper limit of "normal" blood pressure is 140/90 mm Hg, and a goal of "B/P within normal limits" would imply this number. However, for a patient whose B/P is usually 90/50 mm Hg, the "normal" limit is too high.

9. *(Standard: Depth)* **Each goal/outcome statement has all the necessary components.** These include subject, action verb, performance criteria, special conditions (when needed), and target time (usually).

10. *(Standard: Depth)* **Desired outcomes are adequate (e.g., in number) to address each nursing diagnosis.** This is related to Guideline No. 1. Ask, "If these desired outcomes are achieved, will the problem be resolved?" If they are written in very specific terms, several outcomes may be needed for each diagnosis in order to meet this guideline. For the diagnosis of Anxiety, for example, none of the following outcomes by itself would show that anxiety was resolved.

EXAMPLE:

Nursing Diagnosis: Severe Anxiety r/t unresolved role conflicts (mother/wife/attorney)

Outcomes: After one-on-one interaction, will be less anxious, as evidenced by:
1. statements that she feels better.
2. fewer than two episodes of tearfulness in the next 24 hours.
3. smoking no more than one cigarette per hour.

11. *(Standard: Breadth)* **The goal/outcome is valued by the client, family, or community.** The plan of care is more likely to be effective if it is designed to help clients achieve goals that they value. For example, knowing that obesity aggravates hypertension, your goal may be that a client will lose 40 lb. However, if eating is the client's only pleasure, he may not share your goal; he may prefer to accept the risks of hypertension rather than lose his only pleasure. If his goals do not include losing weight, then no matter how good your plan is, it will probably fail.

When nurse and patient goals conflict, it may help to explore the patient's reasoning with him, provide a rationale for your goals, and look for alternative approaches. This will involve the patient in decisions about his care and keep communication open. Involve patients and families to the extent of their interests and abilities. Be sure they agree that the problem is one that requires change and that the outcome is worth achieving. This ensures that your time and energy are spent on plans that meet patient needs and are likely to succeed.

12. *(Standard: Breadth)* **The goal/outcome is congruent with the total treatment plan.** For example, the outcome "Will demonstrate correct technique for bathing baby by postpartum day 2" would not be compatible with the medical treatment plan for a mother whose newborn is too ill to be bathed.

13. *(Standard: Breadth)* **Remember that goals/outcomes can be written for families and communities, as well as individuals.** Refer to preceding discussions of "Family and Home Health Outcomes" and "Community Outcomes."

14. *(Standards: Breadth and Depth)* **The desired outcomes are realistic and achievable** in terms of the client's internal and external resources. Be sure you have considered physical and mental status, coping mechanisms, support system, financial

status, and available community services. The outcome "Will demonstrate desire to comply with treatment by keeping all clinic appointments" is not realistic for a client with no car and no money for cab fare. Clients are not motivated to achieve outcomes they believe to be impossible.

Consider, also, whether the capabilities of the staff and the resources of the agency are adequate to achieve the outcomes. For example, "Uses relaxation techniques to achieve pain relief" is not achievable unless staffing is adequate to allow time for teaching and supervised practice.

6-3 WHAT DO YOU KNOW?

List as many guidelines as you can recall for judging the quality of outcome statements.

See answer to #6-3 What Do You Know? in Appendix A.

Ethical Considerations in Planning

The planning process raises issues about the extent to which patients should be involved in planning their own care and about whether they are truly able to make free and informed decisions about their care. Goals are not value neutral—not even the goals that nurses and patients set together. Merely by stating a goal in the direction of health, we declare that health is something we value. Most people probably do value health, but the situation is not so clear with all goals.

Obligation to Inform

The American Nurses Association code of ethics (2001) states, "The nurse, in all professional relationships, practices with compassion and respect for the inherent dignity, worth, and uniqueness of every individual, unrestricted by considerations of social or economic status, personal attributes, or the nature of health problems." Respect for human dignity derives from the moral principle of autonomy. An autonomous person is one who is both free and able to choose. This suggests that after determining that a client is physically and mentally capable, you should provide the client with information necessary to make informed choices about his care—that is, about the goals for improving health and the means for achieving those goals (interventions and treatments).

Obligation to Respect Choices

It is practical to involve clients in goal setting because it increases their motivation to achieve healthy outcomes. Client motivation is also a moral obligation. Mutual goal setting and care planning demonstrate respect for clients' values and their dignity and worth. Ill persons are vulnerable and dependent. They often believe that health professionals are more capable than they are to make decisions about their care, and their decision-making abilities may be diminished by their illness. When clients are experiencing conflict about choices or when they are too ill to choose, it is appropriate to propose alternatives. In your eagerness to help, however, you can, without even realizing it, impose your own values on the client. Unless you are very sensitive, clients may defer to what they believe you want them to do, without making their true preferences known. Be aware of your power to influence patient decisions and make sure the choices are truly the patient's.

Managed Care and Nursing Values

The prevailing view now is that health care is a business. Treating health care as an item to be bought and sold like furniture is far different from the concept of health care as a human service created by society to meet the needs of the ill. The underlying values in business are economic: cost, efficiency, and effectiveness. Traditional nursing ethical values are respect for persons, advocacy, holistic care, and concerns of justice and fairness (Aroskar, 1995). Managed care and multidisciplinary critical pathways, as well as Medicare and Medicaid guidelines, for the most common and most costly illnesses attempt to balance the business values of cost and quality. Although they may guarantee good care for the majority of patients, they can cause hardship for individuals. Consider the following example:

> **EXAMPLE:** Mrs. Ex, a 65-year-old patient who has diabetes, underwent a quadruple coronary bypass 4 days ago. Before her surgery, she controlled her diabetes with oral hypoglycemic agents, but she now needs insulin injections. She has been discharged home today (Friday), as dictated by the critical path for quadruple bypass. The discharge plan is for a home health nurse to teach her how to administer her insulin. However, the home health nurse does not work on weekends and is not scheduled to see Mrs. Ex until Monday. Who is supposed to administer the insulin twice a day between Friday and Monday? What ethical judgment was used when this patient was assigned to this critical path? A more appropriate hospital stay could have prevented this situation. Or if the family had been involved in the discharge planning, perhaps the husband or one of the children could have been taught (during the hospital stay) to administer the insulin. (Adapted from McGinty, 1997, pp. 267–268.)

When the only outcomes measured in an institution are cost and length of stay, nurses' ethical obligations to care for patients may be compromised (refer to the example of Anna in the section, "Discharge to Home Care"). It is up to nurses to challenge "cookbook" treatment when it is not appropriate or safe. You should understand the need to vary critical pathways in some situations, educate patients, and speak up when this does not happen. If it is not possible to do this where you work, then do so away from work—in churches, schools, and other organizations or by political action. Patients depend on nurses, whether they know it or not, to balance considerations of cost with considerations of care. Nurses know that each intervention is done to a person, not a "case." They must remind politicians and the healthcare industry that this is so.

Legal Issues in Planning

Writing a desired outcome and target time on a nursing plan of care implies that you accept accountability for helping the patient achieve the outcome. Consider this goal/outcome: "Will be able to walk to the bathroom without help by discharge on 8/15."

If the patient goes home without achieving this goal and falls while walking to the bathroom, you could be found negligent unless you have documented good reasons why the desired outcome was not achieved. For this reason, you may wish to write goals for collaborative problems on multidisciplinary care plans only. Recall that for each patient problem you identify, you must decide whether to refer the problem to another discipline or make a nursing plan of care. To help you decide, ask: "Is nursing responsible for initiating the plan to achieve this outcome? Can nursing care produce the outcome (or contribute to it in a major way)?" If not, refer the problem to the professional who is accountable. If you are unsure, consult a more experienced nurse.

Spiritual Planning and Outcomes

Nurses taking a holistic approach ensure that care plans reflect spiritual needs and outcomes. Spiritual care is usually missing from care plans, sometimes because of the nurse's own spiritual uncertainty and sometimes because the nurse fears imposing her own spirituality on the patient. If you have carefully assessed and diagnosed the patient's spiritual needs (see Chapters 3, 4, and 5), you will have a good idea of whether, and what, spiritual care is needed.

Planning should be directed toward helping patients achieve the overall goals of spiritual strength, serenity, and satisfaction. The specific goals you write will, of course, depend on the nursing diagnoses you have made. NOC suggests the following outcomes for a nursing diagnosis of Spiritual Distress (Moorhead et al, 2008, p. 817):

Comfort Status: Psychospiritual: Psychospiritual ease related to self-concept, emotional well-being, source of inspiration, and meaning and purpose in one's life (p. 283)

Coping: Personal actions to manage stressors that tax an individual's resources (p. 314)

Hope: Optimism that is personally satisfying and life supporting (p. 390)

Social Involvement: Social interactions with persons, groups, or organizations (p. 661)

Spiritual Health: Connectedness with self, others, higher power, all life, nature, and the universe that transcends and empowers the self (p. 665)

Using the Omaha System (Martin, 2005), you would apply the Problem Rating Scale for Outcomes to the diagnosis of Spiritual Distress to create desired outcomes. Examples might be:

Spiritual Distress—Goal: Superior knowledge (5)

Spiritual Distress—Goal: Status—minimal signs/symptoms (4)

Using the CCC (Saba, 2006), you would apply the modifiers *improved, stabilized,* and *deteriorated* to the CCC diagnoses of Spiritual State Alteration or Spiritual Distress (e.g., Spiritual Distress, Improved).

Other, nonstandardized, desired outcomes might include that the patient will:

- Fulfill religious obligations.
- Draw on and use inner resources to meet current situation.

- Maintain or establish a dynamic, personal relationship with a supreme being in the face of unpleasant circumstances.
- Find meaning in existence and the current situation.
- Acquire a sense of hope.
- Access spiritual resources.

Cultural Considerations in Planning

The focus for culturally competent planning is to support a client's practices and incorporate them into the plan of care whenever possible and when they are not contraindicated for health reasons. This requires you to be open to learning about different beliefs and values and to not be threatened when they differ from your own. When patients are "noncompliant," it may be because they are complying with their valued cultural beliefs, rather than the caregiver's valued plan of care. Clients are more likely to adhere to an agreed-upon plan that incorporates their cultural perspectives.

Specific outcomes, whether you use standardized language or create your own, depend on the nursing diagnoses you have identified for the patient. For example, for a diagnosis of Impaired Communication r/t foreign language barrier, you might have a goal that the patient "will be able to communicate basic needs to the staff." A culturally sensitive plan of care can promote respectful and excellent care for every patient (Walsh, 2004).

SUMMARY

Planning

- Begins when the patient is admitted and continues until dismissal.
- Can provide a written framework necessary for individualizing care and obtaining third-party reimbursement.
- Helps ensure continuity of care when the patient is discharged.

Care plans

- Can be standardized or individualized.
- Can be multidisciplinary or primarily for nursing care.

Goals or desired outcomes

- Are guides to planning and evaluation that motivate the patient and the nurse by providing a sense of achievement.
- Are stated in terms of specific, observable, achievable patient behaviors.
- Should consist of subject, action verb, performance criteria, target time, and special conditions.
- May be short or long term.
- Can be written for individuals, families, and groups.
- Should be culturally sensitive.

Standardized language for nursing-sensitive outcomes

- Has been developed by NOC, the Omaha System, and the CCC.
- Can be used to write goals in acute-care, home, and community settings.

Ethical and legal considerations in planning

- Are based on the principle of autonomy, and imply a moral obligation to inform and involve clients in their own care.
- Require the nurse to be accountable for outcomes written on the nursing plan of care.
- Require the nurse to carefully balance the values of cost and care.

CRITICAL THINKING AND CLINICAL REASONING: A CASE STUDY

Your patient is a 69-year-old African American man who has had hypertension and diabetes for 15 years. This is his fourth postoperative day after undergoing partial amputation of his foot because of poor circulation. His diabetes is under control, and before hospitalization, he was injecting his own insulin. He is being discharged with a referral to a home health agency. A nurse will be assigned to administer IV antibiotics, change his foot dressings, and monitor his blood glucose levels. (Look up *diabetes* and *peripheral vascular insufficiency* in a medical/surgical textbook, as needed, to answer the questions for this case.)

1. Does this patient actually need a nurse to monitor his blood glucose levels when he returns home? Explain your reasoning, considering the following:
   a. What is the effect of stress (e.g., surgery) on diabetes and blood glucose levels?
   b. What is the relationship between activity and diabetes? What can you say about this patient's activity level?
   c. How predictable is the course of his wound healing?
   d. What is the relationship between food intake and diabetes? How might this patient's intake differ from presurgery days?
   e. Given all that, do you think his insulin needs will decrease, increase, fluctuate, or remain the same?
2. The discharge plan of care contains a nursing diagnosis, "Risk for Delayed Wound Healing related to impaired peripheral circulation." What risk factors are present to support this diagnosis?
3. State a goal that is the opposite, healthy response of delayed wound healing. How will you be able to tell if the goal is being met? What would you assess for?
4. Would you write "delayed wound healing" as a potential nursing diagnosis or as a collaborative problem? Why?
5. Because of the potential for infection of his wound, you need to teach the patient the signs and symptoms of infection, as well as actions to take if symptoms occur.

How will you know that he has mastered this knowledge? Write outcomes you could use on a plan of care.

6. Should the home health agency try to assign an African American nurse to his case? Why or why not? If a male nurse is available, should he be assigned? Why or why not?

7. After returning home, do you think this patient will be able to provide for his:
   - Nutritional needs?
   - Self-care needs (e.g., bathing, hygiene, toileting, dressing)?
     Explain your reasoning.

8. Write goals or desired outcomes that would demonstrate that the patient's nutritional and self-care needs are being met.

9. This is postoperative day 4, and the patient is being discharged tomorrow. What is your highest priority for care today? Explain your reasoning.

10. What is the home health nurse's highest priority for care during the first week of visits to the patient's home? Explain your reasoning.

Remember that answers will vary based on knowledge, experience, and values. The most meaningful learning comes from discussing the case with others.

See suggested responses to Critical Thinking and Clinical Reasoning: A Case Study in Appendix A

Pearson **Nursing Student Resources**

Find additional review materials at **www.nursing.pearsonhighered.com**
Prepare for success with additional NCLEX®-style practice questions, interactive assignments and activities, Web links, animations and videos, and more!

Planning: Interventions

7

Introduction

In the nursing process, the nurse identifies:

1. The patient's nursing diagnoses (present health status)
2. Goals or expected outcomes (the desired health status)

The next logical step is to choose the interventions that are most likely to bring about the desired changes. This chapter focuses on choosing nursing interventions and writing nursing orders. Figure 7–1 presents an overview of the planning interventions phase. Box 7–1 contains professional standards of practice for planning interventions.

Nursing Interventions

A **nursing intervention** is any action based on clinical judgment and nursing knowledge that a nurse performs to achieve patient outcomes. Nursing interventions are also referred to *as nursing actions, activities, measures,* and *strategies.* As a rule, this text will use interventions and the other terms interchangeably except when referring specifically to the Nursing Interventions Classification (NIC), in which the terms *interventions* and *activities* have specific meanings. Regardless of which term is used, nursing interventions include a broad range of activities.

Types of Interventions

Nursing interventions and activities are identified and ordered during the planning phase; however, they are actually performed during the implementation phase. They may be independent, dependent, or interdependent.

LEARNING OUTCOMES

After completing this chapter, you should be able to do the following:

- Define the terms *nursing interventions*, *nursing activities*, and *nursing orders*.
- Recognize nursing interventions for observation, prevention, treatment, and health promotion.
- Given a nursing diagnosis or desired patient outcome, generate alternatives for nursing interventions.
- Name the components of a nursing order.
- Follow specified guidelines for writing nursing orders.
- Use critical thinking standards to evaluate the quality of nursing interventions and orders.
- Describe the use of standardized terminology for nursing interventions.
- Discuss interventions specific to family, home, and community health.
- Describe the ethical, legal, and cultural factors to consider in planning interventions.

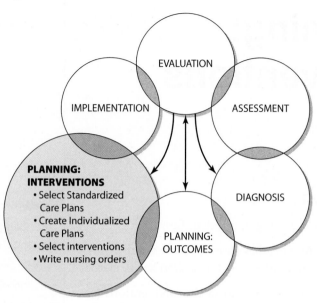

FIGURE 7–1

The planning phase: interventions and nursing orders

BOX 7-1

PROFESSIONAL STANDARDS OF PRACTICE FOR PLANNING INTERVENTIONS

American Nurses Association Standard 4. Planning

The registered nurse develops a plan that prescribes strategies and alternatives to attain expected outcomes.

Competencies

The registered nurse:
1. Develops in partnership with the person, family and others an individualized plan considering the person's characteristics or situation, including but not limited to, values, beliefs, spiritual and health practices, preferences, choices, developmental level, coping style, culture and environment, and available technology.
2. Develops the plan in conjunction with the patient, family, and others, synthesizing patients' values and beliefs, developmental level, and coping style.
3. Includes strategies in the plan of care that address each of the identified diagnoses or issues. These strategies may include, but are not limited to, strategies for promotion and restoration of health and prevention of illness, injury, and disease as well as the alleviation of suffering and provision of supportive care for those who are dying.
4. Provides for continuity within the plan of care.

BOX 7–1

PROFESSIONAL STANDARDS OF PRACTICE FOR PLANNING INTERVENTIONS *continued*

5. Incorporates an implementation pathway or timeline within the plan.
6. Establishes the plan priorities with the patient, family, and others as appropriate.
7. Utilizes the plan to provide direction to other members of the healthcare team.
8. Defines the plan to reflect current statutes, rules and regulations, and standards.
9. Integrates current scientific evidence, trends and research affecting care in planning.
10. Considers the economic impact of the plan on the patient, family, caregivers, or other affected parties.
11. Documents the plan of care in a manner that uses standardized language or recognized terminology, and is understood by all participants.
12. Includes strategies for health, wholeness, and growth from infancy through old age.
13. Explores practice settings and safe space and time for both the nurse and person/family/significant others to explore suggested, potential and alternative options.
14. Modifies the plan based on the ongoing assessment of the patient's response and other outcome indicators.

(*Note:* There are additional measurement criteria for advanced practice RNs.)

Note: This material is from the draft for public comment (ANA, 2010, in press); its wording may be somewhat changed in the final published version (August 2010). For that version of the ANA standards, visit http://www.nursingworld.org.

Source: Reprinted with permission from American Nurses Association (2010, in press). In *Nursing: Scope and standards of practice* (2nd ed.). (Public Comment draft, January). Silver Spring, MD. Available at http:/nursebooks.org.

Canadian Standards (Example)

The following is an example of Canadian standards of practice that apply to planning, excerpted from College and Association of Registered Nurses of Alberta (CARNA) (2003). *Nursing Practice Standards*. Available at http://www.nursingworld.org/DocumentVault/NursingPractice/Draft-Nursing-Scope-Standards-2nd-Ed.aspx.

Standard 2. Knowledge-Based Practice

The registered nurse continually strives to acquire knowledge and skills to provide competent, evidence-based nursing practice.

1. The registered nurse supports decisions with evidence-based rationale.
2. The registered nurse uses appropriate information and resources that enhance patient care and achievement of desired patient outcomes.
3. The registered nurse demonstrates critical thinking in collecting and interpreting data, planning, implementing, and evaluating all aspects of nursing care.
4. The registered nurse exercises reasonable judgment and sets justifiable priorities in practice.
5. The registered nurse documents timely, accurate reports of data collection, interpretation, planning, implementing, and evaluating care.

Independent interventions are those that nurses are licensed to prescribe, perform, or delegate based on their knowledge and skills. NIC refers to these as *nurse-initiated treatments* that are autonomous actions based on scientific rationale (Bulechek et al, 2008, p. xxi). Mundinger uses the term *autonomous nursing practice*: "Knowing why, when, and how to position clients and doing it skillfully makes the function an autonomous therapy" (1980, p. 4). Nurses are accountable, or answerable, for their decisions and actions with regard to independent activities. For example, a nurse may diagnose Impaired Oral Mucous Membranes and plan and provide special mouth care for a patient. The nurse is then accountable for the effects of that action.

Dependent interventions are prescribed by the primary care provider and carried out by the nurse. Medical orders commonly include orders for medications, intravenous (IV) therapy, diagnostic tests, treatments, diet, and activity. Nurses are responsible for explaining, assessing the need for, and administering the medical orders. Nurses may write orders to individualize the medical prescription, based on the patient's status.

EXAMPLE:

Medical Order	Progressive ambulation, as tolerated
Nursing Orders	**1.** Dangle for 5 min, 12 hr post-op.
	2. Stand at bedside 24 hr post-op; observe for pallor, dizziness, and weakness.
	3. Check pulse before and after amb. Do not progress if P <110.

Interdependent interventions (also called *collaborative interventions*) are carried out in collaboration with other health team members, such as physical therapists, social workers, dietitians, and physicians. Collaborative activities reflect the overlapping responsibilities of, and collegial relationships among, health personnel. For example, the physician might order physical therapy to teach the client crutch-walking. The nurse would be responsible for informing the physical therapy department and for coordinating the client's care to include the physical therapy sessions. When the client returns to the nursing unit, the nurse would assist with crutch-walking and collaborate with the physical therapist to evaluate the client's progress.

Theory-Based Planning

Recall from Chapter 3 that theories are used to organize assessment data, and from Chapter 4 that theories provide the perspective for what is likely to count as a problem. This idea carries through to planning, when goals and nursing actions are generated to address the identified problem. For example, if an infant has Pain (Colic), a nurse taking a "gastrointestinal" (GI) perspective might say that the etiology is ineffective peristalsis propulsion of intestinal gas, with overdistention of the GI tract. A logical nursing action, then, might be to decrease gas by burping the infant frequently. A nurse using a "parental anxiety/tension" theory might say that the etiology is overstimulation or unmet needs because of parental anxiety/tension. That nurse might write a nursing order to decrease parental tension by encouraging the parents to relax and spend some time away from the baby (Ziegler, 1993).

7-1 WHAT DO YOU KNOW?

1. Which type of nursing intervention is ordered by the primary care provider: independent, dependent, or collaborative?
2. Which type of nursing intervention is an autonomous action based on scientific rationale: independent, dependent, or collaborative?

See answer to #7-1 What Do You Know? in Appendix A.

Nursing Interventions and Problem Status

Take-away point: Depending on the status of the nursing diagnosis, you will choose nursing interventions for observation, prevention, treatment, and health promotion (Table 7–1).

1. **Observation.** This includes observations to determine whether a complication is developing, as well as observations of the client's responses to nursing, medical, and other therapies. Observation interventions are needed for every problem: actual, risk, and possible nursing diagnoses and collaborative problems.

EXAMPLE:

Auscultate lungs q8h.

Observe for redness over sacrum q2h.

Assess for urinary frequency.

Intake and output, hourly.

TABLE 7–1   Types of Nursing Orders in Relation to Diagnoses

Actual Nursing Diagnosis	Risk Nursing Diagnosis	Possible Nursing Diagnosis	Collaborative Problems
Observation for improvement or complications	**Observation** for change to "actual" status	**Observation** to confirm or rule out diagnosis	**Observation** for onset of complication
			Physician notification of problem onset
Prevention of further complications	**Prevention** Remove or reduce risk factors		**Prevention** Includes physician orders, nursing policies and procedures
Treatment Remove causal and contributing factors Relieve symptoms			**Collaborative Treatments** to relieve or eliminate problem

2. **Prevention.** Prevention activities are those that prevent complications or reduce risk factors. They are used mainly for risk nursing diagnoses and collaborative problems, but they can also be appropriate for actual nursing diagnoses.

EXAMPLE:

Turn, deep breathe, and cough q2hr.   (Prevents respiratory complication)
If fundus is boggy, massage until firm.   (Prevents postpartum hemorrhage)
Refer to county health department for   (Prevents specific disease: measles)
    measles immunizations.

3. **Treatment.** This includes teaching, referrals, physical, and other care needed to treat an existing problem. Treatment measures are appropriate for actual nursing diagnoses. Notice that the same nursing activity may accomplish either prevention or treatment of a problem (compare these examples with the preceding examples).

EXAMPLE:

Turn, deep breathe, and cough q2h.   (Treats respiratory problem)
If fundus is boggy, massage until firm.   (Treats actual postpartum hemorrhage)
Help client plan exercise regimen.   (Treats actual Activity Intolerance)

4. **Health Promotion.** When there are no health problems, the nurse helps the client to identify areas for improvement that will lead to a higher level of wellness. Health-promotion strategies help the client promote positive outcomes rather than avoid negative outcomes. Health promotion is not specific to any disease or problem but aims to encourage activities that will actualize the client's general health potential.

EXAMPLE:

Discuss the importance of daily exercise.
Teach components of a healthy diet.
Explore infant-stimulation techniques.

7-1 THINK & REFLECT!

Describe one activity you have performed (or have seen another nurse perform) in clinical in each of the following categories: observation, treatment, prevention, and health promotion.

See suggested responses to #7-1 Think & Reflect! in Appendix A.

Specific nursing activities for each of the preceding categories might include physical care, teaching, counseling, emotional support, making referrals, and managing the environment.

Teaching Not all teaching requires a separate, formal teaching plan. Informal teaching is an intervention for many, if not most, nursing diagnoses. You will find that you are teaching almost constantly as you explain to clients what you are doing for them and why. Informal teaching may include such activities as explaining the expected effects and side effects of a medication, explaining why the client should not ambulate without help, clarifying the need for fluid restrictions, or teaching patients for self-care (e.g., to use a blood glucose meter).

Counseling and Emotional Support Counseling includes the use of therapeutic communication techniques to help clients make decisions about their health care and perhaps make lifestyle changes. It also involves techniques for helping clients recognize, express, and cope with feelings such as anxiety, anger, and fear. Counseling includes emotional support, but emotional support may occur on a less complex level: it may be given simply by the nurse's touch, presence, or apparent understanding of the client's situation. An example of a counseling strategy would be to help a client to recognize when she is anxious by pointing out symptoms as you observe them.

Referral You should make referrals when the client needs in-depth interventions for which other professionals are specifically prepared. For instance, although a nurse may counsel an anxious patient, long-term treatment of severe anxiety would be referred to a psychotherapist or counselor. Nurses often make referrals for follow-up care after discharge. An example of a referral activity is referring a patient to the Social service department for transportation to a clinic.

Environmental Management Nursing activities are often intended to provide for a safe, clean, therapeutic environment. Environmental management includes removing hazards for clients who are particularly at risk for injury—for instance, children, elderly people, and those with a decreased level of consciousness.

> **EXAMPLE:**
>
> Teach mother to check temperature of formula with back of hand.
>
> Remain at bedside while client is smoking.
>
> Keep crib rails up at all times.

Selection Grid Figure 7–2 is a grid you might use to be sure you have considered all the various types of nursing interventions for a patient. First think of the observations that apply to the problem. For example, if one of your interventions is to auscultate the patient's lungs, place an X in the box under "Observation" and beside "Physical Care." You might wish to teach a patient to assess her own blood glucose levels; if so, place an X in the box under "Observation" and beside "Teaching." Probably none of the other actions in the vertical column would fit under "Observation." Next consider what kind of physical care, teaching, and so on would be involved in preventive nursing orders. Continue to move across the top of the grid in this manner.

7-2 THINK & REFLECT!

When deciding whether to make a referral or deal with a patient's problem yourself, ask (a) What are my knowledge and experience in this area? (b) Does this require in-depth or specialized knowledge that I lack? (c) Do I have any values, beliefs, or biases that could interfere with the quality of care I give for this problem? Which of the following situations would you refer? Why?

1. Mary has come to the clinic for a prenatal visit. When you comment on some bruises, she tells you that her husband beats her. She says, "I'm even afraid for my kids. We need to get out of there, but I don't know where to go or how I'd support the kids."
2. Elaine has just given birth and plans to breastfeed her baby. She is about 25 lb overweight now, and she asks you how she can lose the weight and still maintain her milk supply.
3. A patient's care plan has a nursing diagnosis of "Impaired Gas Exchange r/t changes in alveolar-capillary membranes secondary to chronic lung disease."
4. Would an experienced community health nurse or psychiatric nurse practitioner have addressed the first situation the same way as you did?

See suggested responses to #7-2 Think & Reflect! in Appendix A.

How to Generate and Select Nursing Activities and Interventions

For any given problem, several nursing interventions might be effective. Select the ones that are most likely to achieve the desired goal, taking into consideration the patient's abilities and preferences, the capabilities of the nursing staff, the available resources, and the policies and procedures of the institution. You need creativity for generating new and effective interventions. Even if an intervention has been useful in the past, always rethink it to be sure it is the best way for the patient with whom you are working. The following decision-making process will guide you in selecting the best interventions.

	Observation	Prevention	Treatment	Health Promotion
Physical Care	X			
Teaching	X			
Emotional Support				
Activities of Daily Living				
Environmental Management				
Referrals				

FIGURE 7–2

Grid for identifying nursing interventions

Review the Nursing Diagnosis

Choose nursing strategies that eliminate or reduce the etiology (cause) of the nursing diagnosis. When it is not possible to change the etiological factors, choose interventions or activities to treat the signs and symptoms or the defining characteristics in NANDA International (NANDA-I) terminology. Review the nursing diagnosis to be sure you understand the problem and etiology. Be sure you are familiar with the factors causing or contributing to actual problems and the risk factors that predispose the client to potential problems. You should also know the signs and symptoms associated with any risk diagnoses or collaborative problems. In the following example, the nursing actions should reduce the contributing factor, breast engorgement.

EXAMPLE:

Nursing Diagnosis: Ineffective Breastfeeding r/t breast engorgement

Nursing Actions: **1.** Teach to massage breast before feeding.
                       2. Use hot packs or hot shower before nursing infant.

Nursing interventions are individualized primarily from the second clause (etiology) of a nursing diagnosis. The etiology describes the factors that cause or contribute to the unhealthy response and the nursing activities would specifically target these causal and contributing factors.

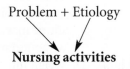

Problem + Etiology

Nursing activities

Any number of factors may contribute to a problem, but it would be inefficient and probably ineffective to address them all. Nursing orders should address the etiological factors specific to a given client. For example, many factors could contribute to Constipation: lack of knowledge, lack of exercise, eating habits, long-term laxative use, or a schedule that causes the client to ignore the urge to defecate. A well-written nursing diagnosis states which factors are causing the client's problem, suggesting nursing interventions that deal directly with those factors. The following example illustrates how different etiologies suggest different nursing actions. Notice that in both cases, the *problem* is the same.

EXAMPLE:

Nursing Diagnosis	*Nursing Orders/Activities*
Constipation *r/t long-term laxative use*	**1.** Work with the client to develop a plan for gradual withdrawal of the laxatives.
Constipation *r/t inactivity and insufficient fluid intake*	**1.** Help client to develop an exercise regimen he can follow at home. **2.** Help client plan for including sufficient fluids in his diet.

You may also need to select interventions for the problem clause of the nursing diagnosis. For a diagnosis of chronic pain related to joint inflammation, nursing orders might include some pain-relief interventions that have nothing to do with relieving joint inflammation; for example:

Observe level of pain before and after activity.

Give back rub (to promote general relaxation of tension).

Instruct client to take analgesic before pain becomes too severe.

Teach slow, rhythmic breathing as a pain control method.

Review the Patient Goals/Outcomes

You should also review the patient outcomes you wish to achieve. They will help you to choose nursing interventions specific to the individual patient.

EXAMPLE:

Nursing Diagnosis: Risk for Ineffective Breastfeeding r/t breast engorgement

Goals:	*Nursing orders suggested by goals:*
1. Infant will be observed to "latch on," suck, and swallow.	**1a.** Observe infant at breast for effective latching on, sucking, and swallowing.
	1b. Teach mother to make these observations.
	1c. When sucking is not long and rhythmic, institute massage of alternate areas of breast without removing infant from breast.
2. Infant will regain birth weight of 8 lb, 6 oz within 14 days after birth.	**2a.** Weigh infant daily at 0600.

Identify Alternative Interventions or Actions

Keeping goals and etiology in mind, think of all the nursing activities that might bring about the desired responses. Include unusual or original ideas. Don't try to predict at this point which ones would be best.

Perhaps you are wondering, "How will I be able to think of interventions to address the etiology? How will I know which actions will achieve the goals?" Principles and theories from nursing and related courses (e.g., anatomy, physiology, psychology) are good sources of ideas for nursing actions. You may also wish to consult resources such as standardized taxonomies (e.g., NIC), model care plans, agency procedure manuals, nursing texts, journal articles, instructors, and practicing nurses. Remember to consult the patient and his family about the care they find to be most helpful.

Ask yourself two broad questions: (a) What patient responses should I watch for? and (b) What should I do? Then branch out to consider all the possible activities that might address the etiology or achieve the goals. Depending on the type of problem, include both independent and collaborative activities from the categories in the Selection Grid, Figure 7–2.

Select the Best Options

Selecting the *best* of the alternative interventions is a matter of hypothesizing that certain actions will bring about the desired outcome. The best options are those you expect to be most effective in helping the client to achieve the goals. To determine this, ask yourself the following questions:

1. What do I know about this patient (health status, knowledge, abilities, resources)?
2. What do I know about the patient outside the hospital (e.g., beliefs, behaviors, feelings)?
3. How would I feel and what would I think if I were in this situation?
4. What have I done in the past for patients in similar situations?
5. Do I have any personal discomfort with this intervention?
6. What does the patient want or request?
7. What potential ill effects might this intervention have on the patient, and how can we manage them?

Your knowledge, experience, and intuition will help you make these judgments, as will the guidelines for writing nursing orders in the section "Reflecting on Interventions," later in this chapter.

Even carefully selected nursing orders do not guarantee success in meeting client goals. A successful intervention for one client may not work at all for another. In fact, for the same client, an intervention may be effective at one time and not at another. Use interventions based on scientific principles and sound research, when possible, to improve the likelihood of success. For example, research indicates that axillary temperatures for newborns are accurate and safer than rectal temperatures.

Take-away point: American Nurses Association (ANA) Standard 17 (Resource Utilization) requires you to "Assess individual patient care needs and resources available to achieve desired outcomes" (2010, p. 55). Keep this in mind as you choose nursing interventions.

Electronic Care Planning

When you use an electronic care planning system, the computer will generate a list of suggested interventions when you enter either a nursing diagnosis or an outcome (Figure 7–3). You can then choose appropriate interventions from the list or enter strategies of your own. Use of computer prompts helps to ensure that a wide range of interventions is considered. However, one danger in using computerized (and standardized) care plans is the temptation to plug in ready-made solutions rather than look for different, more effective approaches for a particular patient.

Take-away point: For standardized and electronic care plans, always think, "What else might work?" and "How should this be adapted for this patient?"

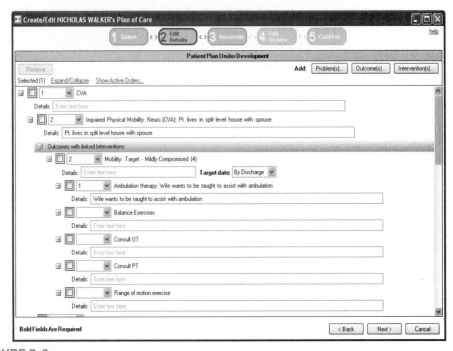

FIGURE 7–3
Computer-generated list of nursing interventions to achieve selected outcomes (*Source:* Copyright 2007–2009 McKesson Corporation and/or one of its affiliates. Used with permission. All rights reserved.)

7-2 WHAT DO YOU KNOW?

List the four steps to follow in generating and selecting nursing interventions.

See answer to #7-2 What Do You Know? in Appendix A.

Writing Nursing Orders

After selecting the appropriate nursing interventions, write them on the plan of care in the form of nursing orders. With computerized care planning, the computer records the interventions as you choose them. You may, however, need to add details specific to your patient. **Nursing orders** are written, detailed instructions for performing nursing interventions. They prescribe the activities and behaviors performed to change present client responses to the desired responses (outcomes). Nursing orders may be something you do for the client or something you help her do for herself. Nursing orders contain more specific, detailed instructions than physician's orders. A physician's prescription relevant to a client's nutritional status might read, "Diet as tolerated." Related nursing orders would specify how the diet is to progress, as well as assessments that need to be made.

EXAMPLE:

1. Auscultate bowel sounds q4hr.
2. Observe for abdominal distention, nausea, or vomiting.
3. Limit ice chips to 1 cup per hour until bowel sounds are auscultated; then give clear liquids as tolerated, for 8 hrs.
4. If no nausea or vomiting, progress to full liquids.

Purpose

Nursing orders provide specific direction and a consistent, individualized approach to the patient's care. They are written as instructions for others to follow, and other nurses are held responsible and accountable for their implementation. Because many different nurses may be involved in caring for a patient, nursing orders must be detailed enough to be interpreted correctly by all caregivers. An order to "force fluids" could be interpreted in many ways. A nurse accustomed to working with young adults might expect this to mean 200 mL/hour; a gerontology nurse might think it means 50 mL/hour; and another nurse might focus on total volume rather than a consistent hourly intake. A better nursing order would be: "Give fluids hourly: Day shift = 1,000 mL total; evening shift = 1,000 mL; night shift = 400 mL."

Components of a Nursing Order

A well-written nursing order contains the following components (see Table 7–2 for examples):

1. **Date the order was written.** The date will be changed to reflect review or revisions.
2. **Subject.** The subject is implied, not written. Nursing orders are written in terms of *nurse* behaviors, so the subject of the order is *the nurse.* As you learn to write nursing orders, think "The nurse will . . ." or "The nurse should . . ." at the beginning of the statement but do not write it.

TABLE 7–2 Examples of Nursing Orders

Subject	Action Verb	Descriptive Phrase	Time Frame	Date and Signature
(Nurse)	(will) Monitor	for verbalization of interest in group activities	with each patient contact	4-14-13 J. Jonas, RN
(Nurse)	(will) Instruct	to avoid drinking liquids with meals if nausea occurs	evening shift 4/14	4-14-13 J. Jonas, RN
(Nurse)	(will) Pad	side rails	during periods of restlessness and confusion	4-14-13 J. Jonas, RN

EXAMPLE:

Goals	*Nursing Orders*
Patient behaviors	**Nurse behaviors**
↓	↓
(*Pt. will*) Walk to the door with help beginning on 2/12.	(*Nurse will*) Assist pt. to ambulate. to the door t.i.d.

3. **Action verb.** This tells the nurse what to do. Examples of action verbs are *offer, assist, instruct, refer, assess, auscultate, change, give, listen, demonstrate,* and *turn.*

   EXAMPLE: *Auscultate* lungs at 0800 and 1600 daily.
               Assist to chair for 30 min. t.i.d.

4. **Descriptive qualifiers.** This is the phrase that tells the nurse how, when, and where to perform the action. It may also describe the action in more detail (what). When one activity depends on another, the descriptive qualifier also includes the sequence in which actions are to be done.

   EXAMPLE: **What**   **When**

   Give   written instructions for incision care   before discharge.

         What   **Sequence/When**

   Take   B/P   before and after ambulating.

5. **Specific times.** State when, how often, and how long the activity is to be done.

   EXAMPLE: Assist to chair *for 30 minutes b.i.d.*
               Change dressing at *0800 and 1400 daily.*

   When scheduling times for the nursing actions, consider the patient's usual rest time, visiting hours, mealtimes, and other activities of daily living. Also coordinate the times with collaborative tests and treatments (e.g., physical therapy).

6. **Signature.** The nurse who writes the order should sign it, indicating acceptance of legal and ethical accountability. A signature also allows other nurses to contact the writer for questions or feedback about the order.

7-3 WHAT DO YOU KNOW?

List the six components of a nursing order.

See answer to #7-3 What Do You Know? in Appendix A.

Standardized Language for Nursing Interventions

Chapter 5 discusses efforts to standardize nursing language and presented vocabularies for describing problems that require nursing care. Chapter 6 presents information about standardized languages for describing patient outcomes. The following is a discussion of standardized terminology for *nursing interventions.* Standardized vocabularies provide a means for nurses to communicate their contributions and participate fully in the multidisciplinary team.

The Nursing Interventions Classification System

The NIC system was developed by a nursing research team at the University of Iowa. The fifth edition includes 542 interventions nurses perform on behalf of patients. NIC classifies nursing interventions into seven *domains*: basic physiological, complex physiological, behavioral, safety, family, health system, and community (Bulechek et al, 2008).

Each NIC intervention has a label, a definition, and a list of activities outlining the key actions of nurses in carrying out the intervention (Box 7–2). The NIC *label* is the standardized terminology used in planning and documenting care. *Activities* are more specific actions a nurse might take in performing an intervention. As you can see in

---

BOX 7–2

NIC INTERVENTION: BATHING

Definition

Cleaning of the body for the purposes of relaxation, cleanliness, and healing

Activities

Assist with chair shower, tub bath, bedside bath, standing shower, or sitz bath, as appropriate or desired

Wash hair, as needed and desired

Bathe in water of a comfortable temperature

Use fun bathing techniques with children (e.g., wash dolls or toys; pretend a boat is a submarine; punch holes in bottom of plastic cup, fill with water, and let it "rain" on child)

Assist with perineal care, as needed

Assist with hygiene measures (e.g., use of deodorant or perfume)

Administer foot soaks, as needed

Shave patient, as indicated

Apply lubricating ointment and cream to dry skin areas

Offer hand washing after toileting and before meals

Apply drying powders to deep skin folds

Monitor skin condition while bathing

Monitor functional ability while bathing

Source: Dochterman, J. M., & Bulechek, G. M. (Eds.). (2008). *Nursing Interventions Classification (NIC)* (5th ed). St. Louis: Mosby, p. 153. Used with permission from Elsevier.

Box 7–2, not all activities would be needed for a particular client, so you would chooses the appropriate activities and individualize them to fit the client's needs and the supplies, equipment, and other resources available in the agency.

Standardized languages are especially useful in computerized care planning systems. Figure 7–4 shows the NIC intervention, Cardiac Care: Rehabilitative; the nurse chooses from the list of activities provided. Use of standardized terminology and computerized planning does not mean that the nurse gives routine, "cookbook" care. Instead, the nurse using NIC chooses which interventions to use for a particular patient (as in Figure 7–4), when to use them, and which activities to adapt to the patient's needs and preferences. Figure 7–5 shows how the nurse can individualize a nursing activity chosen from a computer list. Box 7–3 summarizes the benefits of standardized language for interventions.

Community Nursing Interventions

Community health nurses need terms to describe interventions for individuals, families, and "aggregates" (groups of people or entire communities). An example of a nonstandardized community intervention would be to establish a nurse-managed foot clinic.

The NIC is currently being used in community settings such as schools and public health departments (Parris et al, 1999). "A community (or public health) intervention is targeted to promote and preserve the health of populations. Community interventions

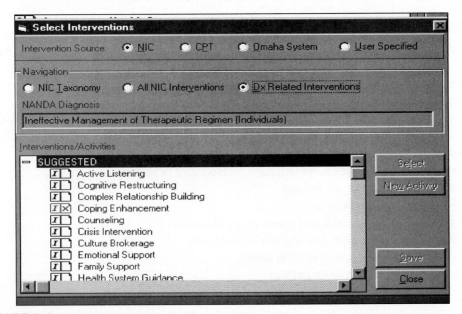

FIGURE 7–4

Computer screen listing standardized (NIC) interventions for a NANDA-I diagnosis (*Source:* Copyright © Ergo Partners, L. C. All rights reserved. Used with permission.)

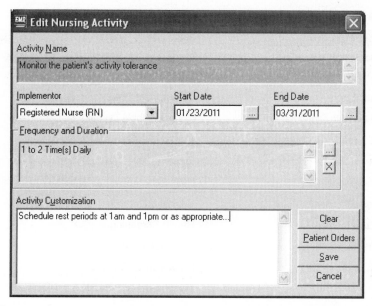

FIGURE 7–5

Computer screen illustrating the customization of an activity chosen from a computer list (*Source:* copyright © Ergo Partners, L. C. All rights reserved. Used with permission.)

emphasize health promotion, health maintenance, and disease prevention of populations and include strategies to address the social and political climate in which the population resides" (Dochterman & Bulechek, 2004, p. 38). The NIC includes 18 interventions to support the health of the community (Table 7–3).

BOX 7–3

BENEFITS OF STANDARDIZED INTERVENTIONS

Standardized language:

- Enhances communication among nurses and between nurses and non-nurses.
- Makes it possible for researchers to determine the effectiveness and cost of nursing treatments.
- Helps communicate the nature of nursing to the public.
- Helps demonstrate the impact that nurses have on health care.
- Makes it easier for nurses to select appropriate interventions by reducing the need for memorization and recall.
- Facilitates the teaching of clinical decision making.
- Contributes to the development and use of computerized clinical records.
- Assists in effective planning for staff and equipment needs.
- Aids in development of a system of payment for nursing services.
- Promotes full and meaningful participation of nurses in the multidisciplinary team.

TABLE 7–3 NIC Community Health Interventions

Community Health Promotion: Interventions that promote the health of the whole community	Community Risk Management: Interventions that assist in detecting or preventing health risks to the whole community
Case Management	Bioterrorism Preparedness
Community Health Development	Communicable Disease Management
Fiscal Resource Management	Community Disaster Preparedness
Health Education	Environmental Management: Community
Health Policy Monitoring	Environmental Management: Worker Safety
Immunization/Vaccination Management	Environmental Risk Protection
Program Development	Health Screening
Social Marketing	Risk Identification
	Surveillance: Community
	Vehicle Safety Promotion

Source: Reprinted from Bulechek, G., Butcher, H., & Dochterman, J. (Eds.). (2008). *Nursing Interventions Classification (NIC)* (5th ed.). St. Louis: Mosby, pp. 90–91. Used with permission from Elsevier.

The Omaha System has four categories of interventions (Martin & Scheet, 1992): (a) health teaching, guidance, and counseling; (b) treatments and procedures; (c) case management; and (d) surveillance. These are used in combination with 63 **targets**—objects of nursing interventions or activities. In addition to physical targets such as bowel care, cardiac care, and nutrition, examples of public health targets are caretaking and parenting skills, day care and respite, durable medical equipment, employment, environment, finances, housing, legal system, and transportation. The following are examples of intervention statements (the italicized portions of the interventions are nonstandardized, client-specific words added by the nurse to individualize the interventions):

"Surveillance: Safety: *basics in home*"

"Health Teaching, Guidance, and Counseling: Nutrition: *normal patterns*"

Even though it was developed specifically for community health nursing, the Omaha System does not include any diagnoses or interventions that are specifically targeted for entire communities or aggregates.

Family and Home Health Interventions

Home health nurses use both individual and family interventions. The NIC taxonomy (Table 7–4) includes three classes of around 75 interventions that support the family (Bulechek et al, 2008). Other NIC interventions can be used with NANDA-I family diagnoses as well. For example, for Compromised Family Coping, an intervention of

TABLE 7-4 NIC Family Interventions Classes

Classes	Examples of Interventions
Childbearing Care: Interventions to assist in the preparation for childbirth and management of the psychological and physiological changes before, during, and immediately after childbirth	Birthing Family Planning: Contraception Newborn Care Preconception Counseling
Childrearing Care: Interventions to assist in raising children	Attachment Promotion Developmental Enhancement: Adolescent Lactation Counseling Teaching: Toddler Nutrition
Life Span Care: Interventions to facilitate family unit functioning and promote the health and welfare of family members throughout the life span	Caregiver Support Family Therapy Home Maintenance Assistance Respite Care

Source: Adapted from Bulechek, Butcher, & Dochterman (Eds.). (2008). *Nursing Interventions Classification (NIC)* (5th ed.). St. Louis: Mosby, pp. 86–88. Used with permission from Elsevier.

"Developmental Enhancement: Adolescent" might be used, although it is not found in the family classes. The NIC is particularly useful because it can be used in all healthcare settings. This helps to bridge the gap between inpatient and home care.

Home care nurses commonly use the Clinical Care Classification (CCC) because it is closely related to the reporting forms required by Medicare. The CCC defines a *nursing intervention* as "a single nursing service—treatment, procedure, or activity—designed in response to a diagnosis to achieve an outcome to a diagnosis—medical or nursing—for which the nurse is accountable" (Saba, 2003). This system includes 198 nursing interventions, each consisting of a label (e.g., Denture Care) and a definition. For each intervention, the nurse must specify the *type of intervention action*—one or more of the following: assess/monitor, care/perform, teach/instruct, or manage/coordinate. For example, a complete intervention statement might be: Denture Care: Assess and Teach. Interventions are linked to the nursing diagnoses they address. Although none are specifically designated as family interventions, some are useful for families (e.g., Caregiver Role Strain; Family Processes Alteration; Home Maintenance Alteration; Terminal Care: Bereavement Support; Terminal Care: Funeral Arrangements; and Stress Control). See Box 7–4 for examples of CCC nursing components and interventions.

The Omaha System can also be used to describe home health interventions for individuals and families. In this system, problems are designated as "family" or "individual," which determines whether the intervention is for the family or an individual.

BOX 7–4

EXAMPLES OF CLINICAL CARE CLASSIFICATION NURSING INTERVENTIONS

M. Role/Relationship Component
    38. Communication Care
    39. Psychosocial Care
        39.1 Home Situation Analysis
        39.2 Interpersonal Dynamics Analysis
        39.3 Family Process Analysis
        39.4 Sexual Behavior Analysis
        39.5 Social Network Analysis

N. Safety Component
    40. Substance Abuse Control
        40.1 Tobacco Abuse Control
        40.2 Alcohol Abuse Control
        40.3 Drug Abuse Control
    41. Emergency Care
    42. Safety Precautions
        42.1 Environmental Safety
        42.2 Equipment Safety
        42.3 Individual Safety
    68. Violence Control

Specify Type of Intervention Action: Assess/Monitor, Care/Perform, Teach/ Instruct, Manage/Coordinate.

    Each Core Intervention must be modified by one of each of the four listed Action Types

Source: Saba, V. K. (2003). CCC Sabacare. Clinical Care Classification (CCC) System. Available at http://sabacare.com.

7-4 WHAT DO YOU KNOW?

1. (True or false) The nurse should choose the NIC intervention labels and activities best suited to your patient's needs.
2. Which classification system was developed specifically for community health: NIC, Omaha, or CCC?

See answer to #7-4 What Do You Know? in Appendix A.

Formal Teaching Plans

Nurses provide a great deal of informal teaching. In fact, at least some teaching interventions may be needed for every one of a patient's nursing diagnoses. Patients with complex teaching needs (e.g., a patient with newly diagnosed diabetes) may need separate, formal teaching plans.

Teaching plans should include the teaching strategies to use in presenting the new information or skill. The appropriate strategy depends on the client's needs and the learning outcome you are working toward. Cognitive content is usually taught through discussion, lecture, printed materials, and audiovisuals. Psychomotor skills need to be demonstrated and discussed and then reinforced with practice. Affective goals generally require role modeling, discussion, and counseling to help the client gain insight. You should write nursing orders for teaching plans in the same format as other orders. They contain the content to be covered, the teaching strategy to be used, and the learner activities assigned or used in the session. An example of a teaching order would be "Demonstrate technique for drawing up insulin."

Teaching orders and strategies should be based on principles of teaching and learning. You may wish to refer to a basic nursing text for more information about teaching strategies, such as role modeling, discussion, demonstration, and use of audiovisual materials. To improve the effectiveness of your teaching plan, keep the following principles in mind:

1. **Assess the learner's knowledge and abilities.** Many factors affect a client's ability to learn, including existing knowledge, previous experience, education, age, and health status. Misconceptions and misinformation may interfere with learning new facts. Illness or sensory-perceptual deficits may make it difficult for the client to process or remember information.
2. **Present content from simple to complex.** This makes the content easier to understand. Learning is a sequential process in which new information builds on previous knowledge and experience.
3. **Use repetition and reinforcement.** Continued practice helps the client to retain new information. Rewards may be internal (personal) or external (praise). Pride in accomplishment can be a good learning incentive.

Wellness Interventions

Wellness interventions stress self-responsibility and active client involvement. The nurse may suggest health-promotion strategies, considering the client's age, sex, lifestyle, education, sociocultural background, and other variables. However, the client is the primary decision maker; the nurse functions mainly as teacher and health counselor. Activities needed for goal achievement may be written in terms of what the nurse is to do or what the client is to do.

Nursing orders on plans for wellness care may take the form of specific behavioral changes the client wishes to make (e.g., "I would like to stop smoking") and strategies for reinforcing the new behaviors. The most effective rewards are self-rewards rather than reinforcement from the nurse.

> **EXAMPLE:** A moderately overweight client wishes to lose weight.
>
> | *Specific Behavioral Changes* | *Rewards* |
> |---|---|
> | I will walk for 45 minutes every day for the next 2 weeks. | I will buy myself a new jogging suit. |
> | I will not eat between meals for 1 week. | I will treat myself to dinner out at my favorite seafood restaurant. |

Most disease-prevention/health-promotion strategies involve lifestyle modifications such as diet changes, regular exercise, stress reduction, or smoking cessation. Motivation for change is sometimes difficult when no actual problem exists. A number of behavior-change strategies are available for helping clients to modify health behaviors—for example, self-reevaluation, cognitive restructuring, modeling, consciousness raising, and reward management. Pender et al (2006) may be useful if you wish to develop detailed nursing strategies to promote high-level wellness.

Standardized Wellness Interventions

Nurses will find the NIC useful in health promotion. It contains all of the interventions nurses use to promote wellness, although they are not all grouped together in one class (Dochterman & Bulechek, 2004). A few CCC interventions also have specific wellness applications. The following are examples of NIC wellness interventions:

Decision-Making Support	Oral Health Promotion
Exercise Promotion	Parent Education
Health Education	Substance Use Prevention
Weight Management	

The following are examples of CCC Wellness Interventions:

Health Promotion	Mental Health Promotion
Nutrition Care: Regular Diet	Mental Health Screening (Saba, 2003)
Safety Precautions	

The Omaha System also works well in health promotion. One of the 75 Omaha intervention *targets* is Wellness. It is defined as "Practices that promote health, including immunization, exercise, nutrition, and birth control" (Martin & Scheet, 1992, p. 83). Using the Omaha System, the nurse would combine a *target* with one of the four *intervention categories* (following) to create wellness interventions for health promotion diagnoses.

EXAMPLE:

Omaha Intervention Categories	*Examples of Wellness Targets*
Teaching, Guidance, and Counseling	Wellness
Treatments and Procedures	Screening Procedures
Case Management	Stimulation/Nurturance
Surveillance	Support System
	Nutrition

Interventions:

Teaching, Guidance, and Counseling: Nutrition

Surveillance: Wellness

For more information about writing interventions using the Omaha System, go to the website at http://www.omahasystem.org.

Spiritual Interventions

Planning should be directed toward helping clients achieve the overall goals of spiritual strength, serenity, and satisfaction. A common intervention is to arrange a visit from a clergy member. Some clients may directly ask to see the hospital chaplain or their own clergyman. Others may discuss their concerns with the nurse and ask about the nurse's beliefs as a way of seeking an empathic listener. However, it is important to ask the client before arranging such assistance. Some people may profess no religious beliefs and may not wish to see a chaplain. The nurse should respect the clients' wishes in this area and not make judgments about whether they are right or wrong.

Spiritual care includes anything that touches a patient's spirit—comforting the family of a dying patient, a late-night conversation with a patient before surgery, or simply sitting quietly at the bedside. If you choose to provide spiritual care and the patient wishes it, interventions can include talking, listening, prayer, reading scripture, fostering hope, and talking to patients about the role of religion in their life (DiJoseph & Cavendish, 2005; Grant, 2004; Laukhuf & Werner, 1998). Interventions used most often by oncology, parish, and hospice nurses to support client spirituality are shown in Box 7–5.

NIC priority interventions for Spiritual Distress are Spiritual Growth Facilitation and Spiritual Support. The other NIC suggested interventions for Spiritual Distress are found in Box 7–6. The Omaha System includes an intervention target of Spiritual Care, defined as "activities directed toward management of religious concerns" (Martin & Scheet, 1992, p. 84). Although not categorized as "spiritual," other standardized interventions could also be used (e.g., Management: Support System in the Omaha System; Meditation Facilitation in the NIC).

Take-away point: Standardized nursing languages can be used to describe wellness and spiritual interventions.

BOX 7–5

SPIRITUAL INTERVENTIONS IMPLEMENTED MOST FREQUENTLY

As reported by 208 oncology, parish, and hospice nurses in the Midwest, in order of frequency.
1. Active listening
2. Conducting a spiritual history and assessment
3. Conveying acceptance, true regard, respect, and a nonjudgmental attitude
4. Therapeutically communicating with clients to facilitate and validate clients' feelings and thoughts
5. Affirming the value of being part of a religious community
6. Touch
7. Conducting self-assessment of own spirituality
8. Presence
9. Prayer
10. Health education

Source: Adapted from Sellers, S. C., & Haag, B. A. (1998). Spiritual nursing interventions. *J Holistic Nurs, 16*(3), 338–354.

Thinking Critically About Planning

Generating interventions is similar to generating hypotheses in the scientific method. Nurses use therapeutic judgment to determine which interventions are most likely to achieve the desired outcomes. This requires critical thinking skills such as generalizing, explaining, predicting, making interdisciplinary connections, and using insights from subjects such as physiology and psychology.

BOX 7–6

EXAMPLES OF NIC INTERVENTIONS FOR SPIRITUAL DISTRESS

Anticipatory Guidance	Grief Work Facilitation
Coping Enhancement	Guilt Work Facilitation
Counseling	Hope Instillation
Crisis Intervention	Presence
Decision-Making Support	Spiritual Growth Facilitation
Dying Care	Spiritual Support
Emotional Support	Support Group
Forgiveness Facilitation	Values Clarification

Source: Adapted from Bulechek, G. M., Butcher, H. K., & Dochterman, J. C. (2008) *Nursing Interventions Classification (NIC)* (5th ed.). St. Louis: Mosby. With permission from Elsevier.

Reflecting on Interventions

Use the following questions to think critically about the interventions you have chosen. The critical thinking standards are in parentheses (review Table 2–3, as needed).

1. *(Accuracy and Relevance)* **Is there research to support the intervention?** If not, do scientific principles or expert opinions provide rationale for the intervention (e.g., ANA or agency standards of care)?

2. *(Clarity)* **Are the nursing orders concise?** Complex statements may be unclear. Do not include complex, routine procedures on the care plan. Instead write, for example, "See Unit 6 Procedure Manual for tracheal suctioning procedure." If the procedure needs to be modified for a client, the procedural changes should be noted in the nursing order (e.g., "Use alcohol; client allergic to Betadine").

3. *(Clarity)* **Are the nursing orders clearly stated?** Would they be interpreted in the same way by other nurses?

4. *(Precision)* **Do the nursing orders give specific directions?** These would include "when," "how often," and so forth. Instead of "Ambulate with help of one person," the orders should specify, "Ambulate length of hall twice a day, with help of one person." A clear, complete order (see Questions 3 and 6) will probably be precise.

5. *(Precision)* **Is the intervention individualized for the patient's unique needs?** For example, "Encourage fluids" is not individualized. A better nursing order would be "Offer fluids every hour; patient likes orange juice."

6. *(Depth)* **Is each nursing order complete—does it contain all the components?** These include date, signature, action verb, descriptive qualifiers, and specific times.

7. *(Depth)* **Does the plan include a variety of interventions and activities? Have I overlooked any approaches?** Does it include (as appropriate) interventions or activities:
   - that are dependent, independent, and collaborative?
   - for monitoring or assessment, prevention, treatment, and health promotion?
   - for physical care, emotional support, teaching, counseling, activities of daily living, environmental management, and referrals?

8. *(Breadth)* **Is the intervention realistic:**
   - *in terms of patient abilities and resources?* For example, it would be unrealistic to order "Refer to home health agency for aide" if the patient could not afford this service.
   - *in terms of institution resources?* For example, "Turn hourly" may not be a realistic order on a unit that is short staffed.

9. *(Breadth)* **Is the intervention safe?** An example would be a nursing order for range-of-motion exercises that specify, "Do not force beyond the point of resistance."

10. *(Breadth)* **Is the intervention acceptable to the patient?** Was the patient given an informed choice? Were the patient's values and culture taken into consideration? For example, even if a vegetarian client were protein deficient, you would not write an order to add meat to the diet.

11. *(Breadth)* **Are the nurses (including myself) capable or competent to carry out the intervention?** An intervention should be used only if the nurse knows the

scientific rationale for the intervention and has the necessary interpersonal and psychomotor skills.

12. *(Breadth)* **Is the intervention compatible with medical and other therapies?** For example, when there is a medical order for bed rest, you would not write an order to assist the patient with ambulation to prevent constipation.

13. *(Logic, Depth)* **Do the interventions address all aspects of the problem etiology?** If the etiology cannot be changed, do the interventions address the symptoms of the problem?

14. *(Significance)* **Which nursing orders must be carried out first or immediately?**

Reflecting on Ethical Factors

The ANA *Code of Ethics for Nurses with Interpretive Statements* (2001), in Appendix B, emphasizes the role of nurses as patient advocates. An **advocate** is one who defends the rights of another. The healthcare system is complex, and patients may be too uninformed or too ill to deal with it. Many need an advocate to cut through the layers of bureaucracy and help them get what they require. In addition to informing and supporting patients (see Chapter 6), nurses can advocate by mediating—by intervening on the patient's behalf, often by influencing others.

> **EXAMPLE:** Ms. Alberghetti is undergoing combined radiation therapy and chemotherapy for cancer. She tells the nurse that she wonders what these treatments are supposed to accomplish and how long she must take them. "I keep forgetting to ask the doctor. He asks me how I'm feeling, and by the time I finish telling him, I just forget." The nurse intervenes by asking the physician to review with Ms. Alberghetti the reasons for the therapies and their expected duration.

Although the nurse's input is important, many people are involved in making ethical (and other) decisions about interventions (e.g., patient, family, other caregivers). Therefore, collaboration, communication, and compromise are important skills for nurses. When nurses do not have the autonomy to advocate for patients, compromise becomes essential. Integrity-producing compromises are most likely to be produced by collaborative decision making. The following mnemonic, LEARN, may remind you how to mediate and collaborate regarding interventions for patients (Berlin & Fowkes, 1983):

L   Listen to others.

E   Explain your understanding of the situation or issue.

A   Acknowledge and discuss differences (e.g., of opinion).

R   Recommend alternative courses of action.

N   Negotiate agreement or compromise.

Refer to Box 7–7 for your professional responsibilities for providing care in an ethical manner.

BOX 7-7

PROFESSIONAL STANDARDS FOR ETHICAL CARE

Standard 7. Ethics

The registered nurse integrates ethical provisions in all areas of practice

Measurement Criteria

The registered nurse:

1. Uses the *Code of Ethics for Nurses with Interpretive Statements* (ANA 2001) to guide practice.
2. Delivers care in a manner that preserves/protects patient autonomy, dignity and rights.
3. Respects the centrality of the patient/family as core members of any healthcare team.
4. Upholds and advocates for patient confidentiality within legal and regulatory parameters.
5. Serves as a patient advocate assisting patients in developing skills for self advocacy and informed decision-making.
6. Maintains a therapeutic and professional patient-nurse relationship with appropriate professional role boundaries.
7. Demonstrates a commitment to practicing self-care, managing stress, and connecting with self and others.
8. Contributes to resolving ethical issues of patients, colleagues, community groups, systems, and other stakeholders.
9. Takes appropriate action regarding instances of illegal, unethical, or inappropriate behavior that can endanger or jeopardize the best interests of the patient or situation.
10. Cooperates in an interprofessional team to make ethical decisions regarding the application of technologies and the acquisition and sharing of data.
11. Demonstrates professional comportment (openness, honesty, integrity, and authenticity). (Mass. Board of Higher Education Nursing Initiative, 2007)
12. Speaks up when appropriate to question health care practice when necessary for safety and quality improvement.

Note: This material is from the draft for public comment (ANA, 2010, in press); its wording may be somewhat changed in the final published version (August 2010). For that version of the ANA standards, visit http://www.nursingworld.org.

Source: Reprinted with permission from American Nurses Association (2010, in press). In *Nursing: Scope and standards of practice* (2nd ed.). (Public Comment draft, January). Silver Spring, MD. Available at http:/nursebooks.org.

Reflecting on Cultural Factors

During planning, you should use information about the client's and family's cultural values, beliefs, and practices to identify interventions that will support client practices and incorporate them into care as much as possible. For example, the nurse considers the client's food preferences and practices; identifies the person responsible for selecting and preparing foods; and then works with the family to teach them how to select and prepare cultural foods that will comply with therapeutic diet prescriptions (e.g., a low-fat diet).

When planning care activities, you should assess language barriers and consider the need for an interpreter. Sometimes culturally diverse clients require information to avoid confusion or embarrassment. For example, the position for bowel evacuation or the norm for the frequency of bowel movements may differ, or the client who is very modest may need much preparation and support before having an enema. When planning client education for clients whose primary language is not English, try to have written materials translated, use pictures to reinforce the written instructions, and have an interpreter give verbal instructions in the client's primary language.

Identify community resources available to assist clients of different cultures. And finally, try to learn from each transcultural nursing situation you encounter in order to improve the delivery of culture-specific care to future clients.

SUMMARY

Nursing interventions

- Are treatments based on clinical judgment and knowledge that a nurse performs to achieve patient goals/outcomes.
- May be independent, dependent, or interdependent.
- May involve observation, prevention, treatment, or health promotion, depending on the patient's health status.
- Include the activities of physical care, teaching, counseling, emotional support, managing the environment, and making referrals.

When selecting nursing interventions, the nurse should choose those that

- Eliminate or reduce the etiology of the nursing diagnosis, or if that is not possible, treat the signs and symptoms of the nursing diagnosis.
- Are most likely to achieve desired outcomes.
- Are based on research, principles, or expert opinion.

Nursing orders

- Provide specific direction and a consistent, individualized approach to patient care.
- Are stated as nurse behaviors—describe what the nurse is to do.
- Are composed of date, subject, action verb, descriptive qualifiers, specific times, and signature.
- Are concise and clearly stated.

Standardized vocabularies for nursing interventions

- Provide a means for nurses to communicate their contributions to patient outcomes and the multidisciplinary team.
- Include NIC, the Omaha System, and the CCC.
- Can be used to describe the individual, family, and community interventions.

A formal teaching plan

- May be needed for patients with complex teaching needs.
- Should be based on principles of teaching and learning (e.g., proceed from simple to complex; use repetition and reinforcement).

CRITICAL THINKING AND CLINICAL REASONING: A CASE STUDY

Dorothy Evans, an obese 40-year-old woman, is recovering from abdominal surgery performed yesterday. Her care plan includes orders for incentive spirometry and regular turning, coughing, and deep breathing. When you prepare to help her with these activities, she says, "You can help me turn, but I'm not doing that breathing stuff. It hurts too much. I'm just so tired. I need rest more than anything."

1. What complication are the breathing exercises designed to prevent?
2. What factors place Ms. Evans at risk for this complication? Explain.
3. What do you need to know before you can decide what to do first? How will you get that information?
4. What is the most important goal in this situation?
5. What will you say and do to respond to Ms. Evans's concerns about pain and rest? Explain your reasoning.
6. What will you say and do to get her to comply with the treatment plan? Why do you think that will help?
7. How will you know if the plan is successful? What specific assessments must you make?

See suggested responses to Critical Thinking and Clinical Reasoning: A Case Study in Appendix A

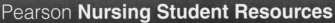

Implementation

8

Introduction

Implementation is the phase in which the nurse performs or delegates the activities necessary for achieving the client's health goals. Described broadly, the activities in this step are (a) doing, (b) delegating, and (c) recording (Figure 8–1). Implementation ends when nursing actions and the resulting client responses have been recorded in the client's chart. Professional standards of practice relating to implementation specifically mention coordination of care and health teaching and health promotion (Box 8–1). For advanced practice nurses, the American Nurses Association (ANA) also describes consultation and prescriptive authority and treatment as aspects of implementation.

You should encourage client participation in implementation, as in all phases of the nursing process. The degree of participation may vary. For example, an infant or an unconscious person cannot participate at all in implementation strategies; all interventions for such patients are carried out by nurses, significant others, or other caregivers. In the case of health-promotion strategies, the client alone might carry out the activities.

> **EXAMPLE:** With the help of his nurse, David Mikos devised a plan for lowering his cholesterol intake. The plan is to follow a low-fat diet at home and reward himself with concert or theater tickets for each month of successful dieting. In this case, the nurse is not involved at all in the implementation phase.

After completing this chapter, you should be able to do the following:

- Discuss the relationship of implementation to the other phases of the nursing process.
- Compare and contrast managed care with case management.
- State ways to enhance patient learning and compliance.
- State guidelines for implementing and delegating safe, effective, and efficient care.
- Explain how to provide ethically, culturally, and spiritually competent care.
- Compare and contrast seven methods of writing nursing progress notes: narrative, SOAP, PIE, PART, Focus® Charting, charting by exception, and integrated plans of care.
- Discuss the pros and cons of computerized documentation.
- Observe guidelines for documenting and reporting patient care and status.
- Explain how documentation in home health and long-term care settings is different from that in institutional settings.
- Describe four common legal pitfalls for nurses and what should be included when documenting them.

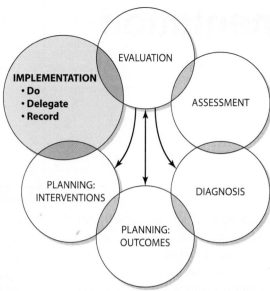

FIGURE 8–1

The implementation phase

BOX 8–1

ANA NURSING STANDARDS OF CARE

ANA Standard 5. Implementation

The registered nurse implements the identified plan.

Competencies

The registered nurse:

1. Partners with the person/family/significant others/caregiver to implement the plan in a safe, realistic, and timely manner.
2. Demonstrates caring behaviors towards patients, significant others and groups of people receiving care.
3. Documents implementation and any modifications, including changes or omissions, of the identified plan.
4. Utilizes technology to measure, record and retrieve patient data, implement the nursing process and enhance nursing practice
5. Utilizes evidence-based interventions and treatments specific to the diagnosis or problem.
6. Provides holistic care that addresses the needs of diverse populations across the lifespan.
7. Advocates for health care that is sensitive to the needs of patients, with particular emphasis on the needs of diverse populations.
8. Applies appropriate knowledge of major health problems and cultural diversity in implementing the plan of care.
9. Applies healthcare technologies to maximize optimal outcomes for patients.

BOX 8–1

ANA NURSING STANDARDS OF CARE *continued*

10. Utilizes community resources and systems to implement the plan.
11. Collaborates with health care providers from diverse backgrounds to implement the plan.
12. Integrates care with other members of the interprofessional healthcare team.
13. Evaluates and assesses the usefulness in integrating traditional and complementary health care practices.
14. Implements the plan in a safe and timely manner in accordance with the National Patient Safety goals.
15. Promotes the person's capacity for the optimal level of participation and problem solving, honoring the person's choices.
16. Coordinates the health care of individuals across the lifespan using principles of interprofessional models of care delivery and case management.

ANA Standard 5a. Coordination of Care

The registered nurse coordinates care delivery.

Competencies

The registered nurse:
1. Coordinates implementation of the plan.
2. Documents the coordination of the care.
3. Coordinates and manages care to meet the special needs of vulnerable populations in order to maximize independence and quality of life.
4. Assists the person to recognize alternatives by identifying options for care choices.

ANA Standard 5b. Health Teaching and Health Promotion

The registered nurse employs strategies to promote health and a safe environment.

Competencies

The registered nurse:
1. Provides health teaching that addresses such topics as healthy lifestyles, risk-reducing behaviors, developmental needs, activities of daily living, and preventive self-care.
2. Uses health promotion and health teaching methods appropriate to the situation and the patient's values, beliefs, health practices, developmental level, learning needs, readiness and ability to learn, language preference, spirituality, culture, and socioeconomic status.
3. Seeks opportunities for feedback and evaluation of the effectiveness of the strategies used.

Note: This material is from the draft for public comment (ANA, 2010, in press); its wording may be somewhat changed in the final published version (August 2010). For that version of the ANA standards, visit http://www.nursingworld.org.

Source: Reprinted with permission from American Nurses Association (2010, in press). In *Nursing: Scope and standards of practice* (2nd ed.). (Public Comment draft, January). Silver Spring, MD. Available at http:/nursebooks.org.

Relationship of Implementation to Other Nursing Process Phases

Implementation depends on the first three phases of the nursing process: assessment, diagnosis, and planning. These steps provide the basis for the autonomous nursing actions performed during implementation. Without them, implementation (and nursing) would reflect only dependent functions—carrying out medical orders and institutional policies. In turn, the implementation step provides the actual interventions and client responses that are reviewed in the evaluation phase.

Implementation overlaps with the other phases. Using data acquired during assessment, the nurse can individualize the care given during implementation, tailoring interventions to fit a specific client rather than applying them routinely to categories of patients (e.g., "All pneumonia patients . . ."). While implementing, you will continue to assess the patient at every contact, gathering data about responses to the nursing actions and about any new problems that may develop. Ongoing assessment is not the same as implementation; it occurs *during* implementation.

EXAMPLE:

Implementation	*Assessment*
While bathing an elderly patient,	the nurse observes a reddened area on the patient's sacrum.
When emptying the catheter bag,	the nurse measures 200 mL and notices a strong odor.

The nurse also implements nursing orders that specifically direct ongoing assessment. For example, a nursing order might read, "Auscultate lungs q4h." When performing this activity, the nurse is both carrying out the nursing order and performing ongoing, focused assessment.

Data obtained during implementation activities are used to identify new diagnoses or to revise existing diagnoses (diagnosis step). These data also enable the nurse to revise and adapt the original goals and nursing orders (evaluation and planning) as the patient's unique needs become more apparent.

Healthcare Delivery Systems

Keep in mind that with the advent of federal healthcare legislation, the healthcare delivery system is likely to change substantially over the next several years. Nursing roles and implementation of care are likely to change as well.

Organizations influence implementation by creating the environment within which nurses provide care. Responding to the demand for healthcare reform, organizations have developed client care approaches that are intended to be cost effective and to provide continuity of care. Two such systems are managed care and case management.

There is a strong movement to incorporate evidenced-based practice into all client care approaches, as mentioned in Chapter 2.

Managed Care

Managed care is used to standardize practice for the most common case types in an agency. For example, case types in a cardiac care unit might be myocardial infarction and cardiac catheterization. The care of a patient is carefully planned from the initial contact to the conclusion of the health problem. Managed care emphasizes cost control, client ("customer") satisfaction, health promotion, and preventive services. Health maintenance organizations (HMOs) and preferred provider organizations (PPOs) are examples of managed care systems. Some hospitals also use managed care approaches.

Third-party payers (e.g., insurance companies, Medicare) usually pay healthcare agencies according to a client's diagnosis or *diagnosis-related group* (DRG), or they pay a fixed amount for each patient treated regardless of the time and resources a client consumes. Therefore, it is essential to achieve specified client outcomes within the length of stay allowed by the client's payer. To this end, managed care systems use standardized multidisciplinary care plans called **critical pathways** for high-volume case types or situations that have relatively predictable outcomes. The critical pathway (a) specifies the time by which each client outcome is to be achieved and (b) outlines crucial activities to be performed by all health team members at designated times. For a discussion of critical pathways, refer to "Multidisciplinary Plans of Care (Critical Pathways)," in Chapter 6. See Figure 10–7 for an example of a critical pathway.

Case Management

Case management is used to coordinate care for high-risk, complex populations who may use a disproportionate share of healthcare resources (e.g., patients with AIDS or chronic obstructive pulmonary disease). Case managers deal with the unusual cases—patients whose condition changes frequently and unpredictably or whose complex needs cannot be addressed by a standardized critical pathway. A case manager—usually a nurse, a nurse-physician team, or a social worker—assumes responsibility for a group of patients from preadmission to discharge or transfer and recuperation. Caseloads may be organized geographically (e.g., clients from all surgical units in a hospital), by diagnosis (e.g., a group of cardiac rehabilitation clients), or by physician. Case managers link patients and families to services (e.g., home health nurse, physical therapy, transportation) in all settings in which the patient receives care. They plan and evaluate the most cost-effective services to meet specified patient outcomes. They also help patients to develop the skills they need to care for themselves and to obtain what they need from the healthcare system.

Take-away point: Implementation activities are doing, delegating, and recording. There is a great deal of overlap among implementation and the other nursing process stages.

> **8-1 THINK & REFLECT!**
>
> Write a scenario illustrating overlapping between implementation and each of the following steps: Assessment, diagnosis, and evaluation. Do not use examples given in your textbook.
>
> **See suggested responses to #8-1 Think & Reflect! in Appendix A.**

Preparing to Act

Preparation for patient-care activities actually begins in the planning phase of the nursing process. When you use time-sequenced planning to set your work priorities and make your daily work schedule, you are actually taking the first step in delivering care to your assigned patients. Box 8–2 is a guide you may wish to use in organizing your nursing care for a clinical day.

Most institutions are concerned about cost and efficiency, so it is important that each nurse–patient encounter be fully utilized. When possible, implement care for several goals simultaneously. For instance, while at the bedside taking vital signs and making physical assessments, you might use the time to talk with the patient, show interest and concern, or do patient teaching.

Preparing the Nurse

Before beginning an intervention, be sure that both you and the patient are prepared. Review the care plan to clarify any details and determine if you need help in performing any of the interventions. You may require assistance under the following conditions:

1. **You lack the skill or knowledge to implement a nursing order.** For example, if you have never taught a patient to crutch-walk, you should ask a colleague for help or review the written procedure before attempting the intervention.
2. **You cannot safely perform the action alone.** For example, you should obtain help when moving a large, immobile patient from a bed to a chair.
3. **Assistance would reduce the client's stress.** For example, having help in repositioning a patient who experiences pain when being moved will minimize her pain.

You are legally and ethically responsible for questioning nursing or medical orders that you believe to be inappropriate or potentially harmful. This should also be done as a part of your preparation.

Preparation includes identifying points in the activity where you need to pause for feedback. The immediate feedback you obtain during an activity guides you in making on-the-spot alterations in the action. For example, when preparing to help a patient ambulate, you might plan to look for responses (feedback) after he sits on the side of the bed for a minute, after standing, after walking to a chair, and again after he has been sitting in the chair for 15 minutes.

BOX 8-2

STUDENT GUIDE FOR ORGANIZING CLINICAL ACTIVITIES

Client profile: Name _____ Age_____

Admitting diagnosis _____ Admit date _____

Name client wishes to be called _____

Significant other(s) _____

Current health status (today):

Has the client's physical or emotional status changed since you received your assignment? Do you need to modify your care plan?

Basic Care Needs:

Hygiene _____

Elimination _____

Feeding _____

Dressing _____

Other _____

Special safety precautions _____

Medications and IVs:

Collaborative tests and treatments (for scheduling and observation)—e.g., physical therapy, radiography:

Prioritized nursing diagnoses and strategies (that you can realistically address today):

New medical orders that need to be implemented (e.g., discontinue IV, ambulate):

Special teaching or counseling needs:

Take-away points:

Are you prepared to act?

Have you reviewed the care plan?

Do you have the necessary skills? Knowledge?

Do you need help to perform the action safely?

Do you need help to reduce stress for the client?

Are there orders that seem inappropriate or potentially harmful?

What are the feedback points?

Preparing the Patient

Do the following to prepare your patient:

- **Reassess whether the intervention is still needed.** Do this just before implementing. Never assume that an order is still necessary simply because it is written on the care plan because the situation or the client's condition may have changed. For example, Gayle Fischer has a nursing diagnosis of Disturbed Sleep Pattern related to anxiety and unfamiliar surroundings. When the nurse makes rounds, she discovers that Gayle is sleeping, so she omits the back rub that was planned as a relaxation strategy.

8-2 THINK & REFLECT!

On the critical pathway for Ms. Fischer, one of the nursing orders for today (postoperative day 2) is "Discontinue IV fluids." However, Ms. Fischer's bowel sounds are infrequent, and she is taking only scant amounts of oral fluids. As her nurse, what would you do?

See suggested responses to #8-2 Think & Reflect! in Appendix A.

- **Assess the client's readiness.** The client's behavioral cues will help you choose a time when the activity will benefit her most. It is a waste of your time to perform interventions when a client is not psychologically ready. For example, when the nurse goes to Ms. Fischer's room to teach her about diabetic foot care, she notices that Ms. Fischer has been crying. Realizing that the patient would probably not be receptive to new information at this time, the nurse decides to postpone the teaching. Do not assume that the patient is ready to progress just because the critical pathway says so.
- **Explain to the client what is to take place.** The client is entitled to an explanation of the action, the sensations he can expect, what he is expected to do, and the results the therapy or procedure is expected to produce. Preparation also includes providing for privacy as well as any physical preparation, such as positioning.

  EXAMPLE: Before administering an enema to Jo Slevin, the nurse explains this will prevent contamination of the surgical area during her bowel surgery. She shuts the door, pulls the curtain around the bed, helps Jo assume a side-lying position, and drapes her with a bath blanket. She tells Jo she will feel pressure and perhaps some cramping as the fluid is instilled, and that she should retain the solution for 5 or 10 minutes until she feels a strong urge to defecate.

Take-away points:

Is the patient prepared?

Determine whether the action is still needed.

Assess the patient's readiness.

Explain what is to be done and what results to expect.

Tell the client what sensations to expect.

Tell the client what she is expected to do.

Provide for privacy.

Preparing Supplies and Equipment

Assemble all necessary equipment and materials before entering the room so you can proceed efficiently and with a minimum amount of stress to the patient. You may need supplies for dressing changes, equipment for removing staples from an incision, linen for a bath and bed change, or pamphlets for a teaching session. The following example demonstrates how inefficient and ineffective it is to stop in midprocedure because the necessary supplies are not at hand.

EXAMPLE: A nurse is inserting a urinary catheter. After draping the patient, opening the sterile kit, and donning sterile gloves, one of the nurse's gloves brushes against the patient's leg. Because she did not think to bring an extra pair of sterile gloves into the room, she is faced with the choice of leaving the patient draped and positioned while she goes for another pair; continuing the procedure with an unsterile glove; or going for new gloves, opening a new cath kit, and redraping the patient to be sure sterility is maintained.

Action: Doing or Delegating

After preparations are complete, action begins. You will apply a wide range of knowledge and skills in performing or delegating planned nursing strategies. The number and kind of specific nursing activities are almost unlimited. They consist of every skill, process, and procedure you will learn as a student and as a practitioner. Cognitive, interpersonal, and technical skills are discussed individually in Chapter 1 in order to facilitate understanding. In practice, however, you will use them in various combinations and with different emphasis, depending on the activity. For instance, when inserting a urinary catheter, you need cognitive knowledge of the principles and steps of the procedure, technical skills in draping the patient and manipulating the equipment, and interpersonal skills to inform and reassure the patient. See Table 8–1 for examples.

TABLE 8–1 Nursing Skills Used in Implementation

Skill	Examples
Cognitive skill	When helping a patient walk, the nurse notices that the IV flow rate is too slow. He quickly checks to see that the tubing is not kinked and that the IV has not infiltrated. When no mechanical problems are noted, he opens the roller clamp to increase the flow. When it is still slow, he raises the bag higher to make use of gravity.
Interpersonal skills	These skills are used with patients, families, and other health team members. The nurse listens actively; conveys interest; gives clear explanations; comforts; makes referrals; delegates activities; and shares attitudes, feelings, and knowledge.
Psychomotor (technical) skills	Performing hands-on skills, such as changing dressings, giving injections, turning and positioning patients, attaching a monitor to a patient, and suctioning a tracheostomy.

The nursing process enables nurses to identify, evaluate, and emphasize their independent activities. However, the full nursing role encompasses dependent and collaborative functions as well. Most nurses provide care for ill clients, whose comprehensive health needs include attention to their medical conditions. In the implementation step, you will implement both the nursing orders on the patient's care plan and the primary care provider's (e.g., physician, nurse practitioner) orders for the medical care plan.

Recall that **dependent interventions** are those performed when following primary care providers' orders or agency policies. Usually they relate directly to the client's medical diagnosis or disease processes.

Collaborative (interdependent) interventions are performed either with other health professionals (e.g., physician, dietitian) or as a result of decisions made jointly with them. **Coordination** of the patient's care is an important nursing activity that is related to, but not the same as, collaboration. This activity involves scheduling the client's contacts with other hospital departments (e.g., laboratory and radiography technicians, physical and respiratory therapists) and serving as a liaison among the members of the healthcare team. As the professionals who are in touch with the patient 24 hours a day, nurses are in the best position to receive all the fragments of information and synthesize a holistic view of the patient. By making rounds with other professionals, reading their reports, and interpreting their findings to patients and families, nurses ensure that everyone gets the "big picture" as well as the specialized one.

Independent (autonomous) interventions are performed when carrying out the nursing orders and often in conjunction with medical orders. In addition to legally conferred autonomy, the nurse's knowledge and critical thinking determine the degree to which an action can be considered autonomous; the same activity can be independent in one situation and dependent in another.

EXAMPLE: Mr. Rauh has a temperature of 100.1°F (37.8°C). The nurse realizes that many things can affect body temperature and asks Mr. Rauh if he had anything to eat or drink before his vital signs were taken. The medical order reads, "V.S. t.i.d;" but because the temperature represents an unusual reading for Mr. Rauh and because the nurse knows he is at risk for infection, she retakes his temperature 1 hour later to establish whether this is a pattern or an isolated cue.

This nurse's actions are independent. If she had been functioning dependently, she would have recorded Mr. Rauh's vital signs without validating their accuracy or questioning their meaning. She might have telephoned the primary provider for instructions or simply passed the data on to the next shift without checking to see if Mr. Rauh's temperature remained the same, continued to rise, or returned to normal.

Accountability is an aspect of autonomy. **Autonomy** implies that the nurse is answerable for her actions and can define, explain, and evaluate the results of her decisions. The nurse in the preceding example is answerable (accountable) for the decisions she made (i.e., to wait an hour and retake Mr. Rauh's temperature before calling the primary provider) and would have been able to provide a rationale for her actions.

Teaching for Self-Care

In this era of early discharge and self-care, patient teaching is an important nursing activity. However, you cannot assume that teaching leads to learning. **Learning** is more likely to occur under the following conditions:

1. The learner has no unmet physical or emotional needs that interfere with learning (e.g., pain, fatigue, hunger).
2. The learner is ready and motivated to learn.
3. The learner is actively involved (e.g., supervised practice with feedback).
4. The environment is conducive to learning (e.g., quiet, appropriately lighted).
5. The emotional climate is favorable (e.g., the client is not angry or anxious).
6. Rapport exists between the patient and nurse.

Even when learning occurs, you cannot assume that the patient will use the information he learns. Patients have many reasons for failing to follow treatment instructions. For example:

- Lack of education for understanding the concepts
- Cultural differences that create a barrier
- Lack of a support system (e.g., lack of money to buy medications)
- Lack of confidence because of past failures (e.g., "I've tried to quit smoking before")
- Reluctance to "bother the doctor (or nurse)" with questions
- A lifestyle that makes adherence difficult (e.g., a salesperson who frequently entertains customers may find it difficult to follow a low-fat, low-salt diet)

You can encourage the patient by assessing his understanding of his illness or injury. This will help you to clear up any knowledge deficits or misinformation. Ask questions and try to discover the patient's viewpoint, priorities, and needs so you can personalize your teaching. For more tips on enhancing adherence, refer to Box 8–3.

8-3 THINK & REFLECT!

Recall a time when you did not follow a doctor's or other health professional's advice. For example, you may have not taken all of the antibiotic capsules, even though the instructions clearly said to do so.
1. List all the reasons you had for not complying.
2. What, if anything, could a nurse have done that would have changed what you did in that situation?

See suggested responses to #8-3 Think & Reflect! in Appendix A.

Delegation and Supervision

Assignment is the transfer of both the responsibility and accountability of an activity from one person to another. For example, when a unit leader assigns a group of patients to an RN for a shift, the RN is both responsible for the care and accountable for the results of that care. **Delegation** is the transfer of responsibility for the performance of a

BOX 8–3

TIPS FOR ENHANCING ADHERENCE

- **Accept the patient as he is.** Respect his values and beliefs. Accept that some attitudes cannot be changed. For example, if a patient does not want to quit smoking, encourage him to reduce the number of cigarettes he smokes each day.
- **Ask the patient what *he* wants to know and what *his* concerns are.** Most patients won't voice their fears unless you ask them. After teaching, ask the patient if there is anything he wants to know that you haven't covered.
- **Be realistic.** Patients may reject big lifestyle or behavioral changes outright. You may need to aim for small changes. No matter how badly he needs to exercise, a patient with overwhelming demands on his time will not be able to exercise every day. It might be better for that person to set a goal to exercise three times a week.
- **Do not assume.** Every patient's situation is different. Don't make the mistake of assuming that the patient understands his disease; that the family is supportive; that the patient has money to buy food or medicine; or that the patient can read, owns a car, or has a phone. Assess carefully.
- **Promote patient confidence,** especially if he has failed in the past. If you can, give examples of other patients who were in similar circumstances and tell how they were able to succeed.
- **Remind the patient that change takes time.** Refer him to a local support or self-help group for ongoing encouragement.

Source: Adapted from London, F. (1998). Improving compliance. What you can do. *RN, 61*(1), 43–46.

task or activity from one person to another while retaining accountability for the outcome (ANA, 2005). For example, the RN can assign an LPN or NAP to take a patient's blood pressure, but if it is inaccurate and the patient becomes seriously hypertensive, it is the RN who must answer for not recognizing that a problem was developing. Because many healthcare institutions use RN extenders (LPNs, NAPs), delegating patient care and assigning tasks is a vital skill. Delegating includes three responsibilities: (a) *appropriate delegation* of tasks, (b) *appropriate communication*, and (c) *adequate supervision* of the RN extender (RNE).

Take-away point: Registered nurses cannot delegate decision-making authority to LPNs or UAPs, but they can delegate the responsibility for performing defined tasks or activities.

Take-away point: You can delegate data gathering duties, such as vital signs or intake and output—but do not confuse these activities with assessment. The RN must be sure the data are accurate and know what the data mean.

Appropriate Delegation

Appropriate delegation means assigning the right activities to the right person. As an RN, when you delegate a task to an RNE, you are essentially guaranteeing that that person is motivated and able to perform the task. This means you must know the RNE's background, experience, knowledge, skills, strengths, and legal scope of practice. You must assess the patient and family to match their needs with the abilities of the various RNEs. Box 8–4 provides suggestions for appropriate delegation, taking into consideration the task, the caregiver, and the patient.

Appropriate Communication

Communication may be oral or written, depending on the circumstances. However, you should leave no room for misinterpretation when giving instructions. For successful delegation, refer to the following guidelines:

1. Set clear boundaries about what to do and what not to do.
2. Be specific in your request (e.g., "Tell me if he seems pale" or "Come get me if he has trouble breathing").
3. Indicate priorities. Explain what must be done immediately and what can be done later.
4. Verify comprehension. Be sure the RNE understands what you want done.
5. Identify and address any of the RNE's concerns.
6. Check your attitude. Be courteous and show respect for each person and the job she does.

Adequate Supervision

The RN is responsible for seeing that delegated tasks are performed adequately. This may mean that you spot check the RNE's work (e.g., retake a blood pressure, check to be sure a patient has been bathed well). How often you need to monitor the RNE's

BOX 8–4

WHAT CAN I DELEGATE?

ACTIVITIES: *You can usually delegate activities that:*

- Are within your scope of practice and the RNE's job description and training.
- Recur frequently in the daily care of a group of patients.
- Require minimal problem solving.
- Have predictable results.
- Have low potential for harm to the patient.
- Are performed according to a standard procedure and require little innovation.
- Do not require the RNE to use nursing judgment.
- Do not require repeated nursing assessments.

PATIENTS: *You can usually delegate care for patients who:*

- Do not need extensive assistance for self-care activities.
- Are relatively stable (i.e., who have a chronic or predictable condition rather than one that has a strong potential for change).

PERSONNEL: *You can usually delegate activities to a caregiver who:*

- Has demonstrated skill in the activity.
- Has performed the activity often.
- Has worked with patients with similar diagnoses.
- Is motivated to perform the activities.
- Has a workload that allows time to do the task properly.

performance will depend on the complexity of the task and how well you know the RNE. You or another RN should be available to observe, facilitate, coach, answer questions, and help as needed. Be sure to speak with the patients after care is given and evaluate both the physical response and the relationship between the patient and the RNE.

Give frequent, positive feedback for good performance. When necessary, communicate privately the specific mistakes that were made and listen to the RNE's view of the situation. Perhaps there were too many tasks to complete in the allotted time, there were unforeseen situations that took priority, or the task took longer than expected. Many RNEs receive minimal training, so be prepared to role model and demonstrate caregiving activities as needed.

?

8-1 WHAT DO YOU KNOW?

List at least three ways you can encourage patients to adhere to treatment regimens.

See answer to #8-1 What Do You Know? in Appendix A.

Thinking Critically about Implementation

In the implementation phase, nurses must use knowledge, experience, and critical thinking as they simultaneously "think and do." As you are giving patient care, you should constantly reassess the patient's responses to care. If the patient does not respond as you expected, try to find out why and then modify what you are doing on the spot. Box 8–5 provides guidelines to use as you prepare to implement safe, effective, and

---

BOX 8–5

GUIDELINES FOR SUCCESSFUL IMPLEMENTATION

Prepare the Nurse

1. Determine whether you need help to perform the action safely and minimize stress to the client.
2. Be sure you know the rationale for the action, as well as any potential side effects or complications. When actions are based on practice wisdom, examine them critically.
3. Question any actions you do not understand or that seem inappropriate or potentially unsafe.
4. Determine feedback points and assess the client's response during the activity.
5. Schedule activities to allow adequate time for completion.
6. Delegate tasks to other team members in order to use your time efficiently.
7. Improve your knowledge base by continually seeking new knowledge.

Prepare the Client

8. Reassess for changes in patient status.
9. Determine that the action is still needed and appropriate.
10. Assess client readiness.
11. Inform the client of what to expect and what is expected of him.
12. Provide for privacy and comfort.

Prepare Supplies and Equipment

13. Gather and organize all necessary supplies.

During Implementation

14. Observe the patient's initial response to the intervention.
15. Continue to observe responses as you implement.
16. Adapt activities to the client's age, values, culture, and health status. Remain flexible and make creative modifications as you work.
17. Encourage the client to participate actively.
18. Perform actions according to professional standards of care and agency policies and procedures.
19. Perform actions carefully and accurately.
20. Supervise and evaluate delegated activities.

CRITICAL REFLECTION: IMPLEMENTATION

The critical thinking standards are in parentheses. Review the Standards of Reasoning table in Chapter 2 as needed.

1. *(Clarity)* Did I explain clearly to the patient what to expect? Did he understand?
2. *(Clarity and accuracy)* Did I communicate what I intended? Could my facial expressions or body language have communicated something different than what I intended?
3. *(Accuracy)* Did I perform the activities or skills accurately (e.g., Did I maintain sterile technique when inserting the catheter)?
4. *(Precision)* Did I follow recommended procedures carefully and exactly (e.g., Did I perform a full 3-minute scrub instead of hurriedly washing my hands)?
5. *(Relevance and significance)* Did I prioritize my care in order to carry out the most important interventions, or did I waste time on trivial activities?
6. *(Depth)* Did I forget to do anything?
7. *(Breadth)* Have I assessed responses from the patient's point of view as well as my own? Did I ask for feedback from the patient?
8. *(Breadth)* Did I convey respect for the patient and the family's cultural and spiritual values, beliefs, and practices?
9. *(Logic)* If the patient's responses to the intervention were not as expected, did I recognize that and make adjustments?

efficient care. After caring for the patient, use the questions in Box 8–6 to reflect on what you have done.

Take-away point: Implementation should be safe, effective, and efficient.

Recording

After doing or delegating, the nurse completes the implementation step by recording the nursing interventions and client responses. These nursing progress notes are a part of the agency's permanent record for the client. The **client record (or chart)** is a permanent, comprehensive account of information about the client's healthcare. It consists of various forms on which information is recorded about all aspects of the client's care (e.g., physician's orders; results of laboratory and diagnostic tests; and progress notes written by physicians, nurses, and other caregivers). Nursing documentation in the permanent record is found on the following forms:

1. The initial, comprehensive nursing assessment (admission database)
2. The individualized nursing care plan
3. Nursing progress notes
4. Flowsheets (e.g., graphic sheets, medication records)
5. The client discharge summary

Functions of Client Records

A client record is usually considered the property of the agency, but as a rule, clients have a right to the information in the record on request. Client records are kept for a number of purposes, such as the following:

- **Communication.** The record provides for communication among health professionals who interact with a client, helping to prevent fragmentation, repetition, and delays in client care.
- **Planning care.** Health team members also refer to the client record when planning care. For example, a nurse may use the social worker's data about the client's home environment when developing the discharge teaching plan.
- **Evaluating and improving patient care.** Patient records provide information used by healthcare agencies to evaluate and improve patient care within an institution (see Chapter 9).
- **Providing information to regulating agencies.** In addition, clinical records are reviewed by accrediting bodies such as The Joint Commission to ensure that the institution is meeting appropriate standards.
- **Reimbursement.** Patient records provide documentation necessary for receiving reimbursement from Medicare, Medicaid, and private insurance companies.
- **Serving as a legal document.** The client's record is a legal document and is usually admissible in court as evidence. The chart may be the only evidence that competent care was given.
- **Research, education, and statistics.** Finally, client records provide data for research; information for educating students in health disciplines; and statistics for local, national, and international data banks.

Documenting Nursing Process

The client record should describe the client's ongoing status and reflect the full range of the nursing process. Regardless of the records system used, nurses document evidence of the nursing process on a variety of forms throughout the clinical record (Table 8–2). This section describes flowsheets, progress notes, and discharge and transfer notes, which reflect various aspects of the nursing process.

Flowsheets

Nurses use **flowsheets** to record assessments and interventions that they perform routinely (e.g., daily hygiene care) or frequently (e.g., hourly position changes). For numerical data (e.g., vital signs), **graphic flowsheets** may be used, as in the top of Figure 8–2. At the bottom of Figure 8–2, a computer-generated flowsheet, is a small section for nurses to record routine interventions. Flowsheets provide a quick, accurate method of recording and make it easy to keep data current and track changes in a client's condition. Intervals for recording data may vary from minutes to months. In a hospital intensive care unit, the nurse may monitor a client's blood pressure by the minute; in an ambulatory clinic, nurses may check a client's blood glucose levels only once a month.

TABLE 8–2 Documenting Nursing Process

Nursing Process Components	Documentation Forms	Comments
Assessment	Initial comprehensive database (nursing history and physical assessment), graphic sheets, flowsheets, nursing progress notes, and discharge and referral summaries	Document initial and ongoing assessments. Frequency is determined by organization policy and client condition.
Diagnosis and Planning	Individualized and standardized care plans and critical pathways, protocols, Kardex, teaching plans, discharge plans, problem lists, SOAP (see Table 8-3) and other progress notes containing nursing diagnoses and intervention plans	Document client problems, nursing diagnoses, and strengths. Plans include desired outcomes and interventions. Care plans may be separate or a part of the chart.
Implementation and Evaluation	Nursing interventions and patient responses recorded in progress notes, flowsheets, graphics, and critical pathways	▪ Document observations, interventions performed, and teaching. ▪ Document client and family responses to nursing and medical interventions and important events; progress toward goals; and questions, comments, or complaints. ▪ Document communication with other disciplines (e.g., physician) and results of the communication.

Progress Notes

Progress notes (also called *nurses' notes*) provide information about the client's progress toward outcome achievement. They should augment but not duplicate flowsheet data. Progress notes should include the following:

1. Assessments of the patient's mental and physical condition
2. Patient activities
3. Both nurse-initiated and physician-initiated treatments and interventions, with patient responses
4. Visits by other caregivers or family members, if relevant.

Various kinds of progress notes are discussed in the following section, "Documentation Methods." For examples, refer to Figures 8–3 and 8–4. Some progress notes (e.g., Table 8–3) also include nursing diagnoses or patient needs.

Discharge and Referral Summaries

A **discharge summary** is a special nursing progress note written at the time a client is discharged from the agency. It should include services provided to the client, status of client outcomes at discharge, and recommendations for further care. Many institutions

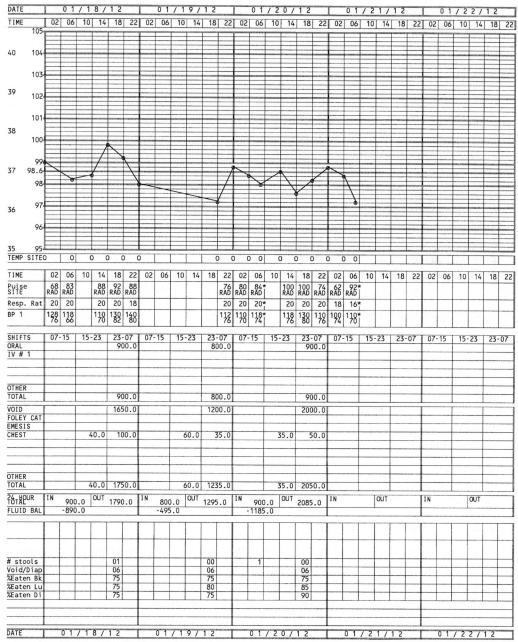

DATE	0 1 / 1 8 / 1 2	0 1 / 1 9 / 1 2	0 1 / 2 0 / 1 2	0 1 / 2 1 / 1 2	0 1 / 2 2 / 1 2

TIME	02	06	10	14	18	22	02	06	10	14	18	22	02	06	10	14	18	22	02	06	10	14	18	22	02	06	10	14	18	22
Pulse SITE	68 RAD	83 RAD		88 RAD	92 RAD	88 RAD						76 RAD	80 RAD	84* RAD		100 RAD	100 RAD	74 RAD	62 RAD	92* RAD										
Resp. Rat	20	20		20	20	18						20	20	20*		20	20	20	18	16*										
BP 1	128 78	118 66		110 70	130 82	140 80						112 76	110 70	118* 74		118 78	130 80	110 76	100 74	110* 70										

SHIFTS	07-15	15-23	23-07	07-15	15-23	23-07	07-15	15-23	23-07	07-15	15-23	23-07	07-15	15-23	23-07
ORAL			900.0			800.0			900.0						
IV # 1															
OTHER															
TOTAL			900.0			800.0			900.0						
VOID			1650.0			1200.0			2000.0						
FOLEY CAT															
EMESIS															
CHEST		40.0	100.0		60.0	35.0		35.0	50.0						
OTHER															
TOTAL		40.0	1750.0		60.0	1235.0		35.0	2050.0						

24 HOUR TOTAL	IN 900.0	OUT 1790.0	IN 800.0	OUT 1295.0	IN 900.0	OUT 2085.0	IN	OUT	IN	OUT
FLUID BAL	-890.0		-495.0		-1185.0					

# stools			01			00	1		00						
Void/Diap			06			06			06						
%Eaten Bk			75			75			75						
%Eaten Lu			75			80			85						
%Eaten Di			75			75			90						

DATE	0 1 / 1 8 / 1 2	0 1 / 1 9 / 1 2	0 1 / 2 0 / 1 2	0 1 / 2 1 / 1 2	0 1 / 2 2 / 1 2

* ADDITIONAL INFORMATION AVAILABLE ONLINE IN OPIS

Shawnee Mission Medical Center
9100 West 74th Street
Shawnee Mission, KS 66204

11:05 01/21/12 FROM *07L,VSPOGSF1

FIGURE 8–2

Graphic flowsheet (*Source:* Courtesy of Shawnee Mission Medical Center, Shawnee Mission, KS).

have a special discharge summary form, which is sometimes combined with the discharge planning form (see Figure 6–2 in Chapter 6). If the client is being transferred to another institution or requires a visit by a home health nurse, the discharge note takes the form of a referral summary. Regardless of format, discharge and referral summaries usually include some or all of the following information:

- Description of client's condition at discharge (including current status of each client problem)
- Current medications and treatments that are to be continued
- Teaching and counseling that was done to prepare the client for discharge
- Instructions for follow-up care given to the client at discharge
- Activity level and self-care abilities
- Support system, significant others
- Mode of discharge (e.g., walking, wheelchair, ambulance)
- Person who accompanied the client
- Where client is going (e.g., home, nursing home)
- Any active health problems

Documentation Methods

Institutional policies and procedures determine the format for documenting progress notes. This section discusses seven documentation methods: narrative, SOAP, PIE, PART, Focus® Charting, charting by exception (CBE), and integrated plans of care (IPOCs).

Narrative, Chronological Charting

Narrative notes (e.g., Figure 8–3), written in paragraph form, are the traditional charting format. Nurses write interventions, client responses, and events in chronological order. To make it easier to find data about a specific problem, specific flowsheets (e.g., 24-hour intake and output record) are often used along with the progress notes. Narrative notes may be combined with flowsheets, as in Figure 8–5, later in the chapter.

SOAP Charting

The SOAP method (Table 8–3) began with the problem-oriented records system in which caregivers from all disciplines write on the same progress notes. However, it is now used in other systems as well. The chart contains a master problem list identified by the whole healthcare team. Each SOAP note refers to a specific problem; multiple problems require multiple notes. SOAP is an acronym for the following (notice that the definitions for "O" and "A" are different from the traditional nursing process definitions):

S—**Subjective data.** This is what the patient tells you. It describes the patient's perspectives, perceptions, and experience of the problem. When possible, quote the patient's words; otherwise, summarize his statement. Include subjective data only when they are important and relevant to the problem.

O—**Objective data.** This is information that can be measured or observed by use of the senses (e.g., vital signs, bowel sounds, radiography results). You will also use this

TABLE 8–3   Comparison of the SOAP, SOAPIER, and APIE Formats

SOAP Format	SOAPIER Format	APIE Format
9/6/12 #5. Nausea 1030 S—Refused breakfast. "I feel too sick." c/o severe nausea during a.m. Stated less severe after IM Compazine. O—Abd. firm but not distended. No bowel sounds heard after auscultating for 5 min. @ quadrant. Vomited × 2: total 300 mL clear, yellow emesis. Closed door; advised to lie still to decrease sensations of nausea. Compazine 5 mg given IM in LVG area at 0930. A—Post-op nausea r/t decreased peristalsis; Compazine somewhat effective. Possible ileus. P—Continue to observe for N&V. If nausea unrelieved by Compazine, notify MD. Continue I&O. Assess hydration q shift. Offer fluids 40 mL/hr if no further emesis.	9/6/12 #5. Nausea 1030 S—Refused breakfast. "I feel too sick." c/o severe nausea during a.m. O—Abd. firm but not distended. No bowel sounds heard after auscultating for 5 min. @ quadrant. Vomited × 2: total 300 mL clear, yellow emesis. A—Post-op nausea r/t decreased peristalsis; Compazine somewhat effective. P—Instruct to lie still to decrease sensations of nausea. Medicate with Compazine. Continue I&O. Continue to assess for N&V. Assess hydration q shift. I—Instructed to lie still to decrease sensations of nausea. Compazine 5 mg given IM in LVG area at 0930. E—States still nauseated but somewhat relieved after Compazine. Lying still most of a.m. No emesis after Compazine. R—Offer fluids 40 mL/hr if no further emesis. If nausea unrelieved by Compazine, notify MD.	9/6/12 #5. Nausea 1030 A—Post-op nausea & vomiting. Refused breakfast. "I feel too sick." Abd. firm, not distended. No bowel sounds heard after auscultating 5 min. @ quadrant. Vomited × 2; total 300 mL clear, yellow emesis. P—Decrease nausea: Instruct to lie still. Compazine per order. Prevent fluid deficit: Continue to assess N&V. Assess hydration q shift. Continue I&O. If nausea and vomiting continue, notify MD. I—Instructed to lie still. Compazine 5 mg given IM in LVG area at 0930. E—Lying still most of A.M. No emesis since Compazine given. States still nauseated, but less severe.

section to record care that has been given (e.g., "Taught procedure for drawing up insulin").

A—Assessment. In this method, *assessment* means an interpretation or explanation of the "S" and "O" data. During the initial assessment, the "A" entry contains statements of the patient's problems (e.g., a nursing diagnosis). In subsequent SOAP notes, the "A" represents evaluation. It describes the patient's condition and level of progress toward goals and is not merely a restatement of the diagnosis.

P—Plan. This is the plan of care designed to resolve the stated problem. The person who enters the problem on the record writes the initial plan (e.g., for a medical problem, the primary provider writes prescriptions for tests and treatments). The plan is continued, updated, or discontinued in subsequent SOAP notes.

SOAPIE and SOAPIER are variations of the SOAP format in which the interventions (I) are written separately from the objective data (O), and an evaluation section (E) is added. The SOAPIER format adds a section for revisions of the plan (R). APIE is a similar format (Groah & Reed, 1983, p. 1184). In this format, the assessment (A) includes both subjective and objective data and the nursing diagnosis; the plan (P) includes predicted outcomes with the nursing orders; and implementation (I) and evaluation (E) are the same as in the SOAPIE format. See Table 8–3 for a comparison of the SOAP, SOAPIER, and APIE formats. Compare these entries with those in Figures 8–3 and 8–4, which contain information about the same incident of nausea.

Take-away point: Narrative notes are organized in chronological order. SOAP notes are organized according to problems.

PIE Charting

PIE charting is similar to SOAP charting. PIE is an acronym for:

P—Problems

I—Interventions

E—Evaluation of patient responses to care

This system supplements the patient progress notes with a flowsheet for assessments and routine care. The nurse keeps a master problem list and rewrites and renumbers it every 24 hours. As in SOAP charting, there may not be a separate care plan.

PART Charting

PART is similar to PIE. However, the problem list is seen as continuous and ongoing, so it is not redone every 24 hours. This method makes use of standards of care, so an individualized plan is not required. However, the nurse records all actual interventions in the chart (Gropper & Dicapo, 1995). PART is an acronym for the following:

P—Problem. This is usually a nursing diagnosis.

A—Actions. This section consists of all interventions actually implemented. It does not contain the plan of care.

R—Response. This section reflects actual patient outcomes. It consists of subjective and objective data describing the patient's responses to the actions or interventions.

T—Teaching. The nurse records all patient and family teaching in this separate section of the progress notes. This is meant to remind the care providers of the importance of this aspect of care.

DATE	TIME	NOTES	SIGNATURE
9-6-12	0800	Refused breakfast. States, "I feel too sick." abd. firm but not distended. No bowel sounds heard p̄ auscultating for 5 min. in ℞ quadrant. Using PCA (morphine) frequently for incision pain (see med. Record).	S. Fried, RN
	0900	200 cc. clear, yellow emesis ———————	S. Fried, RN
	0930	100 cc. clear, yellow emesis. c/o severe nausea. Compazine 5 mg. given I M in LVG area. Closed door & advised to lie still to decrease sensation of nausea.	S. Fried, RN
	1030	States still nauseated, but less severe. No further emesis. T.E.O. hose removed for 15 min & reapplied. No edema or redness on legs. Dangled @ bedside for 5 min. Moves c̄ much reluctance. States, "Hurts too much." ———————	S. Fried, RN

FIGURE 8–3

Patient progress record (nurse's notes)

Date/Time	Focus	Progress Notes
9/6/12 1430	Post-op nausea	**D**—Refused breakfast. Stated, "I feel too sick." C/o severe nausea throughout A.M. Vomited × 2, total of 300 mL clear, yellow emesis. Abd. firm but not distended. No bowel sounds auscultated after listening for 5 min. @ quadrant. **A**—Closed door. Advised to lie still to decrease sensations of nausea. Compazine 5 mg given IM in LVG at 0930 per order. Continue to assess for N&V. If unrelieved by Compazine, notify MD. Continue I&O. Assess hydration × 1 per shift. Increase p.o. fluids to 40 mL/hr if no further emesis. **R**—Nausea somewhat relieved by Compazine. Stated "less severe." No emesis since Compazine administered. See flow sheet for I&O and VS.————————R. Keeler, RN

FIGURE 8–4
Example of a Focus® Charting note

Focus® Charting

Like SOAP notes, Focus® Charting (Lampe, 1985) uses key words to label and organize the progress notes, but the subject of the note is not necessarily a problem (see Figure 8-4). A focus can be a condition, strength, nursing diagnosis, behavior, sign or symptom, significant change in the patient's condition, or significant event. Because the focus should be something requiring nursing care, it should *not* be a medical diagnosis. It can, however, describe needs and conditions associated with a medical diagnosis. For example, foci for a patient with a fractured femur might include preoperative teaching, Acute Pain, Risk for Constipation, and cast or traction assessment. The progress notes column is organized as follows:

D—Data include observations of patient status and behaviors. This might include data from flowsheets (e.g., vital signs). It includes both subjective and objective data, but they are not labeled "S" and "O." This section corresponds to the assessment phase of the nursing process.

A—Action entries include interventions just performed as well as plans for further action. This corresponds to the planning and implementation steps of the nursing process.

R—Response entries describe patient responses to nursing and medical interventions. Data in this section consist of measurements and interventions, many of which will be recorded on flowsheets and checklists. This section corresponds to the evaluation phase of the nursing process.

The focus method is useful for health promotion activities because the nurse can organize around positive headings instead of problems.

Charting by Exception

Charting by exception (CBE) is a system in which only significant findings or exceptions to stated norms are recorded. An agency using CBE must develop its own specific, detailed standards that identify (a) the norms for patient assessments and (b) the minimum criteria for patient care (Murphy & Burke, 1990). The following are examples of standards of care that an agency might develop for hygiene:

The patient will receive or be offered oral care t.i.d.

The patient will receive or be offered a bath and backrub daily and a shampoo once a week.

Figure 8–5 provides an example of a portion of a form used for CBE. The nurse writes a progress note only when patient care or data deviate from the norms printed in the first column. Completed interventions are recorded in the progress notes or flowsheets. Since the initial development of CBE, commercial vendors and healthcare agencies have developed many variations of this system. It has been shown to significantly reduce documentation time as well as costs associated with paper use. It is a legally sound approach if properly implemented and adhered to (Cummins & Hill, 1999).

IPOCs—Charting Integrated into the Plan of Care

As a part of managed care, many agencies have developed critical pathways for common diagnoses and procedures (review Managed Care, earlier in this chapter; Using Nursing Diagnoses with Critical Pathways in Chapter 4; and Multidisciplinary Plans of Care [Critical Pathways] in Chapter 6; as needed). Most critical pathways are "integrated plans of care" (IPOCs) that serve as both a care plan and a form for documenting progress notes (e.g., Figure 8–6). This charting model uses graphics and flowsheets along with the IPOC. For example, Figure 8–6 lists care for the "typical" patient on days 1 to 3 after an open reduction and internal fixation of the femur. The nurse checks each intervention that was done for the patient and fills in applicable blanks. On postoperative day 1, there was no special respiratory care, so nothing is checked in the "RESP" box on Figure 8–6. Under "NEURO/PAIN" the nurse checked "see pain flowsheet," where there would be detailed information about the patient's pain management. She also checked that she had performed a neurosensory assessment. If findings were abnormal, she would have charted them on a different form, or if it required only a few words, in the blank spaces on the IPOC.

Electronic Documentation

Use of computerized nursing care plans is widespread. In addition, electronic documentation is becoming common throughout Canada and the United States. Some agencies have a terminal at each bedside, enabling the nurse to document care immediately after it is given.

Computers make documentation relatively easy. To record nursing actions and client responses, the nurse either chooses from standardized lists of terms or types narrative

THE WESTERN PENNSYLVANIA HOSPITAL

PATIENT CARE
FLOW SHEET

BASELINE PHYSICAL ASSESSMENT: Date _6/9/12_   Time _0800_   RN/GN _J Reed RN_

	NORMALS:	DEVIATIONS:	TIME	PROBLEM/VARIANCE	PROGRESS NOTES
BEHAVIOR-/EMOTIONAL	Behavior and emotions appropriate to situation WNL ☒	☐ Agitated ☐ Depressed ☐ Angry ☐ Anxious ☐ Other ___	08	Neuro	O₂ sat. 70%.
NEUROLOGICAL	Alert & oriented to person, place, time and situation. Speech clear. Follows simple commands. PERL. Sensation intact. WNL ☐	Disoriented to: ☒ Person ☐ Place ☐ Time ☐ Situation ☐ Does not follow commands LOC: ☒ Lethargic ☐ Nonresponsive ☐ Responsive to ___ ☐ Speech deficit ☐ Pupils ☐ R ☐ L ☐ Deficits ___ ☐ Other ___			O₂ admin. per nasal cannula @
					3L/min J Reed RN
			0815	Neuro	O₂ sat. 94% J Reed RN
			0830	Neuro	WNL. J Reed RN
CARDIO-/VASCULAR	Apical regular and HR WNL. Heart tones audible. Peripheral pulses +3. No edema. Capillary refill time <3 secs. WNL ☒	☐ Heart rhythm abnormal ___ ☐ Rate abnormal ☐ Abnormal pulses ___ ☐ Calf tenderness ☐ R ☐ L ☐ Edema (loc/severity) ___ ☐ Other ___			

FIGURE 8–5

Portion of a form used for charting by exception (*Source:* Hill, M., Labik, M., & Vanderbilt, D. (1997). Managing skin care with the CareMap system. *Journal of Wound, Ostomy, and Continence Nursing, 24*(1), 29. Used with permission).

	Date: 3/16/12 **Day 1**	Date: **Day 2**	Date: **Day 3**
MUSCULO SKELETAL / ADL	□☑ **Bedrest** □□ *Buck's Traction #____ □☑ **Turn to injured side for nsg care preop** □☑ **Lock out knees of bed** □☑ **Trapeze to bed** □☑ **Assess knobs of traction, overhead frame & trapeze for tightness** □□ Specialty Bed_____ **Hygiene:** ☑ **Bath**___Help___ □☑ **Oral Care** □□ *Fall/Injury Protocol:* 　□□ Alt in environ___N/A___ 　□□ Diversion_____ 　□□ Physio monitoring_____ 　□□ Pharm Monitoring_____ 　□□ Alarm/alert_____ 　□□ Toileting_____ □□ *Restraint Protocol* See Restraint Flowsheet	□□ **Turn to inoperative side q 2hrs with** 　**pillow between legs** □□ *Buck's Tx #____ □ **Release foot of bed** □□ **Assess knobs of traction, overhead frame & trapeze for tightness** □□ Specialty Bed_____ **Hygiene:** □ **Bath**____ □□ **Oral Care** □□ *Fall/Injury Protocol:* 　□□ Alt in environ_____ 　□□ Diversion_____ 　□□ Physio monitoring_____ 　□□ Pharm Monitoring_____ 　□□ Alarm/alert_____ 　□□ Toileting_____ □□ *Restraint Protocol* See Restraint Flowsheet	□□ **Chair /BSC with assistance** □□ *Weight Bearing Status:____ □□ **Provide egg crate cushion for w/c** □□ **Assess knobs of traction, overhead frame & trapeze for tightness** □□ Specialty Bed_____ **Hygiene:** □ **Bath**____ □□ **Oral Care** □□ *Fall/Injury Protocol:* 　□□ Alt in environ_____ 　□□ Diversion_____ 　□□ Physio monitoring_____ 　□□ Pharm Monitoring_____ 　□□ Alarm/alert_____ 　□□ Toileting_____ □□ *Restraint Protocol* See Restraint Flowsheet
GI / GU	☑☑☑ **Diet:**___Reg.___ □ HS Snack 　□ **NPO after midnight** □☑ **I&O** □□ Cath care □☑ **Last BM**___3/15/12___	□□□ **Diet:**____ □ HS Snack □□ **I&O** □□ Cath care □□ Last BM_____	□□□ **Diet:**____ □ HS Snack □□ **I&O** □□ Cath care □ *DC Cath Time____ □□ Last BM____ □□ If no BM ≥ 72 hrs, RX
RESP	□□ DB q ___ hrs □□ * IS q ___hrs □□ O2 @ ___liters	□□ DB q ___ hrs □□ * IS q ___hrs □□ O2 @ ___liters □ DC O2 if O2 Sat >90% Time____	□□ DB q ___ hrs □□ * IS q ___hrs □□ O2 @ ___liters □ DC O2 if O2 Sat >90% Time____
CIRC	□☑ **VS q 4 hrs** □ **TED hose remove/inspect/replace @ HS** □ **Compression Device remove/replace @HS** 　□ **Foot** □ **Leg** □☑ *Anticoagulant therapy □☑ *IV □□ SL □□ *IV antibiotics □☑ **Assess circ to lower extrem q 2 hrs**	□□ **VS q 4 hrs** □□ **TED hose remove/inspect/replace BID** □□ **Compression Device remove/replace BID** 　□ **Foot** □ **Leg** □□ *Anticoagulant therapy □□ *IV □□ SL □□ *IV antibiotics □□ **Assess circ to lower extrem q 4 hrs** □ * CBC x 3 days	□□ **VS q 4 hrs** □□ **TED hose remove/inspect/replace BID** □□ **Compression Device remove/replace BID** 　□ **Foot** □ **Leg** □□ *Anticoagulant therapy □ *PT/INR □□ *IV □□ SL □□ *IV antibiotics □□ **Assess circ to lower extrem q 12 hrs** □ *CBC x 3 days
SKIN	□□ Start/Change IV/SL Location:① wrist 　Time:___Gauge:___a # attempts:___ t □□ *Skin Integrity Risk Protocol* 　□☑ Instruct / Assist to reposition q 2 　□□ Support surface_____ 　□☑ Buttocks protected/inspected 　□☑ Heels off bed, inspected 　□□ Protectors in place_____ 　□□ Incontinence / moisture care 　□☑ Increase protein / hydration □☑ *Wound Care Protocol* See Wound Care FS	□□ Drain activated/measured q 12 hrs □□ *Bubb*Empty drain when full □□ *Reinforce dressing □□ Change IV/SL Location:_____ 　Time:___Gauge:___a # attempts:___ t □□ *Skin Integrity Risk Protocol* 　□□ Instruct / Assist to reposition q 2 　□□ Support surface_____ 　□□ Buttocks protected/inspected 　□□ Heels off bed, inspected 　□□ Protectors in place_____ 　□□ Incontinence / moisture care 　□□ Increase protein / hydration □□ *Wound Care Protocol* See Wound Care FS	□□ Drain activated/measured q 12 hrs □□ *Bubb*Empty drain when full □□ *Reinforce dressing □□ Change IV/SL Location:_____ 　Time:___Gauge:___a # attempts:___ t □□ *Skin Integrity Risk Protocol* 　□□ Instruct / Assist to reposition q 2 　□□ Support surface_____ 　□□ Buttocks protected/inspected 　□□ Heels off bed, inspected 　□□ Protectors in place_____ 　□□ Incontinence / moisture care 　□□ Increase protein / hydration □□ *Wound Care Protocol* See Wound Care Flowsheet
NEURO/ PAIN	□☑ *Pain Protocol* Assess pain q 4 hrs, after 　each new report and each interventions □☑ See Pain Flowsheet □☑ **Assess neuro-sensory status to effected extremity q 2 hrs**	□□ *Pain Protocol* Assess pain q 4 hrs, after 　each new report and each interventions □□ See Pain Flowsheet □□ *Ice bag □□ **Assess neuro-sensory status to effected extremity q 2 hrs**	□□ *Pain Protocol* Assess pain q 4 hrs, after 　report and each interventions □□ See Pain Flowsheet □□ *Ice bag □□ **Assess neuro-sens status to effected extrem q 2 hrs**
ENDO-CRINE	□□ FSBS q ___ hrs □□ FSBS q AC & HS □□ *Diabetic Protocol*	□□ FSBS q ___ hrs □□ FSBS q AC & HS □□ *Diabetic Protocol*	□□ FSBS q ___ hrs □□ FSBS q AC & HS □□ *Diabetic Protocol*
PSS	□ Obtain Advance Directive □ Verify home meds are reordered	□□ **Encourage verbalization of concerns by pt/SO. Use encouragement, praise & listening skills**	□□ **Encourage verbalization of concerns by pt/SO. Use encouragement, praise & listening skills**
SIGN-ATURE	Shift　Signature　Initial Title Dept 7p-7a　_Jvick_　_Jw_ _RN_ _Ms_	Shift　Signature　Initial Title Dept	Shift　Signature　Initial Title Dept

ORIF FEMUR/HIP PLAN OF CARE
Interdisciplinary Plan of Care
Shawnee Mission Medical Center
Shawnee Mission, Kansas 66204
SMMC # 62069　Revised: 2/18/12　Page 1 of 4

FIGURE 8–6

Portion of a critical pathway or documentation form (*Source:* Courtesy of Shawnee Mission Medical Center, Shawnee Mission, KS).

information into the computer (refer to Figure 8–7 for an example of a computerized progress note). Automated speech recognition technology now allows some nurses to do voice-activated documentation.

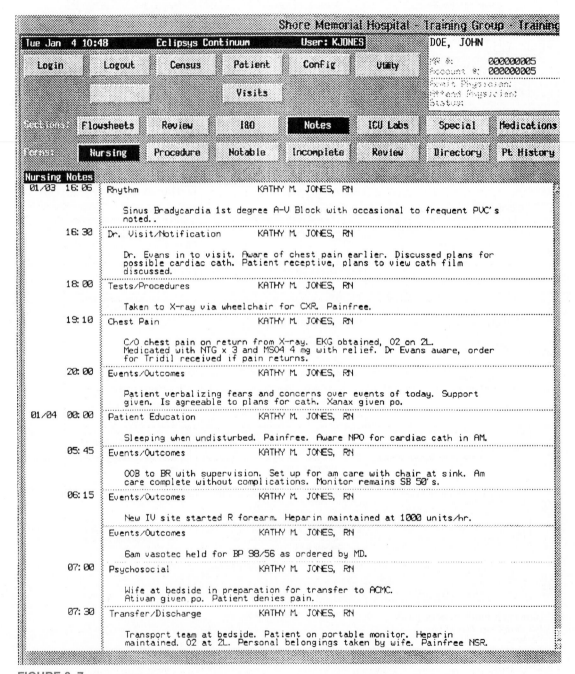

FIGURE 8–7

Computer screen showing nurse's notes (*Source:* Courtesy of Shore Memorial Hospital, Somers Point, NJ. Used with permission).

Because information can be easily retrieved in a variety of forms, multiple flowsheets are not needed in computerized systems. For example, a nurse could obtain the results of a client's blood test, a schedule of all clients on the unit who are to have surgery during the day, a suggested list of interventions for a nursing diagnosis, a graphic chart of a client's vital signs, or a printout of all the progress notes for a client. Selected pros and cons of computer documentation are shown in Box 8-7.

BOX 8-7

SOME PROS AND CONS OF ELECTRONIC HEALTH RECORDS (EHRs)

Pros

Multiple healthcare providers can use the same information at the same time.

Productivity increases; documentation time is reduced.

Accuracy improves, and documentation is more reliable.

Nurse satisfaction and professional practice are increased.

Information can be stored and retrieved easily in a variety of forms; multiple forms are not needed.

Client information, requests, and results are sent and received quickly.

Terminals can record data directly from monitoring equipment.

Bedside terminals eliminate need to take notes on a worksheet before recording.

Information is current.

Information is legible.

Standardized terminology improves communication among care providers.

The system incorporates and reinforces standards of care.

Allows for creation and sharing of huge data files to be used for research and quality improvement.

Medical errors are minimized by programmed alerts that display automatically when a care provider takes an action that could be harmful (e.g., when a provider prescribes a drug to which a patient is allergic or calls for a dose that exceeds the safe range).

Cons

Additional security measures are needed to ensure patients' privacy.

"Downtime" processes must be in place for times when parts of the EHR are not available (e.g., because of power outages, severe weather, and system upgrades).

Initial purchase of hardware and software is very expensive.

Extended training periods may be required.

It is not easy to capture narrative nursing content from paper documentation into an electronic format.

Adapted from Catanzano, F. (1994). Nursing information/documentation system increases quality care, shortens stay at Desert Samaritan Medical Center. *Comput Nurs, 12*(4), 184–185; Kozier et al. (2008). *Kozier & Erb's Fundamentals of nursing: Concepts, process, and practice* (8th ed.). Upper Saddle River, NJ: Prentice Hall; Town, J. (1993). Changing to computerized documentation—PLUS. *Nurs Manage, 24*(7), 44–46, 48. Wilkinson, J., & Treas, L. (2011, in press) *Fundamentals of nursing* (2nd ed) Philadelphia: F. A. Davis.

Documenting with Standardized Language

Chapters 5 to 7 discuss the use of standardized terminology for nursing care plans. Those concepts apply to documenting patient progress as well. For computerized documentation systems, standardized terminology is essential. It is also useful in some pen-and-paper systems. Among benefits described in previous chapters, standardized language allows the nurse to concentrate on the clinical judgment aspects of the nursing process rather than spending time searching for the "right words" to describe interventions and patient responses.

Guidelines for Charting

Requirements for record keeping vary among agencies. Agency policies may describe which personnel are responsible for recording on certain forms, the frequency with which entries are to be made, which abbreviations are acceptable, and the preferred way to handle an error in recording. In addition to legal and policy requirements, you should also observe the following general guidelines (when, what, and how).

When to Chart

1. **Date and time each entry**. Timing guidelines are critical for legal and safety reasons.
2. **Indicate both the time the entry was made and the time the observation or intervention occurred, if different.** For example, in a chart entry timed 1445, you might write, "Drank 150 mL water at 1245, vomited 200 mL clear fluid at 1310."
3. **Record the nursing action or client response as soon as possible after it occurs.** This helps ensure that the client will not be medicated or treated a second time by a different nurse. It is usually acceptable to record routine repetitive nursing actions at the end of the shift (e.g., hourly position changes, mouth care) but keep notes on a worksheet. Don't rely on memory.
4. **Never leave the unit for an extended time unless all important information has been charted.** The rationale is similar to that for Guideline 3.
5. **Do not document interventions before carrying them out.** The client might refuse the treatment or you might encounter an emergency situation that prevents you from carrying out the intervention. Another staff member, seeing it charted, might

conclude the action has been done and would not wish to repeat it. The result would be that the client does not get the proper care.

6. **Document in chronological order.** If you forget to chart something, record it as soon as possible, marking it "Late Entry." If there is a lengthy delay in charting, explain why (e.g., "9/24, 1215—Late entry—Chart not available 9/24 at 1030. Patient c/o shortness of breath. Notified physician").

What to Chart

1. **As a rule, do not chart actions performed by someone else.** In some situations, it is permissible to do so, but your note should identify the person who actually gave the care (e.g., "Assisted to car by nursing assistant. L. Woods, RN").
2. **Progress notes must be accurate and correct.** If you are not absolutely sure about your assessment findings, ask someone else to check before you chart.
3. **Go beyond flowsheet data.** Chart judgments about the data to indicate whether the patient is doing better or worse. Compare the current patient status with previous data (e.g., "Incision becoming redder and beginning to ooze serous fluid").
4. **Progress notes should be factual.** Chart what you see, hear, smell, or observe. To improve the precision of your charting, think, "Exactly what happened, and how, when, and where did it happen?" For example, you would chart, "Talking constantly, pacing the floor; pulse 120," rather than "Patient is anxious."
5. **Progress notes should be clear and specific.** Do not use vague generalities, such as "good," "normal," or "sufficient." It is better to say "a 2×2 cm area of blood" than "a small amount of blood."
6. **Do not use negative, prejudicial terms.** (e.g., uncooperative, noncompliant, unpleasant). Instead, describe what the client did that was uncooperative (e.g., "Yelled, 'Go away!' and threw his tray on the floor").
7. **To organize a narrative entry, include** *D-I-E*. Don't actually label the entry with these letters or words; use them as a memory device.

Data	What did you observe about the patient (S, O)?
Intervention	What actions did you take? What did you do?
Evaluation	What was the patient's response to the actions? What did he say or do? How did his condition change?

8. **Record only appropriate and relevant data.** You do not need to record everything you know about the client. Recording irrelevant data is a waste of time, and it is sometimes an invasion of privacy (e.g., do not chart "slept well" unless this is unusual).
9. **Progress notes should be complete.** This is essential for communication among caregivers, as well as for legal purposes. For example, if there is no record of turning and skin care, nurses may be found negligent if the client develops a dermal ulcer.
10. **Be brief.** Omit unnecessary words, such as *patient*. It is assumed the entry refers to the patient. Progress notes are usually written in incomplete sentences, but be sure to end each thought with a period. For example, write "300 mL clear emesis," rather than, "The patient vomited 300 mL of clear fluid."

11. **Balance conciseness with completeness.** When deciding on the right amount of detail to record:
    - Ask yourself, "What would someone else need to know to understand what is going on with the patient?"
    - Include enough detail to justify any conclusions or judgments you have made (see Item 3).
    - Remember that busy caregivers will not take the time to read a long, wordy note carefully. They will skim over it.

Refer to Box 8-8 for essential information to include in nursing progress notes.

What NOT to Chart

Report the facts. DO NOT chart the following:

- Words suggesting errors (e.g., *accidentally*, *unintentionally*, *by mistake*)
- That an incident report has been filed
- Staff conflicts or critical comments about the behaviors or care given by other team members
- Staffing problems or staff shortages (Use a confidential memo or incident report instead.)

How to Chart

1. **Use dark ink.** Most agencies specify black ink. Erasable ink is not acceptable.
2. **Write legibly or print.** Narcan and Marcaine are different drugs, but they may look almost identical if handwriting is illegible or messy.
3. **Use correct grammar, spelling, and punctuation.**
4. **Use standard symbols, terminology, and abbreviations carefully.** Agencies should have a list of approved abbreviations and terminology. If not, use only those that are standard and used universally. If you are in doubt about an abbreviation, write the term out fully. The Joint Commission (2008) mandates that healthcare organizations not use the following abbreviations. This is referred to as the "do not use" list.

"U" or "u" for unit

"IU" for International Unit

Q.D., QD, q.d., qd (daily)

Q.O.D., QOD, q.o.d., qod (every other day)

Trailing zero (X.0 mg) and lack of leading zero (.X mg)

MS, MSO_4 and $MgSO_4$—could mean morphine sulfate or magnesium sulfate

The following abbreviations and symbols are under serious consideration for inclusion on The Joint Commission's "do not use" list in the future. Some institutions have already stopped using them:

The symbols ">" and "<" (write "greater than" or "less than")

All abbreviations for drug names (write drug names in full)

Apothecary units (use metric units instead)

The symbol "@" (write "at" or "each")

The abbreviation "cc" (write "mL" or "milliliters")

The abbreviation "µg" (write "mcg" or "micrograms")

5. **Sign each entry with your name and title** (e.g., "Kay Wittman, RN" or "K. Wittman, RN").

BOX 8–8

ESSENTIAL DATA TO CHART

1. **A physical symptom that:**
   Is severe (e.g., extreme shortness of breath)
   Recurs or persists (e.g., vomiting after every meal)
   Is not normal (e.g., elevated temperature)
   Becomes worse (e.g., fever increases from 102° to 104°F)
   Is not relieved by prescribed actions (e.g., patient unable to sleep after taking sleeping pill)
   Is a symptom of a complication (e.g., inability to void after surgery)
   Is a known danger signal (e.g., a lump in the breast)
2. **Changes in physical function,** such as loss of balance or difficulty seeing or swallowing.
3. **Behavior changes, such as:**
   Strong expressions of emotion (e.g., crying, yelling, expressing fear)
   Marked changes in mood
   Change in level of consciousness or orientation
   Changes in relationships with family or friends
4. **Nursing interventions,** especially those performed in response to symptoms and changes in patient status. For example:
   Medications administered
   Treatments or therapies (both dependent and independent)
   Patient teaching
5. **Patient responses to nursing interventions; evaluation of outcomes or goal achievement**
6. **Inability to carry out prescribed treatments or patient's refusal of treatments or interventions.** Include your teaching about the need for treatment and the possible consequences of refusal.
7. **Patient's ability to manage care after discharge.**
8. **All medical visits and consultations.** Note time, date, what was discussed, directions given by the physician, and actions you took.
9. **Discussions with the primary provider about your concerns with medical orders.** Note the time; date; what directions the provider gave about confirming, canceling, or modifying the orders; and the actions you took.

6. **The nurse who makes the entry should sign it.** You should not sign someone else's notes. Remember that the person signing the entry is accountable for the entry.
7. **Chart entries on consecutive lines. Never skip a line or leave a line blank.** Draw a line through any blank spaces before or after your signature. For example, "Lungs clear to auscultation. Skin warm and dry. _____ K. Wittman, RN."
8. **Correct errors by drawing a single line through the mistaken entry.** Write the word *error* above it. Initial the error and then rewrite the entry correctly (or follow agency policy). Never try to erase or obliterate the entry; the incorrect entry should still be visible. Do not insert words above the line or between words.
9. **Be sure the client's name and identification number are on every page.**

Home Healthcare Documentation

Home health care is different from institutional care in that fewer caregivers are present to provide and witness the care. The home care record is usually the only evidence of how patient care decisions were made, the only basis for insurance coverage, the only legal record, and the main source of communication among health team members, who do not see each other as frequently as those in a hospital. Home health documentation is often in the form of a **progress summary**—a brief narrative report of a client's health status and needs, nursing interventions performed, and client outcomes and responses. In home health care, progress summaries are used in two ways:

1. They provide the information the physician needs to determine whether to continue medical treatments, to monitor client progress, and to be aware of any new health or treatment problems that develop.
2. They are sent to third-party payers to establish the continuing need for home health care. Medicare regulations, for example, require that progress summaries be written every 60 days to be sure the client meets Medicare requirements. Therefore, the nurse must be sure to address the following in the summary.
   - The client is homebound.
   - The client still needs skilled nursing care.
   - The potential for rehabilitation is good or the client is dying.
   - The client's status is not stabilized.
   - The client is making progress in expected outcomes of care.

The nurse should be certain that the checklists, progress summaries, and other forms also reflect how and why the skills of a professional home care nurse are needed. Documentation should include the following:

- Nursing assessment highlighting changes in the client's condition
- Skilled interventions performed (wound care, dressing changes, teaching, and so on), including the reasons they are needed
- The client's response to interventions
- Any interaction or teaching that the nurse conducted with caregivers
- Any interaction with the patient's primary care provider
- The reasons home care was initiated

- The plan of care (patient outcomes or goals of care)
- Discharge plans (including rehabilitation potential)

A unique problem in home care documentation is that the nurse may need some parts of the client's record in the home while, at the same time, those records are needed in the office. For this reason, many home health agencies provide nurses with laptop computers. In this way, records are available in multiple locations, and nurses can upload new client information to agency records without even traveling to the office.

Long-Term Care Documentation

Documentation requirements for long-term care depend on the level of care the client requires. All residents in long-term care facilities must have a comprehensive assessment at admission. Federal law requires that a resident be evaluated using the Minimum Data Set for Resident Assessment and Care Screening (MDS) within 14 days of admission. The MDS must be updated every 3 months and with any significant change in client condition.

The principles of documentation in long-term care are the same as those explained in this chapter. However, federal and state regulations usually require nurses to document less frequently in long-term care than in acute-care settings. Some long-term care facilities require weekly client progress summaries; others require summaries only every 90 days. Charting should reflect the client's current status (e.g., vital signs, skin condition, status of admitting diagnoses), daily functioning (e.g., mobility, self-care abilities, sleep patterns), and progress toward expected outcomes, with focus on preventive measures and restorative care.

Take-away point: In home care, it is especially important to reflect that the client is homebound and still needs skilled nursing care, that the client's status has not stabilized, and that the client is making progress toward goals.

Take-away point: Nurses usually document less frequently in long-term care; however, the principles of documentation are the same as in other settings.

8-3 WHAT DO YOU KNOW?

1. State two rules relating to *when* to chart.
2. State three rules relating to *what* to chart.
3. State one thing you should *not chart*.
4. State two rules about *how* to chart.
5. List three items of *essential data* to chart (from Box 8-8).

See answer to #8-3 What Do You Know? in Appendix A.

Oral Reports

In addition to written records, nurses use oral reports to communicate nursing interventions and client status. When the client's condition is changing rapidly, physicians and other caregivers must be constantly informed. Oral reports are also given when a client is transferred from one unit to another (e.g., from the emergency department to a medical floor), at change of shift, and when family members request reports of the client's condition. A report is given to communicate specific information about what has been observed, done, or considered. It should be concise but still contain all pertinent information.

A **change-of-shift report** (or **handoff report**) is given to the oncoming nurse by the nurse who has been responsible for the patient. Reports may be given in a meeting, on walking rounds, or on audiotape. Tape-recorded reports are less time consuming but do not allow for questions and clarification. A typical change-of-shift report includes the following:

1. **Basic identifying information for each client.** Name, room number, age, medical diagnosis or reason for admission, admission date, and physicians. This information will vary depending on the setting (e.g., in a long-term care facility, you might omit the admission date).
2. **A description of the client's present condition.** Include only significant measurements. It is not necessary to report that the vital signs are normal unless this is a change for the client (e.g., "After medication, her temperature returned to 98.6°F").
3. **Significant changes in the client's condition.** Report both deterioration and improvement in condition (e.g., "At 1400 her blood pressure was 150/94; baseline was under 130/80 until that time"). When reporting changes, organize your report as follows: state what you observed, its meaning (if appropriate), what action was taken, the client's response, and the continuing plan for the oncoming nurse.

   EXAMPLE: "Her respirations are slow and shallow, and she has weak cough effort. I helped her turn and cough hourly. Her lungs are clear, but she still does not deep breathe well. You should continue to have her cough and deep breathe hourly unless you see improvement."

4. **Progress in goal achievement for identified nursing diagnoses** (e.g., "Mrs. Martin has Risk for Impaired Skin Integrity. We are currently meeting our goal of intact skin.").
5. **Results of diagnostic tests or other therapies performed in the last 24 hours** (e.g., "Blood cultures were negative").
6. **Significant emotional responses** (e.g., "She has been crying since she was told she won't be able to go home").
7. **Description of invasive lines, pumps, and other apparatus** (e.g., Foley catheter).
8. **Description of important activities that occurred on your shift.** This should not be a detailed catalog of the patient's day. Report only significant activities (e.g., there is no need to report that all clients showered and ambulated in the hall).

9. **Description of care the oncoming nurse needs to do.** This does not include routine care, such as the daily linen change or routine vital signs unless it is something you were unable to accomplish (e.g., "Her bed still needs to be changed"). Include laboratory and diagnostic tests and preps that the oncoming nurse should do or special observations that she should make (e.g., "She is scheduled for surgery in the morning and should be NPO after midnight").

10. **Patient-centered information.** This is not a report of the nurse's activities over the shift. Using a shift report sheet such as Figure 8–8 will help to keep your shift reports patient centered.

11. **When your report is finished,** ask the receiving nurse if he has any questions. Get the nurse's full name and then record it along with the transfer date and time in your transfer documentation.

Standardized Formats

It is a good idea for an agency or unit to adopt a standardized format for oral reports. Standardized formats provide an easy-to-remember, concrete mechanism useful for framing conversations with primary care providers or with other nurses at change of shift. Two examples, discussed next, are SBAR and PACE.

SBAR

Because nurses and physicians communicate in very different ways, the SBAR format (situation, background, assessment, recommendation) is useful for interdisciplinary communication, especially critical situations requiring a clinician's immediate attention

BON SECOURS HOSPITAL
GROSSE POINTE, MI 48230

SHIFT:_____

DATE:_____

CHANGE OF SHIFT REPORT

Room No.		Name/Age		Hx / Dx	Problem #1	Problem #2	Problem #3	Special Procedures/ Diet/Abnormal Labs or Diagnostics	Meds	Teaching D/C Prep	Comments
328	1	Marks	81	CVA	Skin – Turn q 2h.			CT-09	9,1,5,11 HS Pre-op		Speech eval.
329	1	Smith	60	Lap. Chole.	Pain: 3 pain	Resp: Lungs clear			9, 1, 5, 11 HS Pre-op	Enc. amb.	probable discharge
329	2	Warren	69	Heart Failure	Cardiac Output	Resp: O2@2L		24 hr. urine	9, 1, 5, 11 HS Pre-op	S.S. to see	
									9, 1, 5, 11		

FIGURE 8–8

Sample handover (change of shift) report (*Source:* Courtesy of Bon Secours Hospital, Grosse Point, MI. Used with permission).

and action. The SBAR technique can be adapted for handoff reports (Haig et al, 2006). The following is a brief summary of SBAR:

First, identify yourself, the patient, and the agency.

Situation—"Here's the situation . . ."

Background—"The supporting background information is . . ."

Assessment—"My assessment of the situation is that . . ."

Recommendation—"I recommend that you . . ."

PACE

You might prefer the PACE template, developed specifically for handoff reports (Schroeder, 2006).

Patient and Problem—Include the patient's name, room number, diagnosis, reason for admission, and recent procedures. State the present problem. Briefly summarize the patient's medical history relevant to the current problem.

Assessment and Actions—Nursing assessments and interventions to address the problem

Continuing Changes—Continuing needs and potential changes, including care and treatments that must be monitored on other shifts (e.g., dressing changes); recent or anticipated changes in the patient's condition or the care plan (e.g., new orders, changes in discharge date)

Evaluation—Evaluation of responses to nursing and medical interventions, progress toward goals, and effectiveness of the plan

8-4 WHAT DO YOU KNOW?

1. What do the letters in the mnemonic SBAR stand for?
2. What do the letters in the mnemonic PACE stand for?

See answer to #8-4 What Do You Know? in Appendix A.

Ethical Issues in Implementation

As client advocates, nurses are obligated to protect clients' humanity. During implementation of care, opportunities exist for humanization or depersonalization of care. Issues of confidentiality and dignity arise frequently in implementation. In addition, Provision 4 of the ANA Code of Ethics for Nurses (2001) indicates that delegation of care has ethical implications (see Appendix A).

Respect for Dignity

Provision 1 of the ANA Code of Ethics emphasizes *respect for human dignity*. Many of the procedures performed during implementation are invasive or require the client to be exposed or assume awkward positions. Nurses are obliged to show respect by providing adequate draping and privacy for such interventions as enemas, catheterizations, and bed baths. These may seem like routine procedures to a busy nurse, but they can be very depersonalizing for the patient. The more skilled you become in technical procedures, the more you will be able to adopt and respect the patient's perspective on what is occurring.

The manner in which you address a patient can also preserve or diminish his dignity. It is easy to fall into the habit of addressing everyone as *dear* or *honey*. Some nurses do this in an effort to express caring; others do it because it is hard to remember patients' names. However, patients lose their individuality when they all have the same name—even if it is a "nice" name. This is a particularly disrespectful practice when the patient is older than the nurse. You should not call a patient by his first name unless you know that he prefers it or you are on a reciprocal first-name basis with him.

Privacy and Confidentiality

Privacy and confidentiality are related to the issue of client dignity. When you provide good nursing care, patients feel comfortable with you. They may trust you enough to disclose important and personal information (e.g., "This baby does not belong to my husband, but he doesn't know"). Do not chart such information unless it is important to the care plan and do not share it with other staff members. Nurses are free to share only information that is pertinent to the client's health.

The law restricts access to the client's written record. Even if it did not, nurses have a moral obligation to protect the confidentiality of the record. This means that insurance companies and other agencies and even the client's family have no right to the information in the record without the client's permission. Legally, the client must sign an authorization for review, copying, or release of information from the chart. When charts are used for educational or research purposes, the student or researcher is obligated to avoid using the client's name or identifying her in any way.

Widespread use of computer-based record systems presents new risks that clients' privacy will be accidentally or intentionally violated. Be aware of the potential for abuse of computer data systems. Angry employees may break through system security to destroy, change, or distribute data or computer hackers may break into the system simply for the challenge. Refer to Box 8–9 for ways to ensure the confidentiality of computer records.

Take-away point: Documentation and oral communication should respect patients' dignity, privacy, and confidentiality.

BOX 8-9

KEEPING ELECTRONIC RECORDS CONFIDENTIAL

1. Follow agency policies and procedures regarding computer documentation.
2. A personal password is needed to enter and sign off computer files. Do not share this password with anyone, including other health team members.
3. After logging on, never leave a computer terminal unattended.
4. Do not leave client information displayed on the monitor where others may see it.
5. Know and follow agency procedures for documenting sensitive material, such as a diagnosis of AIDS.

Legal Considerations

For legal protection, adhere to professional standards of nursing care and follow agency policy and procedures for interventions, delegation, and documentation, especially in high-risk situations. An even more important measure for preventing lawsuits is to develop an attentive, caring relationship with patients. Patients are less likely to sue if they feel you are respectful and attentive to their needs.

The legal purposes of documentation are to show that care was provided and that there was continuity of care. The preceding "Guidelines for Charting" will help you to chart in a legally prudent manner. In addition, the following discussion focuses on some of the more common legal pitfalls for nurses. In some situations, the healthcare agency may require you to fill out an incident report. If so, document the facts of the incident in the progress notes but do not chart that an incident report has been completed.

Falls

Although anyone can fall, infants and older adults are especially at risk for injury from falls. Most falls occur in the home, but they are a major concern in healthcare facilities as well. Falls are among the most common incidents reported in hospitals and long-term care facilities (Institute for healthcare Improvement, n.d.). Hospitals and long-term care agencies have a duty to take reasonable measures to ensure patient safety. Most have policies and routines for identifying patients who are likely to fall and for taking the necessary precautions. All inpatients should be assessed for falls risk on admission. Documentation should include data about level of consciousness, balance, and mobility; precautions taken to prevent falls (e.g., helping with ambulation); and any comments by the family that they have accepted some responsibility for helping to prevent falls.

Restraints

The standard of care is to avoid use of restraints. Use restraints only according to your agency's policies and procedures and only with a medical order (refer to a basic nursing text for information about restraints). Document the reasons the patient is restrained, the method of restraint used, the time and duration of application, the frequency of observation, patient responses, safety outcomes, and assessment of the continued need for restraint.

Questioning Medical Orders

When a primary care provider prescribes an order that you do not understand or that you believe to be incorrect, you must be diligent in getting your questions answered before implementing the order. Ask your nurse manager or supervisor for help and call the prescriber if necessary. Be sure to document the fact that you questioned the order and were assured that it was correct, by whom, and under what circumstances.

Patient Behaviors That May Contribute to an Injury

Risk managers use the phrase **potentially contributing patient acts** to refer to patient behaviors that may contribute to injury. Documenting such acts may help the nurse defend against a malpractice suit, as in the following situations.

Refusal or Inability to Provide Information

When the client refuses to or cannot give accurate, complete information (e.g., about health status, history, or medications), you should try to obtain information from other sources. Document any difficulties in communicating with the client and reflect his understanding of the importance of the information.

> **EXAMPLE OF CHARTING:** When asked how she received the bruises on her face and head, client replied, "I don't have to answer that. It's none of your business." Discussed with her the possibility that her dizziness and blurred vision may be caused by her injuries and that the source of injury may be an important piece of information. She turned her face to the wall and did not reply.
> _____ R. Jones, RN

Nonadherence to Medical and Nursing Interventions

Examples of nonadherence include failure to follow medical prescriptions for medications, diet, or staying in bed. When this occurs, chart instructions given to the patient, what the patient did that specifically contradicts instructions, and actions taken to try to encourage compliance.

> **EXAMPLE OF CHARTING:**
>
> 0700 – Ate all of prescribed diabetic diet. _____ R. Jones, RN
> 0830 – Friends visited. Client found eating sweet rolls and chocolate milk. Reviewed with him the possible effects of not following diet. He stated, "I get tired of the stuff they bring me here." He continued eating. _____R. Jones, RN

Possession or Use of Unauthorized Personal Items

Examples of unauthorized items are heating pad, hair dryer, alcoholic beverages, street drugs, and tobacco. Progress notes should describe what was found, what was done with it, and any persons notified.

EXAMPLE OF CHARTING:

0900 – Client found using hair dryer from home. Sent dryer to biomedical department to be checked before further use. _____ R. Jones, RN

Tampering with Medical Equipment

Examples of tampering with equipment may include changing the intravenous (IV) flow rate, removing traction, and adjusting monitoring equipment. Document any observations that might indicate that the patient or family is manipulating equipment. Describe what was done about the problem (e.g., instructing the patient, notifying the physician).

EXAMPLE OF CHARTING:

0900 – IV infusing at 100 mL/hr with 500 ml. in bag. _____ R. Jones, RN

0930 – IV found barely dripping, 475 mL in bag. Site not inflamed or infiltrated; tubing patent. Rate increased to 100 mL/hr. Pt. and wife deny touching IV tubing; however, their 2 small children have been in the room this am. Roller clamp repositioned high on IV pole; cautioned wife to watch children closely around medical equipment. _____ R. Jones, RN

Take-away point: Documentation is important for legal protection when issues arise involving patient falls, restraints, questioning medical orders, or patient behaviors that may contribute to an injury.

Cultural and Spiritual Considerations

By now, it should be clear that providing holistic, individualized care means including culture and spirituality in every phase of the nursing process. Certainly, it is important to assess, diagnose, and plan for cultural and spiritual needs, but it is during implementation that you have the best opportunity to interact with patients and to demonstrate cultural and spiritual competence.

Cultural Care

To provide meaningful nursing care, you must reflect on and understand your own values, beliefs, and behaviors. This includes your own culture. Box 8–10 offers suggestions for providing culturally competent nursing care.

BOX 8-10

PROVIDING CULTURALLY COMPETENT CARE

- Convey respect for the individual and respect for the individual's values, beliefs, and cultural and ethnic practices.
- Learn about the major ethnic or cultural groups with whom you are likely to have contact.
- Increase your knowledge about different beliefs and values and learn not to be threatened when they differ from your own.
- Analyze your own communication (e.g., facial expression and body language) and how it may be interpreted.
- Recognize differences in ways clients communicate. Do not assume the meaning of a specific behavior (e.g., lack of eye contact) without considering the client's ethnic and cultural background.
- Understand your own biases, prejudices, and stereotypes.
- Recognize that cultural symbols and practices can often bring a client comfort.
- Support the client's practices and incorporate them into nursing practice whenever possible and not contraindicated for health reasons (e.g., provide hot tea to a client who drinks hot tea and never drinks cold water).
- Don't impose a cultural practice on a client without knowing whether it is acceptable (e.g., Vietnamese clients may prefer not to be touched on the head).
- Review your own attitudes and beliefs about health and objectively examine the logic of those attitudes and beliefs and their origins.
- Remember that during illness, clients may return to preferred cultural practices (e.g., a client who has learned English as a second language may revert to the primary language).

Spiritual Care

When orienting patients to the nursing unit, you can provide information about hospital services and arrange for them to participate in these as they are able. Many hospitals have full-time chaplains to assist with spiritual needs, and many nursing units have a list of clergy in the community who are on call for spiritual care.

To intervene effectively for patients with Spiritual Distress, you should have already examined and clarified your own spiritual beliefs and values. If you feel uncomfortable with spiritual interventions (e.g., praying with a patient who requests it), you should verbalize your discomfort and offer to get someone else to help. It is important to respect and support the patient's beliefs, but it is equally important to not feel guilty about your own discomfort.

When there is true conflict between the client's spiritual (or cultural) beliefs and medical therapy, you should encourage the client and physician to discuss the conflict and consider alternative therapies. As a nurse, you should always support the client's right to make informed decisions.

SUMMARY

Implementation:

- Is action focused.
- Occurs in the environments created by healthcare systems such as managed care and case management.
- Requires nurses to perform or delegate dependent, independent, and collaborative actions.
- May use a variety of models of allocating nursing tasks and authority (e.g., functional, team, and primary nursing, and differentiated practice).
- Should preserve confidentiality and client dignity.
- Relies on client readiness and the nurse's cognitive, technical, and interpersonal skills.
- Includes teaching strategies to enhance learning and promote compliance with therapies.
- Includes delegating the right activities to the right person, as well as supervising the activities.
- Requires reflection and critical thinking to ensure safe, effective, and efficient care.
- Is completed when the nursing actions have been carried out and recorded, along with the client's reactions to them. (The client record or chart is a permanent, legal document of the client's health care and status.)
- Is documented in flowsheets and progress notes and reported orally at change of shift and when a client is transferred.
- Is documented on forms and in the format (e.g., narrative, SOAP) determined by individual institutions.
- Must be documented according to accepted guidelines and agency policies and procedures.
- Provides the opportunity for culturally and spiritually competent nursing care.
- Carries some legal risks that can be minimized by prudent documentation.

Take-away point: After implementing an intervention, use these questions to evaluate your performance.

❏ Did I consider the patient's readiness before implementing?
❏ Did I communicate effectively with the patient?
❏ Did I make periodic observations of the patient's condition during the intervention?

CRITICAL THINKING AND CLINICAL REASONING: A CASE STUDY

Brad Williams is a 72-year-old man who had a cerebrovascular accident (stroke) caused by a right cerebral thrombosis 1 week ago. He has been taking antihypertensive medications for 2 years, but his wife says that he often forgets to take them. Mr. Williams is drowsy but responds to verbal stimuli, although he cannot talk. He nods his head to indicate yes or no when asked questions, and he becomes agitated and tearful when he cannot understand or be understood. He cannot move his left arm and leg; flaccid paralysis is present in both (he is left-handed). He does not respond to touch in those extremities. Although he voids when offered a urinal, he is occasionally incontinent of urine. He is receiving heparin sodium by continuous intravenous drip; the dose is adjusted according to the results of a partial thromboplastin time (PTT), which is performed every 4 hours. The nurse has identified the following nursing diagnoses for Mr. Williams:

- Impaired Physical Mobility related to left hemiplegia secondary to neurologic deficits
- Risk for Impaired Skin Integrity related to inability to change position secondary to left-sided paralysis
- Feeding Self-Care Deficit secondary to paralysis of left hand and arm
- Impaired Verbal Communication related to cerebral tissue injury

1. Based just on the information given, what other actual or potential nursing diagnoses should the nurse write?
2. The NANDA International definition of Chronic Low Self-Esteem is long-standing, negative self-evaluating/feelings about self or self-capabilities.
   a. Does Mr. Williams have this diagnosis (yes/no)?
   b. What risk factors exist that may cause Mr. Williams to develop low self-esteem?
3. In addition to "inability to change position," what other etiological factor should be added to the diagnosis Risk for Impaired Skin Integrity? Why?
4. For the nursing diagnosis of Risk for Impaired Skin Integrity related to inability to change position secondary to left-sided paralysis, the nurse wrote the following expected outcome: "Maintains skin integrity." What assessments should the nurse make to evaluate whether this goal is being met? Be specific.
5. For the diagnosis of Risk for Impaired Skin Integrity related to inability to change position secondary to left-sided paralysis, the nurse has included in the care plan the Nursing Interventions Classification (NIC) intervention Pressure Ulcer Prevention. NIC lists the following nursing activities for Pressure Ulcer Prevention (Bulechek, Butcher, & Dochterman, 2008, p. 587).

- Remove excessive moisture on the skin resulting from perspiration, wound drainage, and fecal or urinary incontinence.
- Turn every 1 to 2 hours, as appropriate.
- Inspect skin over bony prominences and other pressure points when repositioning at least daily.
- Provide trapeze to assist patient in shifting weight frequently.
- Use specialty beds and mattresses, as appropriate.

Refer to Box 2–9, in Chapter 2. What questions should you ask about the reassuring intervention before deciding to use it?

6. Which of the three interventions can you probably choose even without knowing the etiology or symptoms?
   a. Underline the activities that are appropriate for Mr. Williams. If some are only partially appropriate, draw lines through the words that do not apply to Mr. Williams.
   b. Which activity needs to have details added to make it more specific? What is needed?
7. What collaborative problem is associated with heparin administration?
8. When delegating bathing and oral care for Mr. Williams, what safety precautions should the nurse give to the aide, keeping in mind that Mr. Williams is receiving heparin (an anticoagulant)?
9. Keeping in mind Mr. Williams's nursing diagnoses, what specific instructions should the nurse give to the aide regarding the linen change?
10. Write a reasonable long-term goal for Mr. Williams's diagnosis of Feeding Self-Care Deficit.
11. There are some safety issues associated with Mr. Williams's Impaired Verbal Communication.
    a. What do you think they might be?
    b. What nursing actions could you take to address these risks?
12. For the nursing diagnoses she identified, what referrals might the nurse need to make? Why?
13. Write a nursing order to address Mr. Williams's Impaired Physical Mobility.

See suggested responses to Critical Thinking and Clinical Reasoning: A Case Study in Appendix A

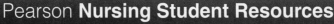

Pearson **Nursing Student Resources**
Find additional review materials at **www.nursing.pearsonhighered.com**
Prepare for success with additional NCLEX®-style practice questions, interactive assignments and activities, Web links, animations and videos, and more!

Evaluation

Introduction

As a nurse, you will make frequent and varied evaluations. Because the client is your primary concern, the most important evaluations involve the following:

1. The client's progress toward health goals
2. The success of the nursing plan of care in helping the client to achieve desired outcomes
3. The overall quality of care given to defined groups of clients

This chapter examines the universal characteristics of evaluation, discusses evaluation as a step of the nursing process (Figure 9–1), and explains the process of quality assurance (QA).

General Characteristics of Evaluation

Before learning how evaluation is used in the nursing process, it may be helpful to analyze a more general definition of the term. In general, **formal evaluation** is a deliberate, systematic process in which a judgment is made about the *quality, value, or worth* of something by comparing it with *previously identified criteria or standards*. Almost anything can be the subject of evaluation (e.g., a painting, a highway system, a teaching method, or a person's character). Furthermore, various aspects or properties of a thing can be evaluated. If you are evaluating a painting, for instance, you can assess the artist's use of color or the extent to which the painting elicits emotion. If you were evaluating teaching methods, you might measure the teacher's ability to hold student

LEARNING OUTCOMES

After completing this chapter, you should be able to do the following:

- Define *evaluation* as it relates to (a) the nursing process and (b) quality assurance.
- State the importance and purpose of evaluation in (a) the nursing process and (b) quality assurance.
- Explain how nurses use critical thinking when evaluating.
- Describe the process of evaluating client progress toward outcome achievement.
- Given predicted outcomes and client data, write two-part evaluative statements.
- Describe a process for modifying the nursing plan of care.
- Explain the relevance of culture and spirituality to evaluation in the nursing process.
- Describe a process for nursing quality assurance.
- Differentiate between criteria and standards.
- Explain how quality-assurance evaluation supports the moral principles of beneficence and nonmaleficence.

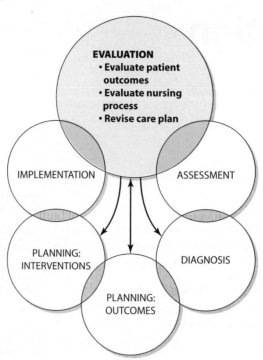

FIGURE 9–1

The evaluation phase

interest or minimize student stress. The important thing to remember is that you must decide *in advance* what properties you are going to consider and how you will measure those properties.

Take-away point: The distinctive characteristics of evaluation are:

- Determination of quality or value
- Use of predetermined criteria or standards

Standards and Criteria

Although *standards* and *criteria* are sometimes used interchangeably, most texts differentiate between these terms. A **standard** is established by authority, custom, or consensus as a model of what should be done. In nursing, standards describe quality nursing care and are used for comparison when evaluating job performance. Some standards, such as those written for routines of care on a nursing unit, are specific enough to serve as criteria. Others are broad and abstract, as in the American Nurses Association's (ANA's) *Nursing: Scope and Standards of Practice* (2nd ed.) (2010, in press). When standards or criteria are broad, as in Box 9–1, more specific criteria must be developed to guide the collection of data for evaluation. **Criteria** are measurable or observable qualities that describe specific skills, knowledge, behaviors, attitudes, and so on. In Box 9–1,

BOX 9–1

AMERICAN NURSES ASSOCIATION STANDARDS OF PRACTICE

Standard 6. Evaluation

The registered nurse evaluates progress towards attainment of outcomes.

Competencies

The nurse:

1. Conducts a systematic, ongoing, and criterion-based evaluation of the outcomes in relation to the structures and processes prescribed by the plan and the indicated timeline.
2. Collaborates with the person and others involved in the care or situation in the evaluation process.
3. Evaluates, in partnership with the person, the effectiveness of the planned strategies in relation to the person's responses and the attainment of the expected outcomes.
4. Documents the results of the evaluation.
5. Uses ongoing assessment data to revise the diagnoses, outcomes, the plan, and the implementation, as needed.
6. Disseminates the results to the patient, family, and others involved, in accordance with federal and state regulations.
7. Actively participates in assessing and assuring the responsible and appropriate use of interventions in order to minimize unwarranted or unwanted treatment and patient suffering.

(*Note:* There are additional measurement criteria for advanced practice nurses.)

Note: This material is from the draft for public comment (ANA, 2010, in press); its wording may be somewhat changed in the final published version (August 2010). For that version of the ANA standards, visit http://www.nursingworld.org.

Source: Reprinted with permission from American Nurses Association (2010, in press). In *Nursing: Scope and standards of practice* (2nd ed.). (Public Comment draft, January). Silver Spring, MD. Available at http:/nursebooks.org.

---

the criteria for ANA Standard 6 are called Competencies. Concrete, specific criteria serve as guides for collecting evaluation data and for making judgments about such data. The patient outcomes you learned to write in Chapter 6 are also examples of criteria.

Criteria should be both valid and reliable. A criterion is **valid** if it actually measures what it is intended to measure. For example, the white blood cell (WBC) count is often used to measure the presence of infection. However, it would not be valid if used alone because the WBC count is not elevated in all infections; in addition, the WBC count is sometimes elevated when there is no infection. More valid indicators might be a blood culture or a bacterial count of a body fluid. A **reliable** criterion yields the same results every time it is used no matter who uses it (e.g., determining a patient's age by asking his friends is less reliable than asking the patient or checking his birth certificate). Box 9–2 presents a comparison of standards and criteria.

BOX 9–2

COMPARISON OF NURSING STANDARDS AND CRITERIA

	Standards	Criteria
Similarities	Describe what is acceptable or desired	Describe what is acceptable or desired
	Serve as basis for comparison	Serve as basis for comparison
Differences	Describe nursing care	Describe expected nurse or client behaviors
	May be broad or specific	Are specific, observable, measurable
Example	ANA standards	Patient outcomes on a care plan

?

9-1 WHAT DO YOU KNOW?

What are three important evaluations nurses make?

See answer to #9-1 What Do You Know? in Appendix A.

Evaluation in Nursing Process

In the nursing process, **evaluation** is a planned, ongoing, deliberate activity in which the client, family, nurse, and other healthcare professionals determine (a) the client's progress toward outcome achievement and (b) the effectiveness of the nursing plan of care. The nurse and client determine the *quality* of the client's health by using as *predetermined criteria* the predicted responses (outcomes) identified in the planning step. They determine the value of the nursing plan of care by using as *standards* the excellent application of each step of the nursing process.

General Definition of Evaluation	**Nursing Process Definition**
Determination of quality or value	**1.** of the client's health.
	2. of the nursing plan of care.
Use of predetermined criteria or standards.	**1.** Use of the outcomes identified in the planning phase.
	2. Use of the nursing process according to guidelines such as those in Table 6–9.

Evaluation begins with the initial baseline assessment and continues during each contact with the client. The frequency of evaluation depends on frequency of contact, which is determined by the client's status or the condition being evaluated. When a patient has just returned from surgery, the nurse may evaluate for signs of change in status every 15 minutes. The following day, the nurse may evaluate the client only every 4 hours. As the client's condition improves and she approaches discharge, evaluation gradually becomes less frequent.

Take-away point: In the nursing process, evaluation is a planned, ongoing, deliberate activity in which the nurse, client, significant others, and other healthcare professionals determine (a) the extent of client outcome achievement and (b) the effectiveness of the nursing care plan

Relationship to Other Phases

Effective evaluation depends on the effectiveness of the steps that precede it. Assessment data must be accurate and complete so the outcomes written in the planning step will be appropriate for the client. The desired outcomes (planning) must be stated in concrete behavioral terms if they are to be useful for evaluating actual client outcomes. Finally, without the implementation step, there would be nothing to evaluate.

Evaluation overlaps with assessment. During evaluation, the nurse collects data (assessment), but for the purpose of evaluating (evaluation) rather than diagnosing. The *act* of data collection is the same; the differences are in when it is collected and how it is used. In the assessment step, the nurse uses data to make nursing diagnoses. In the evaluation step, data are used to assess the effect of nursing care on the diagnoses.

	Assessment Data	**Evaluation Data**
When collected	In assessment phase Before interventions	In evaluation phase After interventions
Purpose or use	Make nursing diagnosis Determine present health status	Evaluate goal achievement Compare "new" health status with desired health status

Although it is the final step in the nursing process, evaluation does not end the process because the information it provides is used to begin another cycle. After implementing the plan of care, the nurse compares client responses with predicted outcomes and then uses this information to review the plan of care and each step of the nursing process.

Evaluating Patient Progress

In the context of the nursing process, outcome evaluation focuses primarily on the client's progress toward achieving health goals. After giving care, the nurse compares the clients' health status (responses) with the predicted outcomes identified during the planning phase and makes a judgment about whether the outcomes have been achieved. Evaluation of client outcomes may be ongoing, intermittent, or terminal.

- **Ongoing evaluation** is done while (or immediately after) implementing an intervention, enabling you to make on-the-spot modifications.
- **Intermittent evaluation**, performed at specified times, shows the amount of progress toward outcome achievement. It enables you to correct any inadequacies in the client's care and modify the plan of care as needed. Evaluation continues until the client's health goals are achieved or until he is discharged from nursing care.

- **Terminal evaluation** indicates the client's condition at the time of discharge. It includes understanding of follow-up care and status of outcome achievement, especially with regard to self-care abilities. Most agencies have a special discharge record for the terminal evaluation, as well as for instructions regarding medications, treatments, and follow-up care. As you work with the client throughout her stay, you should prepare her for eventual discharge by gradually promoting more self-care and talking about the time when she will be leaving.

Professional Standards of Practice

Professional standards of practice (see Box 9–1) identify evaluation as a mutual nurse–client activity. Family and other team members provide data and participate, but the nurse is responsible for initiating and recording the evaluation.

By performing organized, systematic evaluation of client outcomes, nurses demonstrate caring and responsibility. Examining outcomes shows that nurses care not only about planning and delivering care but also about its effect on those whose lives they touch. Without evaluation, nurses would not know whether the care they give actually meets the client's needs.

Evaluation enables the nurse to improve care. It promotes efficiency by eliminating unsuccessful interventions and allowing the nurse to focus on actions that are more effective. Only by evaluating the client's progress in relation to the plan of care can the nurse know whether to continue, change, or terminate the plan.

Finally, by linking nursing interventions to improvements in client status, evaluation can demonstrate to employers and consumers that nurses play an important role in achieving client health.

Process for Evaluating Client Progress

The professional nurse responsible for the plan of care is also responsible for evaluating the client's responses to care. The following discussion provides a six-step guide for evaluating client progress:

1. **Review the desired outcomes (indicators).** Outcomes and indicators identified in the planning phase are the criteria used to evaluate the patient's responses to nursing care. Desired outcomes (indicators or goals) have two purposes: (a) they establish the kind of data that need to be collected and (b) they provide standards against which the data are judged. For example, given the following desired outcomes, any nurse caring for the patient would know what data to collect.

   - Urine output will be at least 50 mL/hr.
   - Oral fluid intake will be at least 2,000 mL per 24 hours.

2. **Collect evaluation data.** Collect data about the client's responses to the nursing interventions. Use the nursing diagnosis and its list of outcomes from the plan of care to guide your ongoing focus assessment. Evaluation data are collected by observing the client's behavior and responses; examining client records; and talking to the client, family, friends, and other health team members. In the example in Table 9–1, in order

TABLE 9–1   Evaluation Example: Sam Rizzo

Nursing Diagnosis: Moderate Anxiety r/t unfamiliar environment and dyspnea		
Compare Desired Outcomes . . .	**with Actual Outcomes (Data) . . .**	**Conclusion**
Broad goal: Will experience reduced anxiety, as evidenced by outcomes:		
1. verbalization of feeling less anxious	When dyspneic, states, "What should I do? Can you help me?"	Outcome not achieved.
2. relaxed facial muscles	Face relaxed except during episodes of dyspnea.	Outcome partially achieved.
3. absence of skeletal muscle tension	No skeletal muscle tension except during episodes of dyspnea.	Outcome partially achieved.
4. verbalization of understanding of hospital routines and treatments	States, "I feel better since you explained about the fire drill. I thought there was a real fire."	Outcome achieved.
	States, "I understand about the hospital routines and the breathing treatments. Those things really aren't causing any anxiety."	

to get the data under "Actual Outcomes" during interactions with Sam Rizzo, the nurse focused on his facial expression and muscle tension and listened for statements reflecting his level of anxiety and his knowledge of routines and treatments.

The nature of the outcome determines the type of information you will collect. Outcomes can be classified as cognitive, psychomotor, or affective or as pertaining to body appearance and functioning.

- For cognitive outcomes, you might ask the client to repeat information or apply new knowledge (e.g., choose low-fat foods from a menu).
- For psychomotor outcomes, you could ask the client to demonstrate a skill, such as drawing up insulin.
- For affective outcomes, you might talk to the client and observe her behavior for cues to changes in values, attitudes, or beliefs.

You can obtain data about body appearance and functioning by interviewing, observing, and examining the client, as well as from secondary sources, such as laboratory results. Some examples of data-collection methods for the different types of outcomes appear in Table 9–2.

3. **Compare the patient status with desired outcomes and draw a conclusion**. If the nursing process has been effective up to this point, it is relatively simple to determine if a goal has been met. Is the client's response (actual outcome) what you wanted it to be (desired outcome)? Is it at least the best you can expect, given the time and circumstances? Include the client in decisions about the level of outcome achievement. Go over the desired outcomes with the client and ask him if he

TABLE 9–2 Evaluation Data-Collection Methods

Type of Outcome	Outcome Statement	Example of Data-Collection Activity
Cognitive	By the end of the week, names foods to avoid on a low-fat diet.	Using a chart of MyPyramid, ask the client to tell you which foods to avoid.
Psychomotor	Within 24 hours after delivery, positions baby correctly at breast.	Observe the mother breastfeeding the infant.
Affective	After orientation to routines and procedures, states he is feeling less anxiety.	Listen for spontaneous statements about anxiety or ask, "How are you feeling?"
Body function and appearance	Heart rate <100 beats/min at all times.	Auscultate apical heart rate.

believes they have been achieved. You can draw three possible conclusions about outcome achievement.

Outcome achieved	The desired client response occurred; that is, the actual response is the same as the desired outcome.
Outcome partially achieved	Some, but not all, desired behaviors were observed or the predicted outcome is achieved only part of the time.
Outcome not achieved	The desired client response did not occur by the target time or the actual outcome does not match the desired outcome.

Table 9–1 shows how actual outcomes would be compared with predicted outcomes in order to draw conclusions about Sam Rizzo's goal achievement.

4. **Write the evaluative statement.** An evaluative statement consists of two parts: (a) the judgment about whether the outcome was achieved ("Conclusion" in Table 9–1) and (b) data to support the judgment ("Actual Outcomes" in Table 9–1). Following are the evaluative statements that would be written for Sam Rizzo using the data and conclusions in Table 9–1.

Desired Outcome	**Evaluative Statement**
Verbalization of feeling less anxious	2/14. Outcome not achieved. When dyspneic, states, "What should I do? Can you help me?" No statements of feeling less anxious.
Relaxed facial muscles	2/14. Outcome partially achieved. Face relaxed except during episodes of dyspnea.
Absence of skeletal muscle tension	2/14. Outcome partially achieved. No skeletal muscle tension except during episodes of dyspnea.

Verbalization of understanding of hospital routines and treatments

2/14. Outcome achieved. States, "I feel better since you explained about the fire drill. I thought there was a real fire." Also states, "I understand about the hospital routines and the breathing treatments. Those things really aren't causing any anxiety."

When using the Nursing Outcomes Classification (NOC) or other standardized outcomes and indicators, evaluative statements may take a different form. Recall from the NOC and Table 6–4 in Chapter 6 that goals may be created by writing the label, the indicator, and the scale number of the desired outcome. Goals and evaluation statements are written in exactly the same manner. For example, for a patient with Impaired Transfer Mobility, the goal might be to transfer independently; after interventions, reassessment shows that the patient can transfer using crutches. The goal and evaluative statements would read as follows:

Goal: Transfer performance: 5
Evaluation Statement: Transfer performance: 4

Figure 9–2 is an example of using NOC outcomes in computerized care planning. It is a screen that provides the definition and indicators for a NOC outcome. Toward the bottom of the screen, it shows the patient's status on admission (Initial scale), the patient goal (Expected scale), and the evaluation statement (Outcome Progress).

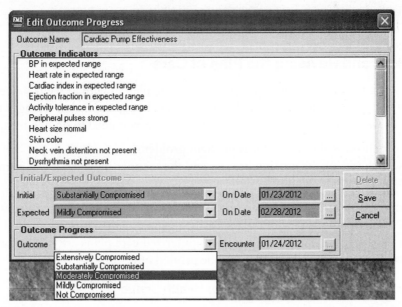

FIGURE 9–2

Computer screen: NOC outcome progress (*Source:* Copyright © Courtesy of Ergo Partners, L. C., Boulder, CO. All rights reserved).

Some plans of care have a special column for the evaluative statement; in other systems, you may record the evaluative statement in the progress notes. In still other systems, you may record the evaluation data but not the conclusion about goal achievement.

5. **Relate nursing interventions to outcomes.** It is important to establish whether the patient outcomes were actually caused by the nursing actions. You should not assume that a nursing intervention was the reason a goal was or was not met. A number of variables can affect outcome achievement, for example:

Actions and treatments performed by other healthcare professionals

Influence of family members and significant others

Client's attitudes, desire, and motivation

Client's failure to give accurate or sufficient information during data collection

Client's prior experiences and knowledge

Other variables are possible; nurses cannot control all the variables that might influence the outcome of care. Therefore, in determining the effect of a nursing action, you should try to identify other factors that might have promoted or interfered with its effectiveness.

9-2 WHAT DO YOU KNOW?

List the five-step process for evaluating client progress.

See answer to #9-2 What Do You Know? in Appendix A.

Evaluating and Revising the Plan of Care

After finishing the outcome evaluation, examine the plan of care to see if it needs to be changed. You will probably modify the plan if the client's condition changes or if the health goals were not met. In evaluating a plan of care, you need to do two things:

1. Draw conclusions about the status of client problems.
2. Review each step of the nursing process and the manner in which it was performed.

Some agencies use a pink or yellow highlighter to mark through discontinued sections of the care plan. Others have a status column in which to write the date of any revisions. These methods do not obliterate the original plans; thus, they can be photocopied or used for reference as needed. Computerized care plans are easily changed on screen, and a copy of the revised plan can be printed out.

Draw Conclusions About the Problem or Health Status

You will use judgments about goal achievement to determine whether the care plan was effective in resolving, reducing, or preventing patient problems. This is important in deciding whether to continue or modify the care plan.

9-1 THINK & REFLECT!

Mrs. Adams needed to lose 60 lb (28 kg). With her input, the nurse included in the care plan a goal to "Lose 6 lb (2.8 kg) by 5/2/12." A nursing order in the care plan was to "Explain how to plan and prepare a 1,000-calorie diet." When Mrs. Adams weighed herself on May 2, she had lost 10 lb. The goal had been met.

1. Does this mean that the nursing order was effective?
2. What do you need to know in order to decide if that nursing action led to the weight loss?
3. What other factors might have caused Mrs. Adams to lose weight?
4. If Mrs. Adams says, "I forgot what you said about the diet, so I just ate out a lot," what conclusion would you draw about the nursing strategy?

See suggested responses to #9-1 Think & Reflect! in Appendix A.

When Goals Have Been Met You can draw one of the following conclusions about the status of the patient's nursing diagnoses:

- **The actual problem has been resolved.** If all the outcomes for the nursing diagnosis have been achieved, you can conclude that the problem has been resolved. This means that nursing care is no longer needed for that nursing diagnosis. Document that the goals were met and discontinue the nursing diagnosis. In Mr. Rizzo's case (see Table 9–1), the Anxiety problem can be considered resolved when Outcomes 1, 2, and 3 have been achieved.

- **The actual problem or wellness need still exists.** Even if a goal has been achieved, the problem may still exist, particularly if the goal was only one of several written for the problem. The Anxiety diagnosis in Table 9–1 illustrates this point. Mr. Rizzo did verbalize understanding of hospital routines and treatments. However, other goals were not met, so the nursing diagnosis of anxiety should remain in the plan. Nursing orders related to explaining routines and treatments could be discontinued, but other interventions for Anxiety should be continued or changed to make them more effective.

- **The potential problem has been prevented.** If the risk factors have been removed, the nursing diagnosis can be removed from the plan of care. However, risk factors may still be present even though the problem still has not occurred. This means that nursing care is still required, so you would not remove the diagnosis from the plan.

  EXAMPLE: Tamara Jordan's nursing diagnosis is Risk for Puerperal Infection r/t membranes having ruptured several days before delivery of her baby. The goal is that she will not develop puerperal infection. When the home health nurse evaluates her progress on postpartum day 3, Tamara's temperature is normal, and she has no other signs of infection. However, she could still develop an infection, so the nurse keeps the nursing diagnosis in the plan of care and will continue to assess for it.

- **A possible problem has been ruled out.** In that case, you would discontinue the problem, goals or outcomes, and nursing orders.

■ **All problems have been resolved; there are no new problems.** When this is the case, the patient is discharged from nursing care. In an acute-care setting this is not likely to occur before dismissal from the institution.

When Goals Have Been Partially Met You may have some, but not enough, evidence that the outcome has been achieved or perhaps it is being demonstrated at one time and not another. Mr. Rizzo, for instance, demonstrates absence of muscle tension at times but not when he is dyspneic. In such instances, you can draw the following conclusions about the nursing diagnosis:

■ **The problem has been reduced and the plan of care needs revisions.** As in Mr. Rizzo's case, nursing interventions are still needed. Because the goal is not being fully met, you may need to modify the plan of care to make it more effective.
■ **The problem has been reduced; continue with the same plan but allow more time for goal achievement.** Perhaps the interventions are effective, but the client needs more time to achieve the outcome. To decide, you must assess why the outcome has not been fully demonstrated.

When Goals Have Not Been Met This means that the problem still exists. Even so, you cannot assume that the plan of care needs revision. Recall that patient, family, and other variables also influence outcome achievement. Therefore, you must reexamine the entire plan of care and each step of the nursing process and decide whether to continue with the same plan or revise the plan.

Evaluating Collaborative Problems The evaluation process is slightly different for collaborative problems and nursing diagnoses. For both, the nurse collects and evaluates data about changes in the patient's condition. However, in the nursing process, the nurse compares patient responses with the desired outcomes (goals) on the plan of care and concludes "goal met" or "goal not met." For collaborative problems, the nurse compares data with established norms (e.g., normal blood glucose) and concludes that the data are or are not within an acceptable range. If the collaborative problem is becoming worse, the nurse notifies the physician.

Take-away point: Patient goals may be met, partially met, or not met. If all goals for an actual problem have been met, you can conclude that the problem is resolved. If only some of the goals are resolved, it is likely the problem still exists.

Critically Review All Steps of the Nursing Process

As you can see, whether or not desired outcomes (goals) have been achieved, there are several decisions to make about continuing, modifying, or terminating nursing care for each problem. Before making specific changes, you must first determine why the plan was or was not effective. This requires that you review the entire plan of care and the nursing process steps involved in its development. This section provides a checklist of questions and actions for use in your review of each step of the nursing process. Table 9–3 provides questions to help you review each step of the

TABLE 9–3 Evaluation Checklist

Assessment Review

1. Were the assessment data complete and accurate?
   - ❏ Yes. No action.
   - ❏ No. Reassess client. Record the new data. Change care plan as indicated.

2. Have all data been validated, as needed?
   - ❏ Yes. No action.
   - ❏ No. Validate with client (by interview and physical examination), significant others, or other professionals. Record validation (or failure to validate). Change care plan as indicated.

3. Have new data become available that require changes in the plan (e.g., a different problem etiology, new goals or outcomes, new medical orders)?
   - ❏ No. No action.
   - ❏ Yes. Record the new data in the progress notes; redefine the problem, goals, and nursing orders, as needed.

4. Has the patient's condition changed?
   - ❏ No. No action.
   - ❏ Yes. Record data about present health status. Change care plan as indicated.

Move to a review of the diagnosis step.

Diagnosis Review

1. Is the diagnosis relevant and related to the data?
   - ❏ Yes. No action.
   - ❏ No. Revise the diagnosis.

2. Is the diagnosis well supported by the data?
   - ❏ Yes. No action.
   - ❏ No. Collect more data. Support or revise diagnosis.

3. Has the problem status changed (actual, potential, possible)?
   - ❏ No. No action.
   - ❏ Yes. Relabel the problem.

4. Is the diagnosis stated clearly?
   - ❏ Yes. No action.
   - ❏ No. Revise the diagnostic statement.

5. Does the etiology correctly reflect the factors contributing to the problem?
   - ❏ Yes. No action.
   - ❏ No. Revise the etiology.

6. Is the problem one that can be treated primarily by nursing actions?
   - ❏ Yes. No action.
   - ❏ No. Label as collaborative and consult appropriate health professional.

7. Is the diagnosis specific and individualized to the patient?
   - ❏ Yes. No action.
   - ❏ No. Revise the diagnosis. Revise outcomes and nursing orders as suggested by the new nursing diagnosis.

(continued)

TABLE 9–3 Evaluation Checklist *(continued)*

---

8. Does the problem (diagnosis) still exist?
   - ❑ Yes. No action.
   - ❑ No. Delete diagnosis and related outcomes and nursing orders.

Proceed to a review of client goals.

Planning Review: Outcomes

1. Have nursing diagnoses been added or revised?
   - ❑ No. No action.
   - ❑ Yes. Write new outcomes.

2. Are the outcomes realistic in terms of patient abilities and agency resources?
   - ❑ Yes. No action.
   - ❑ No. Revise outcomes.

3. Was sufficient time allowed for outcome achievement?
   - ❑ Yes. No action.
   - ❑ No. Revise time frame.

4. Do the outcomes address all aspects of the client's problem?
   - ❑ Yes. No action.
   - ❑ No. Write additional outcomes.

5. Do the expected outcomes, as written, demonstrate resolution of the problem specified in the nursing diagnosis?
   - ❑ Yes. No action.
   - ❑ No. Revise outcomes.

6. Have client priorities changed or has the focus of care changed?
   - ❑ No. No action.
   - ❑ Yes. Revise outcomes.

7. Is the client in agreement with the goals?
   - ❑ Yes. No action.
   - ❑ No. Get client input. Write outcomes valued by the client.

Proceed to review of nursing orders

Planning Review: Nursing Orders

1. Have nursing diagnoses or outcomes been added or revised in previous review steps?
   - ❑ No. No action.
   - ❑ Yes. Write new nursing orders.

2. Are the nursing orders clearly related to the stated patient outcomes?
   - ❑ Yes. No action.
   - ❑ No. Revise or develop new nursing orders.

3. Is the rationale sufficient to justify the use of the nursing order?
   - ❑ Yes. No action.
   - ❑ No. Revise or develop new nursing orders.

4. Are the nursing orders unclear or vague so that other staff may have had questions about how to implement them?
   - ❑ No. No action.
   - ❑ Yes. Revise nursing orders. Add details to make more specific or individualized to the patient.

5. Do the nursing orders include instructions for timing of the activities?
   - ❑ Yes. No action.
   - ❑ No. Revise nursing orders—add times or schedules.

6. Was an order clearly and obviously ineffective?
   - ❑ No. No action.
   - ❑ Yes. Delete it.

TABLE 9–3   Evaluation Checklist *(continued)*

---

7. Are the orders realistic in terms of staff and other resources?

   ❏ Yes. No action.   ❏ No. Revise orders or obtain resources.

8. Have new resources become available that might enable you to change the goals or nursing orders?

   ❏ No. No action.   ❏ Yes. Write new goals or nursing orders reflecting the new capabilities.

9. Do the nursing orders address all aspects of the client's health goals?

   ❏ Yes. No action.   ❏ No. Add new nursing orders.

   Proceed to review of implementation step.

Implementation: Review

1. Did the nurse get client input at each step in developing and implementing the plan?

   ❏ Yes. No action.   ❏ No. Obtain client input and revise plan and implementation as needed.

2. Were the nursing interventions acceptable to the patient?

   ❏ Yes. No action.   ❏ No. Consult patient; change nursing orders or implementation approach.

3. Did the nurse prepare the patient for implementation of the nursing order (e.g., explain what the patient should expect or do)?

   ❏ Yes. No action.   ❏ No. Continue same plan but prepare the patient before implementing. Reevaluate.

4. Did the nurse have adequate knowledge and skills to perform techniques and procedures correctly?

   ❏ Yes. No action.   ❏ No. Continue same plan. Have someone else implement or help the nurse to acquire the needed knowledge or skills. If neither of these is possible, delete nursing order.

5. Did the client or family comply with the therapeutic regimen? Were self-care activities performed correctly?

   ❏ Yes. No action.   ❏ No. Reassess motivation, knowledge, and resources. Add outcomes and nursing orders aimed at teaching, motivating, and supporting the patient in carrying out the regimen. Set time for reevaluation.

6. Did other staff members follow the nursing orders?

   ❏ Yes. No action.   ❏ No. Implement the omitted nursing orders or ensure that others will do so. Set time for reevaluation. Find out why order was not carried out.

7. Was the plan of care implemented in a manner that communicated caring?

   ❏ Yes. No action.   ❏ No. This is a problem that must be addressed by personal and staff development.

After making the necessary revisions to the plan of care, implement the new plan and begin the nursing process cycle again.

nursing process and make decisions about revising the plan of care. For in-depth evaluation of each step, refer to the guidelines and critical thinking standards in Chapters 3, 4, 6, 7, and 8.

Assessment Review Examine the initial and ongoing assessment data in the client's chart (e.g., database, progress notes). Errors or omissions in data influence subsequent steps of the nursing process and may require changes in every section of the plan of care. You may find that new data have become available since the client's initial assessment, or perhaps the client's condition has changed.

> **EXAMPLE:** Wasumita Singh answers the nurses in brief phrases; she does not initiate conversation. Her nurses initially believed her communication problem was caused by her difficulty with English. When evaluating her progress, the nurse concludes that her impaired verbal communication problem still exists. However, on reviewing Ms. Singh's chart, she finds new data: a psychiatric consultation note indicating that Ms. Singh is deeply depressed. The nurse realizes now that Ms. Singh's communication problem is more than simply a language barrier.

Diagnosis Review If your examination of the assessment step results in a revision of the database, you may need to revise or add new nursing diagnoses. Even if data were complete and accurate, you must still analyze the diagnostic process and each of the diagnostic statements. The nursing diagnosis could be incorrect because of errors in the diagnostic process, or the diagnostic statement may have been poorly written. Perhaps the nurse who wrote the statement had a clear idea of the client's problem but was unable to communicate the idea when writing the diagnostic statement. Other nurses might therefore have focused their interventions inappropriately.

Planning Review: Outcomes or Goals If you have made additions to the data or changed the nursing diagnosis, you will need to revise the desired outcomes. If the data and the diagnostic statement are satisfactory as initially written, the reason for lack of goal achievement may lie in the outcomes themselves. Perhaps they were unrealistic, or perhaps the target time was too soon.

Planning Review: Nursing Orders If you have revised the nursing diagnoses or desired outcomes, you will need to change the nursing orders as well. You may wish to revise them anyway for clarification or to add more effective strategies.

Implementation Review If all sections of the nursing plan of care appear to be satisfactory, perhaps the lack of outcome achievement is due to the manner in which the plan was implemented. To find out what went wrong in the implementation step, consult the progress notes, the client, significant others, and other caregivers.

Reflecting Critically about Evaluation

After you have reviewed each step of the nursing process (e.g., using Table 9–3), you should also reflect on the thinking you used in evaluating the plan of care and the patient's health status. The following questions will guide your reflection (critical thinking standards are shown in parentheses):

1. **Clarity**—Is my evaluation statement clear: Goal met plus supporting data?
2. **Accuracy**—Have I compared reassessment data with the goals on the care plan? Is the patient being honest about goal achievement or is he trying to please?
3. **Precision**—Is my evaluation statement precise, using patient statements and behaviors rather than such statements as: "Tolerated well"?
4. **Relevance**—Did I collect reassessment data that relate to the stated goals?
5. **Depth**—Am I missing anything? Have we covered all the bases? If interventions did not produce desired outcomes, do I need consultation?
6. **Breadth**—How does the patient describe the outcomes or goal achievement?
7. **Logic**—In what way did the interventions contribute to goal achievement? Could we have done better?
8. **Significance**—Is there still a need for nursing care? Do we need to make a plan to prevent further problems?

9-2 THINK & REFLECT!

Explain the difference between relevance and significance when evaluating the plan of care.

See suggested responses to #9-2 Think & Reflect! in Appendix A.

Evaluation Errors

Probably the most common evaluation error is failure to perform systematic evaluation of patient outcomes. Many nurses are more action oriented than analytic and reflective. It is relatively easy in the press of a busy day to make a plan and act; however, you may have to make determined efforts to find time to observe and record the client's responses to the actions. Remember that quality care is not guaranteed by simply implementing nursing orders. Only when you evaluate client outcomes can you be assured that the care has met the client's needs.

Nurses usually do, in fact, observe the client's response, but they may not document it or consciously use it in an evaluation process that would enable them to modify interventions. You must be sure to document the evaluative statements so other nurses will be able to judge the effectiveness of your interventions. Otherwise, they might continue with approaches you have already discovered to be ineffective.

Another error occurs when a nurse uses irrelevant data to judge the level of goal achievement. Consider only data that are clearly related to the predicted outcome. Box 9–3 provides examples of both relevant and irrelevant data related to Mr. Rizzo's anxiety problem from Table 9–1.

BOX 9–3

RELEVANT AND IRRELEVANT DATA: SAM RIZZO

Relevant data When dyspneic, states, "What should I do?
Can you help me?"
Face relaxed; no skeletal muscle tension except during episodes
of dyspnea.
States, "I feel better since you explained about the fire drill. I thought
there was a real fire."
States, "I understand about the hospital routines and the breathing
treatments. Those things really aren't causing any anxiety."

Irrelevant data Temperature 98.6°F.
Watching television except when wife is here.

Errors are also possible in judging the congruence between actual and predicted client outcomes; actual outcomes may be measured inaccurately or data may be incomplete. In the example of Table 9–1, if the nurse observed Sam Rizzo only during periods when he was not dyspneic, she might erroneously conclude that his anxiety was relieved.

Ethical Considerations

The moral principle of **beneficence** holds that we ought to do good things for other people, that is, to benefit them. A nurse who holds the hand of a dying patient honors this principle. The principle of **nonmaleficence** holds that we should not harm others. For example, a nurse upholds this principle when she withholds morphine from a client whose respirations are already depressed. You can think of these principles as being on a continuum, with the duty to do no harm taking precedence over the other duties. It is easy to see how the first situation is a stronger duty than the last one.

QA evaluation (to be discussed later) and evaluation of client progress fulfill the obligation of beneficence by enabling nurses to improve the quality of care they deliver. QA can also produce changes in the total healthcare system and improve communication and collaboration between healthcare disciplines. The ANA code of ethics (2001) in Appendix B includes at least four items that imply that evaluating care is a nursing responsibility:

Provision 3. The nurse promotes, advocates for, and strives to protect the health, safety, and rights of the patient.
3.4 Standards and review mechanisms

Provision 4. The nurse is responsible and accountable for individual nursing practice and determines the appropriate delegation of tasks consistent with the nurse's obligation to provide optimum patient care.

Provision 6. The nurse participates in establishing, maintaining, and improving healthcare environments and conditions of employment conducive to the provision of quality health care and consistent with the values of the profession through individual and collective action.

Provision 7. The nurse participates in the advancement of the profession through contributions to practice, education, administration, and knowledge development. 7.2 Advancing the profession by developing, maintaining, and implementing professional standards in clinical, administrative, and educational practice

Cultural and Spiritual Considerations

When desired outcomes have not been achieved, review the client's cultural values, beliefs, and practices to determine what effect they may have had. Consider these factors in addition to other physiological, psychological, social, and developmental factors when you review the nursing process and revise the treatment plan. Thorough evaluation includes evaluating your own ability to provide culturally competent care and to determine whether you need to improve your ability to work with clients from culturally diverse backgrounds.

When evaluating whether clients have accomplished spiritual goals, you will need skill in observation, helping relationships, and communication. You will need to observe the client when he is alone and when he is interacting with others, and listen to what the client says and does not say. The following are characteristics that indicate spiritual well-being and achievement of spiritual goals: a sense of inner peace, compassion for others, reverence for life, gratitude, appreciation of unity and diversity, humor, wisdom, generosity, ability to transcend the self, and the capacity for unconditional love (Carson, 1989).

Some indicators for the NOC (Moorhead et al, 2008, p. 665) outcome of Spiritual Health are as follows:

- Meaning and purpose in life
- Feelings of peacefulness
- Ability to love
- Ability to forgive
- Participation in spiritual rites and passages
- Connectedness with others

Quality Assurance and Quality Improvement

In addition to evaluating goal achievement for individual patients, nurses are involved in evaluating and improving the overall quality of care for groups of patients (e.g., in a hospital). Government programs (e.g., Medicare), regulatory agencies (e.g., The Joint Commission), and state boards of nursing require institutions to provide documentation that nursing care is being given according to nursing standards. Various programs exist for this purpose, including QA, quality improvement (QI), continuous quality improvement (CQI), total quality management (TQM), and persistent quality improvement (PQI).

TABLE 9–4 Comparison of Quality Assurance and Nursing Process Evaluation

	Nursing Quality Assurance	The Nursing Process
Scope of evaluation	Groups of clients	Individual clients
Subject of evaluation	Overall quality of care	1. Progress toward achieving client outcomes 2. Review of nursing care plan
Type of evaluation	Structure, process, outcome	1. Outcome evaluation of patient progress 2. Process evaluation of nursing care plan
Responsibility for evaluation	Chief nurse in the institution	Nurse caring for client

Although focuses and approaches may vary, all such programs involve the evaluation of care provided in the agency. Table 9–4 compares QA and nursing process evaluation.

QA programs make use of **peer review**, which means that members of the profession who are delivering the care develop and implement the process for evaluating that care. This usually involves a **nursing audit**, in which patient records are reviewed for data about nursing competence. A committee establishes standards of care (e.g., for safety measures, documentation, preoperative teaching), and charts are randomly selected and reviewed to compare nursing activities against these standards.

Electronic Health Records and Standardized Nursing Languages

In agencies with electronic patient records, the laborious task of manual chart audits can be avoided; information is simply retrieved in the form of reports. When records systems make use of standardized nursing languages (e.g., NANDA-I, NIC, NOC), specific data about nursing care can be retrieved from the database. This means that data about individual patients can be combined to create data about groups of patients (e.g., all the patients on a unit). Such data can be used to support unit, organizational, and national policy decisions and to compare the care given in different institutions.

Types of Quality-Assurance Evaluation

QA requires evaluation of three components of care: structure, process, and outcome (Table 9–5). Each type of evaluation requires different criteria and methods, and each has a different focus. All three must be considered because they work together to effect care.

Structure evaluation focuses on the setting in which care is given. It asks the question, What effect do environmental and organizational characteristics have on the quality of care? To answer that question, it uses information about policies, procedures, fiscal

TABLE 9–5 Comparison of Structure, Process, and Outcome Evaluation

Aspect of Care	Focus	Criterion Examples
Structure	Setting	Exit signs are clearly visible. A resuscitation cart will be housed on each unit. There is a family waiting room on each floor.
Process	Caregiver activities	Initial interview is completed within 8 hours after admission of client. Client responses to medications are charted. Patients will receive oral hygiene on each shift. Nurse introduces self to client before giving care.
Outcome	Patient responses	B/P <140/90 mm Hg at all times. Walks to bathroom unsupported by day 3. Abdomen will be soft and nontender by day 5.
	Grouped patient responses	Temperature <100°F 24 hr after surgery *(Expected compliance = 90%)* Patient will not fall during hospital stay *(Expected compliance = 95%)*

resources, facilities, equipment, and the number and qualifications of personnel. The following are examples of criteria that might be written for structure evaluation:

- Call light is within reach
- Narcotics are kept in double-locked cabinet
- Policies for medication errors are written and easily accessible

Although adequate staff and resources do not guarantee high-quality care, they are certainly important factors. Without them, it is difficult to meet process and outcome criteria.

Process evaluation focuses on how the care was given—on the activities of the nurses. It answers questions such as: Is the care relevant to the patient's needs? Is the care appropriate, complete, and timely? The ANA *Nursing: Scope and Standards of Practice* (2nd ed) (2010, in press) provides examples of process standards. Other examples include the following:

- Checks client's identification band before giving medication
- Explains procedures (e.g., catheterization) before implementing
- Administers medications on time

Of course, even perfect processes do not guarantee good outcomes. For example, a patient's health or the agency infection rate may become worse no matter how expertly nurses perform. But overall, good nursing care should improve patient and agency outcomes.

Outcome evaluation focuses on demonstrable changes in client's health status as a result of care. Currently, outcomes evaluation is extremely important because accreditation and certification agencies and managed care companies are demanding outcomes data. For example, the Health Care Financing Administration (HCFA) requires home health agencies to use their OASIS tool (Centers for Medicaid and Medicare, 2005) to measure and report changes in patient status at various times. In an effort to standardize patient outcomes that are sensitive to nursing care, the ANA developed a Nursing Care Report Card for use by healthcare organizations. It includes the following outcome measures: nosocomial infection rate, patient fall rate, patient satisfaction with nursing care, patient satisfaction with pain management, nursing job satisfaction, maintenance of skin integrity, and total nursing care hours provided per patient day (ANA, 1995).

For agency evaluation, criteria are written in terms of client responses or health states, just as they are for evaluation of individual client progress. In addition, for QA evaluation the criterion states the percentage of clients expected to have the outcome when nursing care is satisfactory.

> **EXAMPLE:** Skin over bony prominences is intact and free from redness.
> *Expected compliance: 100%*

Taken alone, this means that you would expect that with good care, no clients in the institution will develop redness over a bony prominence. However, that fails to consider the effect of variables other than nursing care—some clients' nutritional and mobility status may be so compromised that no amount of care could prevent redness. For example, a process evaluation for a client might show that a plan to turn the client hourly was written and implemented; this would indicate that nursing care was adequate even though the outcome was poor. A structure evaluation might also show that the nursing unit was chronically understaffed, which would validate a process evaluation that reveals that the client often went for more than 2 hours without being repositioned. That would explain the reason for the poor outcome and processes.

It is not easy to demonstrate the relationship between nursing care and client outcomes. Medical, or disease-related, outcomes are easy to observe. For instance, a temperature of 98.6°F (37°C) and a WBC count of 8,000/cmm provide good evidence that there is no infection, and it is relatively easy to attribute these results to the effects of the antibiotic that was prescribed. The nursing perspective is more holistic, so it is sometimes difficult even to define the outcomes desired. Emotional, social, or spiritual responses, for instance, are hard to state in measurable terms. It is also difficult to measure the degree to which the outcome was caused by the nursing care. Many variables contribute to improvement (or deterioration) in the client's health (e.g., the nature of the illness, medical interventions, quality of nursing care, availability of resources, client motivation, and family participation).

However, studies have demonstrated nursing's impact on selected patient outcomes, such as the following (ANA, 1997; Agency for Healthcare Research & Quality, 2007):

- Higher nurse staffing was associated with shorter patient lengths of stay.
- A high ratio of RNs to non-RNs was related to patients having fewer preventable conditions (e.g., pressure ulcers, pneumonia, postoperative infections, and urinary tract infections).

9-3 THINK & REFLECT!

In the past 3 months, several medication errors have been made on your nursing unit. The unit has instituted some policies and procedures to improve the safety of this task. Develop criteria to use to evaluate whether this practice problem has been solved. Include criteria to measure structure, process, and outcomes. To begin, answer these questions:

- What is the purpose of the evaluation?
- What is being evaluated; what is the function of the "thing" being evaluated?
- What different points of view may exist?

See suggested responses to #9-3 Think & Reflect! in Appendix A.

A Procedure for Quality-Assurance Evaluation

The quality-assurance process is similar to the nursing process; it involves data collection, comparison of data with criteria, identification of problems, generation and implementation of solutions, and reevaluation. It is different in that it focuses on nurses and institutions rather than patients and is concerned with groups of clients rather than individuals. The following steps are included in the quality-assurance models of most organizations:

1. **Decide the topic to be evaluated.** The topic might be the care for a group of clients with a particular medical diagnosis, care for all clients in a hospital, or record keeping on a nursing unit.
2. **Identify standards of care.** Determine whether structure, process, or outcome standards are appropriate. Recall that standards are broad guidelines and are not measurable or useful in data collection. Therefore, this step is sometimes omitted, and only the criteria are actually written.
3. **Establish criteria for measuring the standards of care.** Process and outcome criteria are specific, observable characteristics that describe the desired behaviors of the nurse or client.
4. **Determine expected compliance or performance levels.** A performance level is the percentage of times you would expect the criterion to be met. This may vary from 0% to 100%, depending on how the criterion is stated. For example, you might expect that 95% of the time, an admission database would be completed within 4 hours after the client was admitted.
5. **Collect data related to the criteria.** Data may be obtained from client interviews, chart audits, direct observation of nursing activities, questionnaires, or special evaluation tools, depending on the criterion being evaluated.
6. **Analyze the data.** Identify discrepancies between the data and the criteria. Using information about structures, processes, and outcomes, determine the reasons for the discrepancies. Identify problems. In the example in Item 4, if fewer than 95% of the admission databases were completed in the specified time, it would be important to find out why this is happening.
7. **Generate solutions for correcting discrepancies and solving problems.** For instance, more in-service education may be needed for nurses, perhaps the staffing pattern should be changed, or maybe a new data collection form should be used.

8. **Implement the solutions.** The purpose of evaluation is to maintain the quality of care being delivered. After problems have been identified, action must be taken to see that they do not recur.
9. **Reevaluate to determine if the solutions were effective.**

QA enables nursing to demonstrate accountability to society for the quality of its services. Consumers, administrators, and bureaucrats do not always clearly see the relationship between good nursing care and improved patient outcomes. Professional survival requires that nurses demonstrate this link. Additionally, the current payment systems encourage agencies to keep patients for as short a time as possible, raising both professional and consumer concerns about quality. Providing adequate care is difficult under these circumstances, and nurses are challenged to monitor and promote good care.

SUMMARY

Evaluation:

- Is a deliberate, systematic process in which the quality, value, or worth of something is determined by comparing it with previously identified criteria or standards.
- Considers *structure* (focusing on the setting in which care is given), *process* (focusing on nursing activities), and *outcomes* (focusing on the changes in client health status that result from nursing care).
- In nursing process, is a planned, ongoing, deliberate activity in which the nurse, client, significant others, and other healthcare professionals determine the client's progress toward goal achievement and the effectiveness of the nursing care plan.
- Does not end the nursing process because the information it provides is used to begin another cycle.
- Involves five steps: (a) *review* of the stated client goals or predicted outcomes, (b) *collection* of data about the client's responses to nursing interventions, (c) *comparison* of actual client outcomes with the desired outcomes and drawing a conclusion about whether the goals have been met, (d) *recording* of evaluative statements, and (e) *relating* the nursing interventions to the client outcomes.
- Requires the nurse to consider all variables, including cultural and spiritual, that may have influenced goal achievement and to modify the care plan as needed.

Quality-assurance evaluation:

- Is an ongoing, systematic process designed to evaluate and promote excellence in health care.
- Is usually concerned with the care given to groups of clients.
- Frequently refers to evaluation of the level of care provided in an agency; it may be as limited in scope as an evaluation of the performance of one nurse or as broad as the evaluation of the overall quality of care in an entire country.
- Commonly uses the methods of retrospective chart audit and peer review.
- Reflects the moral principles of beneficence and nonmaleficence.

Take-away point: As a quick check on your thinking when evaluating, you can use the following four questions:

❑ Do the data indicate goal achievement?
❑ Which nursing interventions did or did not contribute to goal achievement?
❑ Have I reexamined each step of the nursing process?
❑ Did I get patient input during evaluation?

CRITICAL THINKING AND CLINICAL REASONING: A CASE STUDY

Carla Jackson, a 55-year-old widow, has come to the clinic for her annual check-up and mammogram. Her history indicates that she has not worked outside the home in more than 30 years. She tells the nurse that since the death of her husband a few months ago, she has lost interest in her usual physical activities. She no longer attends her swimming and yoga classes, and she does not see the couples she and her husband had as mutual friends. Carla says she is bored, depressed, and "I hate how I'm beginning to look." Her height is 5 ft 2 in, and she weighs 160 lb. She says, "I've gained 15 lb just in the last 2 months!" She says that her eating habits have changed: "It doesn't seem worth the trouble to cook a meal now. I just snack on whatever is handy—chips, cookies, ice cream. If I crave 'real' food, I buy a fast-food burger or something." Ms. Jackson's lab results are all normal. She asks the nurse to help her find a way to lose weight. The nurse diagnoses a nutrition problem and together they make the following plan:

Nursing Diagnosis: *Imbalanced Nutrition: More than Body Requirements r/t excess calorie intake and decreased activity expenditure.*

1. Has the nurse omitted any important nursing diagnoses (refer to a nursing diagnosis handbook, such as Wilkinson (2009) or NANDA (2009) to check Ms. Jackson's defining characteristics)?
2. What do you think about the nursing diagnosis of Imbalanced Nutrition for Ms. Jackson?

[handwritten: Risk for? Dx = Depression]

Goals or Desired Outcomes	Nursing Interventions and Activities

Weight Maintenance Behavior (NOC #1628).
1. Maintains optimal daily caloric intake
2. Develops an exercise plan that gradually engages her in 30 minutes of daily exercise (by next appointment, which is in 1 month)
3. Identifies eating habits that contribute to weight gain by day 2.
	1. **Weight Reduction Assistance** (NIC #1280)
	  a. Determine eating patterns by having pt. keep a diary of what, when, and where she eats.
	  b. Help pt. to develop a daily meal plan with a well-balanced diet, reduced calories, and reduced fat.
	2. **Nutritional Counseling** (NIC #5246)
	  a. Use accepted nutritional standards to assist Ms. Jackson to evaluate the adequacy of her dietary intake.
	  b. Discuss food likes and dislikes.
	3. **Behavior Modification** (NIC #4360)
	  a. Identify the specific behaviors to be changed.
	  b. Have pt. choose rewards that are meaningful to her for motivation to follow her plans.

3. How could you make it more descriptive of Ms. Jackson's situation?

4. How could the desired outcomes for Weight Control be improved? When you are deciding the desired amount of weekly weight loss, which of the following principles is essential to apply?

   a. Goal setting provides motivation, which is essential for a successful weight-loss program.

   b. A combined plan of calorie reduction and exercise can enhance weight loss because exercise increases calorie utilization.

   c. Intake must be reduced by 500 calories to obtain a 1 lb/week weight loss.

   d. Overweight people are often nutritionally deprived.

5. Look at Nursing Activity 1b. Which of the preceding principles provides the rationale for this nursing activity?

6. What referrals might be helpful for the nurse to make?

   When Ms. Jackson comes to the clinic the following month, she has lost 3 lb. She brings with her a dietary log. Using nutritional standards to evaluate her diet, she and the nurse determine that she has been planning well-balanced, nutritionally sound meals. Ms. Jackson verbalizes awareness that she feels hungry and eats when she is bored and depressed— "but I'm not keeping junk food in the house now, so when I can't resist snacking, at least it is more nutritious food now." She says she has been walking about 20 minutes each day.

7. Discuss the extent to which each of the desired outcomes has been met.

8. Which of the planned nursing activities does the nurse still need to implement at this visit? Why?

9. Ms. Jackson says, "I realize that a lot of my snacking is done while I watch TV. This is one of the behaviors I need to change." Consider this principle: It is easier to increase (or add) a behavior than to decrease (or stop) one.

   a. What specific suggestions can you make using this principle to help her change her snacking behavior?

   b. What has Ms. Jackson already done that uses this principle?

10. Ms. Jackson's specific plans are to (a) decrease her calorie intake by 500 calories per day, (b) engage in 30 minutes of exercise a day, (c) keep a food diary, and (d) stop snacking in front of the TV. Try to imagine you are Ms. Jackson.

    a. How would you reward yourself for modifying these behaviors? Indicate which behaviors you would reward, how often you would reward yourself, and with what (e.g., would you reward yourself every day you decreased your intake by 500 calories or only after you do it every day for a week?).

    b. Explain why each of these rewards would be meaningful to you.

Creating a Plan of Care

10

Introduction

Chapters 3 through 9 presented the six phases of the nursing process and illustrated how each step is applied using nursing models as frameworks for collecting, organizing, and analyzing data. Figure 10–1 is a reminder of the two planning phases of the nursing process, in which the nurse creates the patient plan of care. The nursing process phases are summarized in Figure 10–2.

This chapter describes each component of a comprehensive plan of care. The Luisa Sanchez case, begun in Chapter 3, is used to demonstrate how to create a comprehensive plan of care by combining standardized (preprinted) and individually written plans. And finally, a step-by-step Care-Planning Guide summarizes how the nursing process is used to create plans of care.

Most healthcare organizations (e.g., hospitals) and regulating bodies (e.g., The Joint Commission) require evidence of care planning. However, the plan of care may not all be found in one place. For example, the nursing assessment may be in one place, a critical pathway with outcomes and interventions in another, medical orders in another, and an individualized nursing diagnosis care plan in another. Sometimes an individualized plan can be found only in the progress notes.

Comprehensive Plans of Care

Nurses use the term *plan of care* (or *care plan*) in two ways: (a) when referring to the outcomes and nursing orders for a single problem or nursing diagnosis and (b) when referring to the total plan of care for a patient. To avoid confusion, this text uses **nursing diagnosis care plan** for the first meaning and **comprehensive plan of care** for the second.

LEARNING OUTCOMES

After completing this chapter, you should be able to do the following:

- Describe the content of a comprehensive patient plan of care.
- Compare and contrast standardized and individually written plans of care.
- Explain how critical pathways, model care plans, standards of care, protocols, and policies are used in creating a patient plan of care.
- Compare and contrast individualized nursing care plans with multidisciplinary care plans or critical pathways.
- List guidelines for writing patient plans of care.
- Explain how a well-written plan of care supports two conventional ethical principles of nursing.
- Describe the steps necessary in using the nursing process to develop a comprehensive patient plan of care.

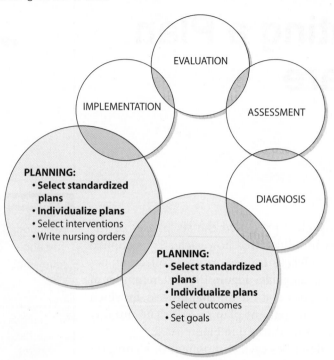

FIGURE 10–1
Creating a plan of care

Components of a Comprehensive Plan of Care

A comprehensive plan of care is made up of several different documents that cover all aspects of the care needed by the patient. Any nurse, even one who does not know the patient, should be able to find in the plan the instructions needed to provide competent care. The plan may consist of a combination of preprinted and handwritten documents, including the following:

1. A brief client profile
2. Instructions for meeting basic care needs
3. Nursing responsibilities for the medical plan
4. The care plan for the patient's identified nursing diagnoses and collaborative problems.

Many care plans also include special sections for discharge and teaching plans. Figure 10–3 illustrates the components of a comprehensive plan of care.

Client Profile

The client profile includes the client's name, age, admitting diagnosis, support people, and other pertinent personal or demographic data. This should be a brief summary, available at a glance, to give a quick overview of the client. On a computer care plan (see Figure 10–12), some profile data appears at the top of each page. The Kardex

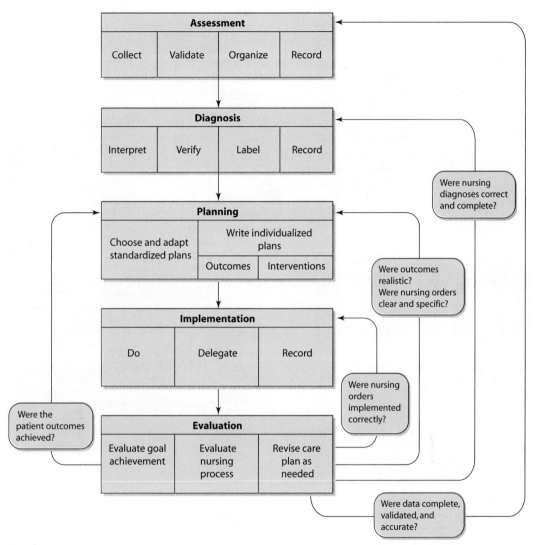

FIGURE 10–2

The interdependent steps of the nursing process

(Figure 10–4) shows Luisa Sanchez's profile data, taken from Figure 3–2 in Chapter 3. The profile data are grouped in a section at the bottom of the Kardex. Notice that even if the nurse is not acquainted with Mrs. Sanchez, she can quickly find out how to reach Mr. Sanchez in case of an emergency. She can also see the date and type of surgery, as well as the physician to call if she needs medical orders.

Instructions for Meeting Basic Needs

Regardless of the client's nursing diagnoses, the nurse must know what routine assistance is needed for hygiene, nutrition, elimination, and other basic needs. Most comprehensive plans of care have a separate section for these instructions, often on a

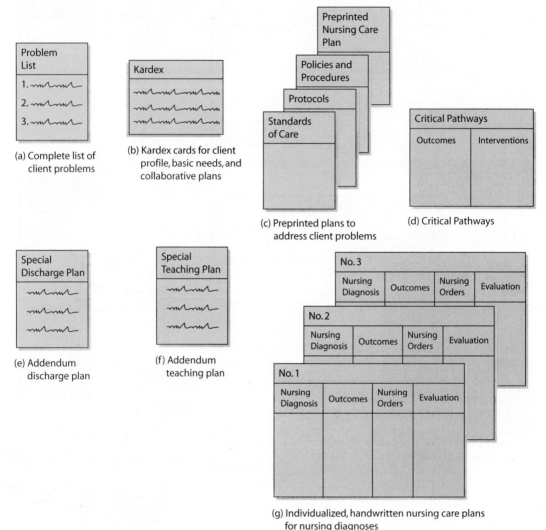

(a) Complete list of client problems

(b) Kardex cards for client profile, basic needs, and collaborative plans

(c) Preprinted plans to address client problems

(d) Critical Pathways

(e) Addendum discharge plan

(f) Addendum teaching plan

(g) Individualized, handwritten nursing care plans for nursing diagnoses

FIGURE 10–3

Components of a comprehensive plan of care

Kardex or basic care flowsheet, where they can be found quickly and conveniently. From Figure 10–4, the nurse can quickly determine that Mrs. Sanchez can feed herself, can have clear liquids and then solid foods as she can tolerate them, can get out of bed to go to the bathroom, has an intravenous (IV) line, and should have 3,000 mL of fluids per day. Because instructions for meeting basic needs change rapidly as the client's condition changes, this section of the care plan is usually marked with pencil so it can be easily altered.

You may need to write individualized nursing diagnosis care plans for clients who have special basic needs requirements (e.g., those with Bathing/Hygiene Self-Care

SHAWNEE MISSION MEDICAL CENTER

Date ord.	Radiology	Date Sch	DONE	Date ord.	Laboratory	Date Sch	DONE	Date ord.	Special Procedures	Date Sch	DONE
4/16/12	Chest X ray PA + lateral	4/16	✓	4/16	Blood Culture	4/16	✓	4/16	C+S sputum		✓
				4/16	urine specific gravity			4/16	24-hr urine		
				4/16	Blood gases	4/16	✓				
				4/16	serum Electrolytes	4/16	✓				
				4/16	CBC with diff	4/16	✓				
									Daily Tests		
	Ancillary Consults										
									Daily Weight		

Diet: Clear liquid, then as tol.

Food Allergies: none

Hold:

Feeding/Fluids
- ☒ Self
- ☐ Assist
- ☐ Feeder
- ☒ Force 3,000 ml/day
- ☐ Restrict c̄ IV

	meal	Ext	IV
7-3			
3-11			
11-7			

☒ I&O
☒ IV O₅ LR, 100/hr
☐ Other

Safety Measures
- ☐ Siderails
- ☐ Restraints
- ☐ Other

Activities
- ☐ Bedrest
- ☒ BRP
- ☐ Dangle
- ☒ Chair
- ☐ Commode
- ☐ Up ad Lib
- ☐ Turn
- ☐ Ambulate

Transportation
per _____

Hygiene
- ☐ Bedbath
- ☒ Assist
- ☐ Self Bath
- ☒ Shower
- ☐ Tub
- ☐ Vanity
- ☐ Oral Care

Bowel/Bladder
- ☐ Foley   IN ____ OUT ____
- ☐ Cath care Bid
- ☐ Incontinent
- ☐ Colostomy
- ☐ Ileostomy
- ☐ Urostomy

Communication

Fowlers or semi-Fowlers position

V.S. q̄ 4h

Physical Therapy	Date	Treatments
Cardio-Pulmonary		4/16 Postural drainage 0900 daily
		4/16 Incentive spirometer q̄ 3 hrs
		4/16 O₂ per cannula at 5 L
		4/16 Nebulizer q4h

Drug Allergies: Penicillin

Isolation: In   Out

Emergency Instructions: Out of town until 4/17.
Relatives: Michael Sanchez
Phone: 641-1212

Clergy: None
Religion: Catholic

Religious Rites: Last Rites only

Code Blue: Yes

Diagnosis: Pneumonia

Surgery & Dates:

Consults & Dates:

Room	Name	Adm Date	Age	Physician
416	Luisa Sanchez	4-16-12	28	R. Katz

FIGURE 10–4

Kardex: client profile, basic needs, and medical plan (*Source:* Courtesy of Shawnee Mission Health System, Shawnee Mission, KS).

Deficit, urinary incontinence, or impaired nutrition). These would be written in the nursing diagnosis care plan section (see Figure 10–3).

Aspects of the Medical Plan to Be Implemented by the Nurse

A comprehensive plan of care includes nursing activities necessary for carrying out medical orders such as dressing changes and IV therapy. It also includes a section for scheduling prescribed diagnostic tests and treatments to be carried out by other departments (e.g., physical therapy). In Figure 10–13, this type of information is listed under "Active Physician Orders" and "Active Ancillary Orders." In Figure 10–4, it appears mainly in the top section of the form.

It is better to have a separate section for these activities, but you may also see them included as a part of the nursing plan of care for a nursing diagnosis or collaborative problem—for example, in the section for "Laboratory" in Figure 10–4, a physician prescribed a "blood culture." However, if you were creating a student care plan, you might not have a Kardex form to work with. So, for Mrs. Sanchez, you might write a collaborative problem: Potential Complication of Pneumonia: Sepsis. The medical prescription for a blood culture would then be incorporated into the nursing interventions for that problem.

EXAMPLE: Medical order (in bold print) included in student plan of care.

Problem	*Nursing Orders*
Potential Complication of Pneumonia: Sepsis	1. **Blood cultures today, per order.** Explain reason for blood cultures
	2. Temperature q4hr. Hourly if > 101°F

Nursing Diagnoses and Collaborative Problems

The **nursing diagnosis care plan** is the section of the comprehensive plan of care that prescribes the outcomes and nursing interventions for the patient's nursing diagnoses and collaborative problems. A comprehensive plan of care usually contains several single-problem care plans. The nursing diagnosis care plan reflects the independent component of nursing practice and is the part of the comprehensive plan that best demonstrates the nurse's clinical expertise. Figure 10–5 is an example of a plan of care for a single nursing diagnosis. Note, too, that Luisa Sanchez's plan of care (see Figure 10–13) also contains nursing diagnosis care plans.

Addendum Care Plans

In many institutions, the comprehensive plan of care includes separate sections (addendum plans) for discharge planning and special teaching needs. Figure 6–2, in Chapter 6, is an example of a discharge plan.

Teaching needs may be addressed in standards of care, in critical pathways (as in Figures 10–7 and 10–8), or by individually written nursing diagnoses. It is usually better to include teaching interventions as a part of the nursing orders for every nursing

PATIENT PLAN OF CARE Genesis Medical Center – Davenport, Iowa

GAS EXCHANGE IMPAIRMENT: Excess or deficit in oxygenation and/or carbon dioxide elimination at the alveolar-capillary membrane.

SIGNS & SYMPTOMS: Observed or reported (select at least 2)

☐ Abnormal arterial blood gases	☐ Irritability	☐ Hypercapnea	☐ Somnolence
☐ Restlessness	☐ Vision disturbances	☐ Hypoxemia	☐ Dyspnea
☐ Confusion	☐ Nasal flaring	☐ Cyanosis (Neonates)	☐ HA upon awakening

OUTCOME SCORING

RELATED FACTORS:	OUTCOMES	ADM			DC	INTERVENTIONS
☐ Alveolar-capillary membrane changes 1A00250001 ☐ Ventilation/ perfusion alterations 1A00250002	☐ **Respiratory Status: Gas Exchange** - Neurological Status IER - Ease of Breathing - Restlessness Not Present - O$_2$ Saturation WNL - PaO$_2$ WNL - PaCO$_2$ WNL - CXR Findings IER ☐ **Respiratory Status: Ventilation** - Respiratory Rate, Rhythm IER - Dyspenea & Rest Not Present - Adventitious Breath Sounds Not Present					☐ Respiratory Monitoring 1E00253350 ☐ Oxygen Therapy 1E00253320 ☐ Ventilation Assistance 1E00253390 ☐ Acid-Base Monitoring 1E00251920 ☐ Acid-Base Management 1E00251910 ☐ Airway Suctioning 1E00253160 ☐ Mechanical Vantilation 1E00253300 ☐ Airway Management ☐ Artificial Airway Management ☐ Cough Enhancement ☐ Mechanical Ventilatory Weaning ☐ Embolus Care: Pulmonary ☐ Resuscitation: Neonate ☐ Aspiration Precautions

Definition of Scoring Scales	1	2	3	4	5
Respiratory Status: Gas Exchange Alveolar Exchange of CO$_2$ to Maintain Arterial Blood Gas Concentration. **Respiratory Status: Ventilation** Movement of Air In and Out of the Lungs.	Extremely Compromised	Substantially Compromised	Moderately Compromised	Mildly Compromised	Not Compromised

Diagnosis _____

Date Initiated _____ RN Initials _____

Date Resolved _____

469-028G 12/99 _____

FIGURE 10–5

Standardized care plan for a single nursing diagnosis, using NANDA-I, NOC, and NIC (*Source:* Courtesy of Genesis Health System [Genesis Medical Center and Illini Hospital], Davenport, IA).

diagnosis rather than to use a Knowledge Deficit problem to address all the patient's various learning needs. However, when a patient has complex learning needs (e.g., a new mother without a support system), you may wish to develop a special teaching plan to ensure efficient use of nursing time and maximize the patient's learning. Figure 10–6 is an example of a section of an individualized teaching plan.

		Nursing Diagnosis: Risk for Ineffective Health Maintenance r/t lack of knowledge of insulin therapy		
Met	**Learning Objective**	**Content**	**Teaching Strategy**	**Learning Strategy**
	1st Session Client will describe the basic pathophysiology of diabetes mellitus (cognitive).	Location and function of pancreas How cells use glucose Function of insulin Effects of insulin deficiency (e.g., elevated blood sugar, mobilization of fats and proteins, ketones)	Explain. Use a transparency of the pancreas.	Read pamphlet, "Your Pancreas."
	2nd Session Client will demonstrate ability to draw up correct amount of insulin (psychomotor).	Syringe markings Sterile technique Preparation	Point out on enlarged drawing then on actual syringe. Demonstrate and discuss. Demonstrate and discuss: How to mix insulin. Read label carefully; be sure syringe and label concentrations match. Clean top of bottle with alcohol. Withdraw correct amount.	Practice with syringe and vial of sterile water.

FIGURE 10–6

Sample teaching plan (partial) for diabetes mellitus

10-1 WHAT DO YOU KNOW?

1. List the five components of a comprehensive plan of care.
2. In which component of the care plan would you expect to find a patient's religious preferences listed?
3. Where would you look to find the plan of care for a patient with special teaching needs?

See answer to #10-1 What Do You Know? in Appendix A.

Standardized Approaches to Care Planning

Obviously, it would be inefficient to handwrite every bit of nursing care needed for all patients for whom a nurse provides care. For predictable or routine problems, the outcomes and nursing orders are often available in standardized, preprinted instructions in critical pathways, standards of care, standardized nursing diagnosis care plans, protocols, and agency policies and procedures. Regardless of the system used, it is up to the nurse to modify standardized plans or handwrite an individualized plan for unique patient needs. The problem list you develop for the patient (see Chapters 4 and 5) will help you to individualize care because each patient, regardless of medical diagnosis, will have a different set of problems and etiologies.

Take-away point: Use standardized care planning for routine or predictable problems, but modify these plans, as needed, to individualize care for each patient.

Critical Pathways

As discussed in Chapters 4 and 6, a **critical pathway** is a standardized form of the multidisciplinary plan that outlines the care required for patients with common, predictable conditions (e.g., a patient undergoing a renal transplant). It is organized with a column (or sometimes a page) for each day of hospitalization. There are as many columns (or pages) on the plan as the preset number of days allowed for the client's diagnostic-related group (DRG). For example, if the expected length of stay for a renal transplant patient is 5 days, the renal transplant critical pathway would have five columns (or five pages). See Figure 10–7 for a portion of a critical pathway. Patients often receive a modified form of their critical pathway so they will know what to expect (see Figure 10–8 for an example).

Critical pathways can result in cost savings and increased patient satisfaction, and the communication that occurs in creating them tends to enhance collaborative practice. Nevertheless, they are time consuming to develop, and there is concern that individualized care may be lost in this system. The focus of such plans is usually more medical than holistic, and the need to achieve outcomes within rigidly specified time frames creates the danger of focusing on efficiency more than quality of care.

HOSPITAL OF THE UNIVERSITY OF PENNSYLVANIA

TOTAL LOWER JOINT (HIP/KNEE)
CLINICAL PATHWAY

ELIGIBILITY CRITERIA: All primary unilateral total hip or total knee replacements

EXPECTED LOS: 3 Days

ADDRESSOGRAPH

CLINICAL KEYS:
1. Pain managed ≤ midpoint on painscale
2. Transfer to chair/commode with assistance POD 1; Ambulate in room, bathroom POD 2
3. DVT precautions
4. Discharge plan completed by POD 2
5. Patient verbalizes knowledge of hip or knee precautions
6. Knee motion 10° to 70° or better (TKA patients only)

	PACU	IMMED. POST-OP	POD 1	POD 2	POD 3–4
ASSESSMENTS	• NV checks with VS q 1h x 4 • Pain • Effects of narcotics/ tolerance • I & O × 24hr • Pulse O× q8 if on O2	• NV check/VS q 4 hr → → • S/S DVT →	→ → → → • Pulse Ox x1 on RA • Dsg/Wound status q4	• NV check/VS q 8 hr → → → • D/C pulse Ox If O2 D/C • Dsg/Wound status q8	→ → → → →
CONSULTS		• PT • PMR	→(If not done already) →(If not done already)		
TESTS	• A/P Hip X-ray (THA) • A/P knee X-ray (TKA)		• CBC	→ • INR (If on warfarin)	• A/P hip X-ray →
TREATMENTS	• O2	• D/C O2 if set ≥ 94% • Incentive spirometry • Order walker (hip chair, elevated commode if needed) • Pneumatic compression device (ankle for knees, calf for hips)	→ → • D/C foley • Dressing change (1st dsg change by MD) →	→ → • Dressing change q day and pm	→ → →
MEDICATIONS/IVS	• PCA or epidural	→ • Anticoagulation	• IV heplock → • Consider conversion to oral pain meds	• D/C heplock → • D/C PCA/PCEA • PO pain meds	→
ACTIVITY/ FUNCTIONAL LEVEL	• Bedrest • Hip precautions if THA • CPM for total knee	→ → →	• OOB to chair BID → → • Weight bear per order • Ambulate with assistive device	• OOB TID → → → • PT x2	→ → → → → →
NUTRITION/ ELIMINATION	• NPO	• NPO → Ice → advance to full as tolerated	• Regular	→	→
EDUCATION/ DISCHARGE PLANNING	• Deep breathing exercises	• Pain management • Initiate d/c plan	→ • Home vs Rehab decision • Anticoagulation if Indicated	→ • S/S wound infection • Medications • Activity level • D/C plan in place	→ → → • Car transfer

Transfer to Rehab when:	Discharge to Home when:
1. Able to participate in care 2. Tolerating 2 Physical Therapy sessions 3. Not requiring IV pain medicine 4. Blood values are stable 5. Motivation is commensurate with projected functional status	1. Mobility and ADL's appropriate for degree of assistance at home and home environment 2. Appropriate assistive device and necessary adaptive equipment is used 3. Independent with hip/knee precautions 4. Independent with home exercise program or ongoing PT in the home or outpatient **IF D/C TO HOME, ENSURE APPROPRIATE CONSULTS TO ARRANGE HOME CARE FOLLOW-UP AND EQUIPMENT

FIGURE 10–7

Portion of a total lower joint critical pathway (*Source:* Courtesy of the Hospital of the University of Pennsylvania, Philadelphia, PA).

Patient's Overview for Total Knee Replacement

NOTE: This is a guide *only*. Your plan of care may vary depending on doctor orders, your individualized needs, and/or your response to treatment.

Category	Operative Day	Post-Op Days 1–2	Post-Op Day 3–Discharge
Exercise/Rest	• You will be on bed rest. • You may be started on gentle knee movement using continuous passive motion machine (CPM). • You will be assisted to turn from side to side approximately every 2 hours after surgery, unless you have a CPM machine.	• Out of bed activity progresses from sitting on side of bed to sitting in chair. • Physical Therapy starts with exercises and progresses to walking with walker/crutches. The amount of weight you can put on your operative leg may be limited according to your doctor. • If you have a CPM, the degree of bend will be increased daily.	• Your activity will continue to progress from sitting in a chair to walking in halls. • You will continue to walk with walker/crutches. The amount of weight you can put on your operative leg may remain limited. • Your goal is 90° bend by discharge with Physical Therapy and/or CPM. • Your CPM will continue to be increased daily.
Nutrition/Fluids	• You will have an IV. • Liquids are allowed upon arrival to the nursing unit following surgery. • Solid foods may be permitted for the evening meal if you are not nauseated.	• IV continued. • Diet as tolerated.	• IV stopped on third day.

FIGURE 10–8

Portion of a critical pathway given to patients (*Source:* Courtesy of Shawnee Mission Medical Center, Shawnee Mission, KS. Used with permission).

Unit Standards of Care

Unit standards of care are standardized, preprinted directions for care developed by nurses for groups of clients rather than for individuals. They are detailed guidelines for the care to be given in defined situations, for example:

- A medical diagnosis (e.g., abdominal hysterectomy)
- A treatment or diagnostic test (e.g., colonoscopy)
- A nursing diagnosis (e.g., anticipatory grieving)
- A situation such as relinquishment of a newborn

Standards of care describe achievable rather than ideal nursing care, taking into account the circumstances and client population of the institution. They do not contain medical orders. They are different from critical pathways in that they are not time sequenced and they define only interventions for which nurses are held accountable. Standards of care are usually not placed in the client's medical record but are reference documents that are stored as permanent hospital records. They are either filed on the unit or in the computer for easy reference. When they are not a part of the comprehensive plan of care, the problem list (see Table 10–1 later in the chapter) should indicate which standards of care apply to the patient. Standards of care may or may not be organized according to nursing diagnoses. Figure 10–9 is an example of standards of care that list only the nursing interventions without identifying the problems to which they apply. Clearly, though, it focuses on the collaborative problem of Potential Complication of Thrombophlebitis: Pulmonary Embolus.

Model (Standardized) Care Plans

Do not confuse **standardized care plans** with *standards of care*. To avoid confusion, some nurses prefer to call them **model care plans**. Although they have some similarities, there are important differences between standards of care and model care plans:

1. Model care plans are kept with the client's active care plan (in the Kardex or computer). When no longer active, they become a part of her permanent medical record. This is not usually true of standards of care.
2. Model care plans provide more detailed instructions than standards of care. They contain deviations (either additions or deletions) from the standards for the agency.
3. Unlike standards of care, model care plans take the usual nursing process format:

Problem → Outcomes → Nursing orders → Evaluation

4. Model care plans allow you to add addendum care plans. They usually include checklists, blank lines, or empty spaces to allow you to individualize goals and nursing orders. This is not usually true for standards of care.

Model care plans are similar to standards of care in that they are preprinted guides for nursing interventions for a specific nursing diagnosis or for all the nursing diagnoses associated with a particular situation or medical condition. They are developed by nurses, and although they are not standards of care, following them ensures that acceptable standards of care are provided. Refer to Figure 10–10 for a portion of a preprinted model care plan. Figure 10–5 is a printout of an electronic model care plan for a single nursing diagnosis. Both of these examples use NANDA-I, NIC, and NOC.

Many commercial books of model care plans are available. You can use them as guides when developing plans of care, but remember that they do not address the client's individualized needs, and they can cause you to focus on predictable problems and miss cues to important special problems the client is experiencing. If you use a model care plan as a student, do the following:

1. Consult your instructor to be sure you are using a reliable source.
2. Perform a nursing assessment and make your own list of all the client's actual and potential problems. You can then consult the model care plan to be sure your list is complete.
3. Using client input, establish specific, individualized goals before consulting the model care plan. Consulting the model plan first may inhibit your creativity.

4. Be sure the nursing interventions in the model plan are appropriate for your client and are possible to implement in your institution. Delete any that do not apply.

5. Individualize the outcomes and nursing orders to fit your client.

STANDARDS OF CARE: Patient with Thrombophlebitis

Goal:
1. To monitor for early signs and symptoms of compromised respiratory status
2. To report any abnormal signs and/or symptoms promptly to the medical staff
3. To initiate appropriate nursing actions when signs and/or symptoms of compromised respiratory status occur
4. To institute protocol for emergency intervention should the client develop cardiopulmonary dysfunction

SUPPORTIVE DATA: The purpose of these standards of care is to prevent, monitor, report, and record the client's response to a diagnosis of thrombophlebitis. Thrombophlebitis places the client at risk for pulmonary embolism. The hemodynamic consequences of embolic obstruction to pulmonary blood flow involve increased pulmonary vascular resistance, increased right ventricular workload, decreased cardiac output, and development of shock and pulmonary arrest.

CLINICAL MANIFESTATIONS: Nursing assessments performed q3–4h should monitor for the following signs/symptoms:

- Dyspnea (generally consistently present)
- Sudden substernal pain
- Rapid/weak pulse
- Syncope
- Anxiety
- Fever
- Cough/hemoptysis
- Accelerated respiratory rate
- Pleuritic type chest pain
- Cyanosis

PREVENTIVE NURSING MEASURES:

- Encourage increased fluid intake to prevent dehydration.
- Maintain anticoagulant intravenous therapy as prescribed (see Protocol for Anticoagulant Administration).
- Maintain prescribed bed rest.
- Prevent venous stasis from improperly fitting elastic stockings; check q3–4h.
- Encourage dorsiflexion exercises of the lower extremities while on bed rest.

INDIVIDUALIZED PLANS/ADDITIONAL NURSING/MEDICAL ORDERS

_____Do not massage lower extremities._____

_____Intake and output q8h._____

Initiated by: _____S. Ibarra, RN_____ Date: _4-9-12_

FIGURE 10–9

Example of non–problem-oriented standards of care

Patient Name: _____

PLAN OF CARE   Medical Record Number: _____

NURSING DIAGNOSIS	INTERVENTION	OUTCOME		
Impaired Physical Mobility Related To:	**Exercise Therapy: Ambulation**	Outcome	Indicators	Scale
☐ Intolerance to activity/ decreased strength and endurance	**ACTIVITIES** Medicate with prescribed analgesic prior to Physical Therapy session to enhance level of mobility.	**Mobility Level** (Ability to move purposefully)	Transfer performance Ambulation: walking	(circle one) Date: _____ Initials: _____ 1 2 3 4 5
☐ Pain/discomfort	Gait training per Physical Therapy.			Date: _____ Initials: _____ 1 2 3 4 5
☐ Perceptual/cognitive impairment	Transfer training per Physical Therapy.			Date: _____ Initials: _____ 1 2 3 4 5
☐ Neuromuscular impairment ☐ Depression/severe anxiety	Bed mobility / activity training per Physical Therapy.			Date: _____ Initials: _____ 1 2 3 4 5
	Monitor patient's use of walking aids/ adaptive devices.			Date: _____ Initials: _____ 1 2 3 4 5
	Instruct patient about safe transfer and ambulation techniques.			Date: _____ Initials: _____ 1 2 3 4 5
	Place side rails (upper and/or lower) to assist patient with mobility and aid patient in turning and repositioning.			Date: _____ Initials: _____ 1 2 3 4 5
	Ensure post-operative hip precautions are followed, as appropriate.			Date: _____ Initials: _____ 1 2 3 4 5
	Active exercise per Physical Therapy: _____			Date: _____ Initials: _____ 1 2 3 4 5
	Passive exercise per Physical Therapy: _____			Date: _____ Initials: _____ 1 2 3 4 5
	CPM per Physical Therapy: _____			Date: _____ Initials: _____ 1 2 3 4 5
	E Stim per Physical Therapy: _____			Date: _____ Initials: _____ 1 2 3 4 5
	Other: _____			Date: _____ Initials: _____ 1 2 3 4 5
Self-Care Deficit:	**Self-Care Assistance**	**Self-Care: Activities of Daily Living** (Ability to perform the most basic physical tasks and personal care activities)	Dressing	Date: _____ Initials: _____
☐ Bathing/Hygiene Self-Care Deficit	**ACTIVITIES** Monitor patient's ability for independent self-care.		Eating	1 2 3 4 5 Date: _____ Initials: _____
☐ Dressing/Grooming Self-Care Deficit	Monitor patient's need for adaptive devices for personal hygiene, dressing, grooming, toileting and eating.		Toileting	1 2 3 4 5 Date: _____ Initials: _____ 1 2 3 4 5
☐ Toileting Self-Care Deficit	Provide assistance until patient is fully able to assume self-care.			Date: _____ Initials: _____ 1 2 3 4 5
Related To: ☐ Decreased or lack of motivation	Assist patient in accepting dependency needs.			Date: _____ Initials: _____ 1 2 3 4 5
☐ Perceptual or cognitive impairment	Encourage patient to perform normal activities of daily living to level of ability.			Date: _____ Initials: _____ 1 2 3 4 5
☐ Neuromuscular impairment ☐ Musculoskeletal impairment ☐ Discomfort				Date: _____ Initials: _____ 1 2 3 4 5

Scale Descriptors: **1** = Dependent, does not participate, **2** = Requires assistive person and device, **3** = Requires assistive person,
4 = Independent with assistive device, **5** = Completely independent

FIGURE 10–10

Portion of a model care plan (using standardized nursing language) (*Source:* Courtesy of Grant Medical Center, Columbus, OH).

EXAMPLE:

Standardized Nursing Order

Force fluids as ordered or as tolerated by patient.

Individualized Nursing Order

Force fluids to 2400 mL per 24 hours:

7–3: Offer 200 mL water or apple juice hourly.

3–11: Offer 200 mL water or apple juice hourly while awake.

11–7: Offer water or juice when awakening patient for VS or meds.

Pt. prefers ice in his water or juice.

Protocols

Protocols are standardized and preprinted (see Figure 10–11 for an example). Like standards of care and model care plans, they cover the common actions required for a particular medical diagnosis, defined situation, treatment, or diagnostic test. For example, there may be a protocol for admitting a patient to the intensive care unit or a protocol covering the administration of magnesium sulfate to a preeclampsia patient. Protocols are different, however, because they may include both medical orders and nursing orders. When a protocol is used, it can be added to the comprehensive plan of care and become a part of the patient's permanent record. An alternative is to keep all protocols in the hospital's file of permanent records and write "See protocol" on the nursing plan of care, as in Table 10–1, later in the chapter.

Policies and Procedures

When a situation occurs frequently, an institution is likely to develop a **policy** to govern how it is to be handled. For example, a hospital may have a policy that specifies the number of visitors a patient may have. Policies and procedures may also be similar to protocols and specify, for example, what actions are to be taken in the case of cardiac arrest. As with protocols and standing orders, the nurse must recognize the situation and then use judgment in implementing the policy. Hospital policies must be interpreted to meet patient needs.

EXAMPLE: While on a business trip, Fred Gonzalez was in an automobile accident. He has been hospitalized in serious condition for several days. It is 8:55 P.M., and Mr. Gonzalez's wife has just arrived on the unit for her first visit. Even though hospital policy requires that visitors leave at 9 P.M., the nurse decides that implementing the policy would not meet Mr. Gonzalez's needs.

If a policy covers a situation pertinent to the patient care plan, it is usually simply noted on the plan of care (e.g., "Make Social Service referral per Unit Policy"). Hospital policies and procedures are institution records, not patient records, so they are not actually placed in the plan of care.

Expected Outcome: The patient's amniotic fluid level will be increased in attempt to eliminate variable decelerations or to dilute the amount of meconium in the amniotic fluid.

Supportive Data:

Contraindications:	**Possible Complications:**
Late decelerations	Prolapsed cord
Fetal tachycardia	Elevation of intrauterine pressure
Absence of variables	Polyhydramnios
Bleeding	Abruption
Fetal presentation other than vertex	Infection

Policy:

The physician will place the IUPC.

When the fetus is premature the fluid will be warmed through a blood warmer during administration.

When the fetus is at term the fluid may be at room temperature.

Preparation/Administration:

1. Connect 1000ml normal saline to infusion pump tubing. Flush the tubing.
2. Zero and assist the physician with insertion of the IUPC.
3. Attach infusion tubing to the amnio port on the IUPC.
4. To treat variable decelerations:
   a. Bolus infusion of 250ml–500ml in 10 min before connecting to infusion pump.
   b. Place the tubing on the pump after the bolus and run @ 3ml/min or 180ml/hr.
5. To prevent variable decelerations:
   a. Infuse @ 10ml/min for 1 hr (Set infusion pump @ 600ml/hr).

Intervention:

Assess/Document:

1. FHR per standards of practice
2. Intrauterine pressure q 30 min
3. Character/amount of leakage
4. Amount of NS infused
   Note: Amount of fluid infused must not exceed amount leaked by 500ml/1000ml to maintain amniotic fluid volume at all times.

Maintain lateral recumbent position (right/left side).
CAUTION! If resting tone is >25mmg or no uterine relaxation—STOP and notify the physician.

Initiated by: _____

Date: _____

FIGURE 10–11

Protocol for amnioinfusion (*Source:* Courtesy of Shawnee Mission Medical Center, Shawnee Mission, KS).

Electronic Care Plans and Standardized Language

Computers are used to create both standardized and individualized plans of care. Figure 10–5 is a printout of a standardized plan of care for Gas Exchange Impairment that is stored in the computer and individualized by checking the signs and symptoms, outcomes, and interventions that apply to a particular patient. Figure 10–12 shows how a section of a care plan might look on the computer screen. Both of these examples use standardized nursing language (i.e., NANDA-I, NIC, and NOC) to label problems, outcomes, and interventions. Figure 10–13 (later in the chapter) is a printout of a computer-generated care plan, but it does not use standardized language for outcomes

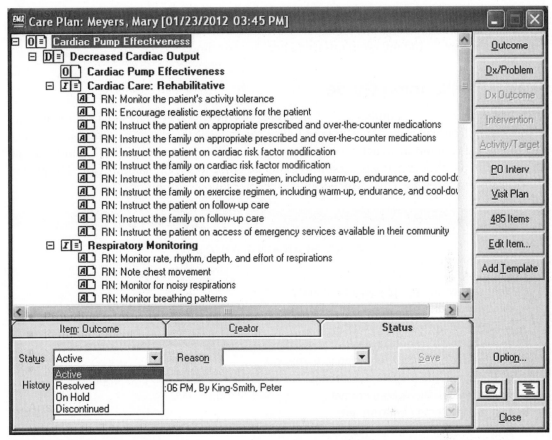

FIGURE 10–12

Computerized plan of care (one screen) using NANDA-I, NOC, and NIC (*Source:* Courtesy of Ergo Partners, L.C. All rights reserved).

10-1 THINK & REFLECT!

You have the following standardized documents:

   a. Critical pathway

   b. Protocol

   c. Agency policy

1. Which one would you probably use to find out how long a patient's friend may visit him in the intensive care unit?

2. Which one would you probably use when a physician is coming to your unit to insert chest tubes in a patient for whom you are providing nursing care?

3. A patient is being admitted for a hip replacement, and you need a map of the collaborative care to be provided during the patient's stay. Which one would you use?

See suggested responses to #10-1 Think & Reflect! in Appendix A.

and interventions. It is an individualized plan created specifically for Luisa Sanchez, for the two nursing diagnoses of Anxiety and Disturbed Sleep Pattern. The nurse typed in the outcomes and interventions using her own wording.

Care-Planning Guide

Now that you are familiar with the various documents that make up a comprehensive plan of care, you should be able to follow the steps of the nursing process and create a plan of care for an actual patient. The Care-Planning Guide in Box 10–1 compresses all the steps of the nursing process into a concise guide to use in planning care. The plan of care developed for Luisa Sanchez in this chapter follows this guide.

BOX 10–1

CARE-PLANNING GUIDE

1. **Collect data.**
   a. Interview, conduct physical examination.
   b. Validate data.
   c. Organize according to framework.
2. **Analyze and synthesize data.**
   a. Group related cues according to framework.
   b. Form new cue clusters as needed.
   c. Identify deviations from normal.
3. **List all problems (working list).**
   a. Human responses that need to be changed.
   b. Medical, nursing, collaborative.
   c. Actual, risk, possible.
4. **Make formal list of labeled problems.**
   a. Label nursing diagnoses (Problem + Etiology)
      1. Problem: Compare patient data to defining characteristics, definitions, and risk factors.
      2. Etiology: Related factors (risk, causal, contributing factors).
   b. Label Collaborative Problems (Potential complications of . . .).
5. **Determine which problems can be addressed by the following:**
   a. Critical pathways
   b. Standards of care
   c. Model care plans
   d. Protocols
   e. Policies or procedures (e.g., note on formal problem list: Risk for Pulmonary Embolus—See Standards of Care.)
6. **Individualize model care plans, protocols, and so forth, as needed.**

BOX 10–1

CARE-PLANNING GUIDE *continued*

7. **Transcribe medical, collaborative, activities of daily living, and basic care needs to Kardex or electronic plan.**
8. **Develop individualized plan of care for remaining nursing diagnoses and collaborative problems.**
   a. Develop individualized outcomes.
      1. State desired client responses.
      2. State opposite of problem response.
      3. Ensure outcomes are measurable and realistic.
   b. Write nursing orders. They should consider the following:
      1. Etiology: reduce or remove related factors.
      2. Problem: relieve symptoms.
      3. Outcomes: how to bring about desired behaviors.
      4. Health promotion, prevention, treatment, and observation.
      5. Physical care, teaching, counseling, environment management, referrals, emotional support, and activities of daily living.
      6. For complex orders, refer to policies and protocol (See "Unit Procedure for IV Therapy").
   c. Include any special or complex teaching or discharge plans.
9. **Implement care plan (do or delegate; document).**
10. **Evaluate results of care.**
    a. Compare patient progress to original goals.
    b. Revise care plan as needed.
       1. Collect more data, if needed.
       2. Revise, discontinue, or continue problem.
       3. Change outcomes if unachievable.
       4. Revise, discontinue, or keep nursing orders.

Each chapter in this book has included a detailed guide for carrying out a particular step of the nursing process. If you need to review any of the steps in the Care-Planning Guide, refer to the appropriate chapter in this book, where the step is expanded for you. In addition to proceeding step by step through the Care-Planning Guide, you should refer to the guidelines in Box 10–2 when writing plans of care.

Creating a Comprehensive Plan of Care

Read the following case study, which describes the course of Luisa Sanchez's hospitalization. Then follow the steps of the Care-Planning Guide in Box 10–1 and the guidelines in Box 10–2 to develop a comprehensive plan of care for Ms. Sanchez.

BOX 10–2

GUIDELINES FOR WRITING PLANS OF CARE

1. **Include each of these components:**
   a. Client profile
   b. Basic needs
   c. Aspects of medical plan
   d. Nursing diagnoses and collaborative problems
   e. Special or complex teaching or discharge needs

2. **Date and sign the initial plan and any revisions.** The date is important for evaluation; the signature demonstrates nursing accountability.

3. **List or number the nursing diagnoses in order of priority.** Priorities can be changed as the client's needs change.

4. **List the nursing orders for each problem in order of priority** or in the order in which they should be done. For instance, you would assess the client's level of knowledge before you teach him to log-roll.

5. **Write the plan in clear, concise terms.** Use standard medical abbreviations and symbols. Use key words rather than complete sentences. Leave out unnecessary words, like *client* and *the* (e.g., write "Turn & reposition q2h" rather than "Turn and reposition the client every 2 hours").

6. **Write legibly and in ink.** When the plan cannot be erased, accountability is emphasized, and more importance is placed on what is being written. If a nursing diagnosis is resolved, write "Discontinued" and a date beside it, highlight it, or date a special "Inactive" column. Outcomes and nursing orders can be discontinued similarly.

7. **For detailed treatments and procedures, refer to other sources** (e.g., standards of care) instead of writing all the steps on the care plan. You might write, "See unit procedure book for diabetic teaching," or you might attach a standard nursing care plan for a problem (e.g., "See standard care plan for ineffective breastfeeding"). This saves time and focuses the written part of the care plan on the unique needs of the client.

8. **Be sure the plan is holistic.** It should consider the client's physiological, psychological, sociocultural, and spiritual needs.

9. **Be sure the plan is individualized** and addresses the client's unique needs. Include the client's choices about how and when care is given. For example, "Prefers evening shower."

10. **Include the collaborative and coordination aspects of the client's care.** You may write nursing orders to consult a social worker or physical therapist, or you may simply coordinate tests and treatments. The medical plan should be incorporated into the nursing care plan so that the two plans do not conflict.

11. **Include discharge plans** (e.g., arrangements for follow-up by a social worker or community health nurse).

CASE STUDY   Luisa Sanchez

Framework: Functional Health Patterns, Gordon

Medical Diagnosis: Pneumonia

Luisa Sanchez, a 28-year-old married attorney, was admitted to the hospital with an elevated temperature; a productive cough; and rapid, labored respirations. During the nursing interview, she told Mary Medina, RN, that she has had a "chest cold" for 2 weeks and has been short of breath on exertion. She stated, "Yesterday I started having a fever and pain in my lungs." Mrs. Sanchez's complete assessment data appear in Figure 3–2 in Chapter 3, so they are repeated here only in part. Admission medical orders included:

CBC with differential	PA and lateral chest X-ray
Arterial blood gases	Blood culture (repeat ×2
Urine specific gravity	if temp over 101°F [38.3°C])
Sputum C&S	24-hour urine
Postural drainage daily	Serum electrolytes
Pulse oximeter	Incentive spirometer q3h
IV of D₅ LR, 100 mL/hr	Nebulizer q4h
Tylenol 650 mg q4h p.o. for	Vancomycin 0.5 g IV q6h
temp >101°F (38.3°C)	O₂ per cannula, 5L

Assessment

Step 1: Collect Data

To begin collecting Mrs. Sanchez's data, you could use a data collection form such as Figure 3–2 in Chapter 3, which is organized by body systems and specific nursing concerns rather than one based on a single nursing model. Next you would organize the data according to a nursing model (e.g., Gordon's Functional Health Patterns) in order to have a worksheet to use during data analysis. Box 4–4 in Chapter 4 summarizes the admission data collected in each of the patterns.

Diagnosis

Step 2: Analyze and Synthesize Data

Next underline all the cues that seem significant or outside the norm (see Box 4–4 in Chapter 4). For example, in the Role-Relationship pattern, the nurse underlined "husband out of town" and "child with neighbor." Next, think about how the abnormal (significant) cues in one group might be related to cues in another group—inductively forming new cue clusters (refer to Table 4–7 in Chapter 4). For instance, in the

Coping/Stress-Tolerance pattern, Luisa shows signs of Anxiety (e.g., tense facial muscles, trembling). You might wonder if the data in the Role/Relationship pattern might be related to that anxiety. Perhaps part of Mrs. Sanchez's anxiety might be caused by worry about her child or by her need for emotional support from her husband, who is away. Because those cues seem related, they are inductively grouped, together with other related cues, into a new cue cluster (Cluster 9 in Table 4–7). Cluster 9 represents a problem that is essentially psychological and fits best in the Self-Perception/Self-Concept pattern.

Notice in Box 4–4 (Chapter 4) that the cues "urinary frequency and amount decreased ×2 days" and "diaphoretic" cannot be interpreted accurately using only the cues in that pattern. To interpret their meaning, you need to think how those abnormal cues relate to the cues in the Nutritional-Metabolic pattern. Notice, too, that even in the new, inductively formed groupings, a single piece of data may appear in more than one cluster. For example, in Table 4–7 (Chapter 4), "Can't breathe lying down" appears in Clusters 4 and 6. In Cluster 4, it is one of the causes of Sleep Pattern Disturbance; in Cluster 6, it indirectly causes Self-Care Deficit by causing Mrs. Sanchez to lose sleep and become too tired and weak to perform self-care activities. Examine Box 4–4 and Table 4–7 to see if you can follow the reasoning for each of the cue clusters. If you need to review Functional Health Patterns, refer to Table 3–10 in Chapter 3.

Step 3: Make a Working Problem List

In this step, you make a judgment about the most likely explanation for each cue cluster; then decide whether it represents an actual, potential (risk), or possible problem. Also decide whether the problem is medical, collaborative, or a nursing diagnosis. Tentative explanations for Luisa Sanchez are listed in Table 4–7 in Chapter 4.

Cluster 1—no abnormal cues in the Health Perception/Health Management pattern. The pattern represents patient strengths: a healthy lifestyle and understanding of and compliance with treatment regimens (e.g., taking her Synthroid as directed).

Cluster 2—problem of inadequate nutrition. A likely explanation is that Mrs. Sanchez's poor appetite is a result of her disease process. Her appetite will probably return on successful medical treatment of the pneumonia. In the meantime, Mrs. Sanchez will need nursing care to assess for and encourage adequate nutrition.

Cluster 3—nursing diagnosis, Deficient Fluid Volume. It is probably caused by excess fluid loss secondary to fever and diaphoresis, as well as inadequate fluid intake because of nausea and poor appetite. Mrs. Sanchez's poor skin turgor, decreased urinary frequency, dry mucous membranes, and hot skin are defining characteristics that help to identify the problem.

Cluster 4—a nursing diagnosis in the Sleep/Rest pattern. Apparently, when she lies down to sleep, she is unable to breathe. In addition, her cough and pain keep her awake. Undoubtedly, her fever, diaphoresis, and chills (in Clusters 3 and 7) also keep her awake. As a result, she feels weak and is short of breath on exertion.

Cluster 5—a medical problem, hypothyroidism, for which Mrs. Sanchez is already receiving medication. Therefore, the problem requires no nursing intervention and would not be included in the care plan. The medication order would appear in the medication record and would be given to Mrs. Sanchez routinely while she was in the hospital.

Cluster 6—nursing diagnosis, either Activity Intolerance or Self-Care Deficit. Both are being caused by cues and problems in other clusters. For example, the Sleep-Rest problem in Cluster 4 and the oxygenation problem in Cluster 11 are both contributing to the overall pattern of weakness in Cluster 6.

Cluster 7—problem, Mrs. Sanchez is uncomfortable because she is having chills. The chills are being caused by fever secondary to the pneumonia and will stop when her illness is treated. The fever will be treated medically (by the order for Ibuprofen); however, nursing interventions can be used to increase Mrs. Sanchez's comfort.

Cluster 8—contains risk factors for a potential nursing diagnosis, Risk for Interrupted Family Processes. However, there are not enough data to indicate an actual problem. In any event, the problem will resolve itself the next day as soon as Mr. Sanchez returns home. You might decide to include it in the care plan to be sure that the necessary follow-up assessments are made.

Cluster 9—nursing diagnosis, Anxiety. Mrs. Sanchez expressed anxiety, but she had no other signs of Anxiety, such as trembling and tense facial muscles. She said she was worried about leaving her child with a neighbor and about getting behind at work. In addition, her Anxiety is obviously caused by periodic difficulty breathing. This is a nursing diagnosis with more than one etiology.

Cluster 10—nursing diagnosis of Acute Chest Pain, which is caused by the pneumonia-induced cough. Until the antibiotic therapy can treat the pneumonia, nursing measures will be needed to promote comfort.

Cluster 11—nursing diagnosis, Ineffective Airway Clearance. Cues are productive cough, shallow respirations, decreased chest expansion, and inspiratory crackles. The other cues (e.g., pale mucous membranes) are signs of pneumonia, the medical problem creating the ineffective airway clearance. You can infer that problems in other patterns are contributing to the oxygenation problem as well: deficient fluid volume creates thick, tenacious mucus, and pain and weakness contribute to shallow respirations and decreased chest expansion.

In addition to the problems identified from the cue clusters, you should identify collaborative problems that exist for Mrs. Sanchez because of her disease process and her IV and medical therapies. Recall that collaborative problems are potential problems for which nursing care focuses on assessment and prevention. The following is a working problem list for Luisa Sanchez before being put into standard NANDA-I terminology:

Cue Cluster	Probable Explanation
1	No problem. Strength: Healthy lifestyle; understanding of and compliance with treatment regimens.
2	Actual nursing diagnosis. Imbalanced Nutrition: Less than Body Requirements. Probably caused by nausea and poor appetite and by increased metabolism secondary to fever and pneumonia.
3	Actual nursing diagnosis. Deficient Fluid Volume caused by excess fluid loss (diaphoresis) secondary to fever and inadequate intake secondary to nausea and loss of appetite.
4	Actual nursing diagnosis. Difficulty sleeping; probably NANDA-I label of Disturbed Sleep Pattern caused by cough, pain, orthopnea, fever, and diaphoresis.
5	No problem as long as patient takes Synthroid. Be sure it is in the medical administration record.
6	Actual nursing diagnosis. Probably Self-Care Deficit (perhaps Activity Intolerance). Lack of oxygen and sleep loss are causing weakness and fatigue. As a result, she is unable to perform self-care activities.
7	Actual nursing diagnosis. Chills are causing discomfort.
8	Potential nursing diagnosis. There could be a problem with child care if Mr. Sanchez's return is delayed. Probably Interrupted Family Processes because both parents are unavailable to care for child; probably self-limiting (tomorrow).
9	Actual nursing diagnosis. Anxiety. Caused by difficulty breathing, worry about child, and of "getting behind" at work.
10	Actual nursing diagnosis. Acute chest pain from cough. Medical treatments will help alleviate.
11	Actual nursing diagnosis. Airway clearance problem. Unable to cough up thick sputum, which has been created by infection, fever, weakness, pain, and fluid deficit.

Collaborative Problems

Potential Complication of pneumonia: septic shock
Potential Complication of pneumonia: respiratory insufficiency
Potential Complications of IV therapy: infiltration, phlebitis
Potential Complications of antibiotic therapy: allergic reaction, GI upset

Step 4: Write Problem Statement in Standardized Language

To make the formal list of nursing diagnoses and collaborative problems, refer to the list of NANDA-I diagnostic labels (see the inside back cover for the list of diagnostic labels organized by Functional Health Patterns). Compare the data in the cue clusters with the defining characteristics in a nursing diagnosis handbook to be sure you have chosen the correct NANDA-I label for each nursing diagnosis. After verifying the diagnoses with Mrs. Sanchez, you would write them on the plan of care in order of priority (Table 10–1). Note that in addition to listing all the problems identified for Mrs. Sanchez on the day of her admission, Table 10–1 indicates changes that a nurse might make to the list after implementing the care plan and evaluating the outcomes.

TABLE 10–1   Formal Prioritized Problem List for Luisa Sanchez

Prioritized Problems	Type of Plan Used
1. Ineffective Airway Clearance related to viscous secretions and shallow chest expansion secondary to pain, fluid volume deficit, and fatigue	See "Unit Standards of Care for Pneumonia"
2. Deficient Fluid Volume Deficit to intake insufficient to replace fluid loss secondary to fever, diaphoresis, and nausea. Resolved 4/17/12 JW	See Standard Care Plan for Deficient Fluid Volume
3. Anxiety related to difficulty breathing and concerns over work and parenting roles	Individualized nursing diagnosis care plan
4. Disturbed Sleep Pattern related to cough, pain, orthopnea, fever, and diaphoresis	Individualized nursing diagnosis care plan
5. Self-Care Deficit (Level 2) related to Activity Intolerance secondary to Ineffective Airway Clearance and Disturbed Sleep Pattern	See "Unit Standards of Care for Pneumonia"
6. Chest Pain related to cough secondary to pneumonia Risk for 4/17/12 JW	See "Unit Standards of Care for Pneumonia"
7. Altered Comfort: Chills related to fever and diaphoresis	Individualized nursing diagnosis care plan
8. Risk for Altered Family Processes related to mother's illness and temporary unavailability of father to provide child care. Resolved 4/17/12 JW	Individualized nursing diagnosis care plan
9. Imbalanced Nutrition: Less than Body Requirements related to decreased appetite and nausea and increased metabolism secondary to disease process	See Standardized Care Plan for Imbalanced Nutrition: Less than Body Requirements
10. Potential Complications of Pneumonia: Septic shock and respiratory insufficiency	See "Unit Standards of Care for Pneumonia"
11. Potential Complications of IV Therapy: Infiltration, phlebitis	See Unit Procedures: "IV Insertion and Maintenance"
12. Potential Complications of Vancomycin Therapy: Ototoxicity, Hepatotoxicity, Allergic reaction, GI upset	See "Protocol for Administration of Intravenous Vancomycin"

Planning

Step 5: Determine Which Problems Can Be Addressed by Critical Pathways and Other Standardized Plans

After developing the formal problem list, decide how each of the problems is to be addressed (i.e., with preplanned interventions or individualized plans). For each problem, ask the following series of questions:

A. **Is there a *critical pathway* or *standard of care* for this medical diagnosis or situation?** Mrs. Sanchez was admitted to 2-South, a medical unit that has written standards of care for patients having pneumonia. These standards describe all the care necessary for Problems 1, 5, 6, and 10 (Ineffective Airway Clearance, Self-Care Deficit, Acute Chest Pain, and Potential Complications of Pneumonia). Most patients with pneumonia experience these problems, so it is possible to plan in advance the care these patients are expected to need. Because no special plan is necessary, you would simply list the problems and write beside them, "See Unit Standards of Care for Pneumonia." (See the instructions as shown in the Care-Planning Guide in Box 10–1.)

B. **Is there a *model nursing care plan* for the client's medical diagnosis or condition?** In Mrs. Sanchez's case, because there were standards of care for pneumonia patients and because her needs did not exceed the standards, you would not look for a model care plan for this medical diagnosis.

C. **For the *collaborative problems* not completely covered by the standards of care, do any of the following exist to direct your interventions?**

> Physician's orders (you may need to call to obtain these)
> Standing orders
> Protocols
> Policies and procedures

   Mrs. Sanchez has two collaborative problems not addressed by standards of care: Problems 11 and 12. For Problem 11, the physician's orders specify the type of IV fluid and prescribe the rate of flow. You would note this information on an IV flowsheet or a Kardex form (Figure 10–4). The 2-South procedure manual contains a section on IV therapy, which specifies how often IV tubing is to be changed, what focus assessments to make, and so forth. This resource is noted on the formal problem list beside Problem 11 (in Table 10–1).

   Because vancomycin is not routinely given to all pneumonia patients, it would not be included in the unit's Standards of Care for Pneumonia. However, because it is often given to patients who are allergic to penicillin, it would not be unusual to give it. Furthermore, the nurses must be aware of assessments and interventions that apply to vancomycin that are over and above those routinely performed when administering penicillin. Therefore, 2-South developed a preprinted multidisciplinary protocol that specifies how the drug is to be administered—for example, that the drug is to be given no faster than 100 mL/hour and that it is never given intramuscularly. It also specifies the important nursing observations to make—for example, monitor for tinnitus, oliguria, hypotensive reaction, rash, chills, and itching. You would simply note on the formal problem list the reference to the protocol (see Table 10–1, item 12).

If there are collaborative problems that are not covered by any of these documents, they must be written on the plan of care, and individualized nursing orders must be developed for them. This is not needed for Mrs. Sanchez.

D. **For the *nursing diagnoses* not covered by the standards of care, determine the following:**

1. *Which nursing diagnoses really need individualized nursing plans of care?* Remember that an individualized plan is needed only if the care is not completely covered by standards of care, protocols, or other routine nursing care. For Luisa Sanchez, Problems 2 through 4 and 7 through 9 need care beyond that specified in the standards of care and unit procedures. You would not expect all pneumonia patients to have these problems (Deficient Fluid Volume, Anxiety, Sleep Pattern Disturbance, Risk for Interrupted Family Processes, and Imbalanced Nutrition). Therefore, they would not be found on the standardized care plan or on unit standards of care for pneumonia.

2. *Is there a preprinted model care plan for the nursing diagnosis?* Recall that model care plans may exist for a medical diagnosis or for a single nursing diagnosis. For Problem 2, Deficient Fluid Volume, 2-South has a standardized (model) nursing diagnosis care plan. You would indicate that resource on the formal problem list (Table 10–1).

For beginning student plans of care, you might not use the procedure in Step 5 (Planning step), but you will certainly use it when you develop working care plans as a professional nurse. While you are learning to write plans of care, your instructors may ask you to make a complete list of the client's nursing diagnoses and collaborative problems and to write your own outcomes and nursing orders for each problem, even the ones that are routine. You may not have the option of using standards of care, standing orders, protocols, and model care plans.

Step 6: Individualize Standardized Documents as Needed

Besides the handwritten plans of care for the three nursing diagnoses, you would use the following documents to direct Mrs. Sanchez's care:

"Unit Standards of Care for Pneumonia"

"Standardized Care Plan for Deficient Fluid Volume"

"Standardized Care Plan for Imbalanced Nutrition: Less than Body Requirements"

"Unit Procedures: IV Insertion and Maintenance"

"Protocol for Administration of Intravenous Vancomycin"

Assume that the "Unit Standards of Care for Pneumonia," the "Unit Procedures for IV Insertion and Maintenance," and the "Protocol for Administration of Intravenous

Vancomycin" are all in the 2-South files and require no alterations for Mrs. Sanchez. Because they are a part of the permanent agency records and reflect the care given to all patients with those conditions and therapies, you would not add copies of them to Mrs. Sanchez's comprehensive care plan. However, the standardized care plans for fluid volume deficit and imbalanced nutrition are meant to be individualized to a specific patient. Therefore, you would individualize them and place copies with Mrs. Sanchez's comprehensive plan of care.

Step 7: Transcribe Medical, Collaborative, Activities of Daily Living, and Basic Care Needs to Special Sections of the Kardex or Computer

Because 2-South uses computerized care planning, you would type the medical orders into the computer. Each day you can obtain a list of orders in effect for that day (see Figure 10–13, "Active Physician Orders"). Instructions for Mrs. Sanchez's diet, activity, hygiene needs, IV therapy, and so on, are also found on the care plan; some appear under "Active Ancillary Orders." (*Note:* Mrs. Sanchez's Problem List is not shown in Figure 10–13.)

Step 8: Develop Individualized Plan of Care for Remaining Nursing Diagnoses and Collaborative Problems

Examining the formal problem list (Table 10–1), you can see that you would need to develop desired outcomes and nursing orders for Problems 3 (Anxiety), 4 (Disturbed Sleep Pattern), 7 (Altered Comfort: Chills), and 8 (Risk for Interrupted Family Processes). You would type these into the computer or in some systems, you would be able to choose appropriate outcomes and nursing orders from a list provided by the computer. See Figure 10–13 for an example of what a printout of an electronic plan of care for two of Mrs. Sanchez's nursing diagnoses might look like.

Implementation

Step 9: Implement the Plan of Care (Do or Delegate)

On the day of admission, care was instituted immediately for Mrs. Sanchez's two highest priority problems, Ineffective Airway Clearance and Deficient Fluid Volume. Medical orders for oxygen and IV antibiotics were begun, diagnostic tests were performed, and routine nursing care was given according to the Unit Standards of Care for Pneumonia, as well as other documents listed in Table 10–1. Problems 3 and 4 (Anxiety and Disturbed Sleep Pattern) were addressed by nursing orders on the nursing diagnosis care plan, and constant monitoring was done for the collaborative problems (10, 11, and 12). As a part of the Implementation step, all of this care would have been charted and passed on to other caregivers in oral reports.

```
                         DAILY CARE ACTIVITY SHEET


WILKINHIAM REGIONAL MEDICAL CENTER                      04/16/0717:15
Patient: SANCHEZ, LUISA
Location: 221A        Sex: F   Age: 28    Birthdate: 1/25/79    Wt.: 125 lbs
Account #: 8-37838-1  MRN: 299333  Vst#: 00279 3   Admitted date: 04/16/12
Discharge Date: / /                        Admitting Diagnosis: PNEUMONIA
Surgical Procedure: NONE
Drug Allergies: PENICILLIN    Admitting Dr.: KATZ, R
Food Allergies: NONE          Consult Dr. 1:
Other Allergies: NONE         Consult Dr. 2:
Religion: CATHOLIC            Consult Dr. 3:
Marital Status: MARRIED       Pri Care Phy: KATZ, R
Diabetic? N     Pregnant? N    Smoker? N     Infectious? Y     Fasting? N
Hygiene? Help bath 4/15/12
```

ACTIVE PHYSICIAN ORDERS

```
                              Start          Stop        Entered by
ACTIVITY
  BRP, CHAIR                   04/16/12                   MLM
  INTAKE & OUTPUT              04/16/12                   MLM
  ROUTINE
IV THERAPY/FLUIDS
  PERIPHERAL - D5LR @ 100CC/HR 04/16/12                   MLM
PULSE OXIMETER                 04/16/12                   MLM
MEDICATIONS
  VANCOMYCIN 0.5 GM IV q6HR    04/16/12                   MLM
  TYLENOL 650 MG Q4HR PO FOR TEMP>101°  04/16/12          MLM
  OXYGEN PER CANNULA, 5L       04/16/12                   MLM
```

ACTIVE ANCILLARY ORDERS

```
                       Ord#  Freq   Priority  Ord Dt    Status    Entered by
LABORATORY
  CBC WITH DIFF        1     X1     ROUT      04/16/12  ORDERED   MLM
  ABG'S                2     X1     STAT      04/16/12  ORDERED   MLM
  BLOOD CULTURE        10    X2IF   STAT      04/16/12  ORDERED   MLM
                             TEMP>101
  SERUM ELECTROLYTES   12    X1     ROUT      04/16/12  ORDERED   MLM
  URINE SPEC GRAVITY   3     X1     ROUT      04/16/12  ORDERED   MLM
  24-HOUR URINE        11    X1     ROUT      04/16/12  ORDERED   MLM
  SPUTUM C&S           4     X1     ROUT      04/16/12  ORDERED   MLM
DIAGNOSTIC RADIOLOGY
  PA & LATERAL CHEST XRAY 9  X1     STAT      04/16/12  ORDERED   MLM
RESPIRATORY THERAPY
  POSTURAL DRAINAGE    5     DAILY  ROUT      04/16/12  ORDERED   MLM
  INCENTIVE SPIROMETER 13    q3HR   ROUT      04/16/12  ORDERED   MLM
  NEBULIZER            14    Q4HR   ROUT      04/16/12  ORDERED   MLM
```

FIGURE 10–13

Initial plan of care for Luisa Sanchez

```
                      DAILY CARE ACTIVITY SHEET                        PAGE 2

Patient: SANCHEZ, LUISA
Location: 221A       Sex: F   Age: 28     Birthdate: 1/25/79     Wt.: 125 lbs
Account #: 8-37838-1  MRN: 299333  Vst#: 00279 3    Admitted date: 04/16/12
```

NURSING PLAN OF CARE

```
Prob.
No.                                                  Start     Stop   Status
3. Nursing Diagnosis: ANXIETY (MODERATE)             04/16/12         IN PROGRESS
   Related to:        DIFFICULTY BREATHING AND
                      CONCERNS OVER WORK AND
                      PARENTING ROLES


   Outcomes:          • LISTENS TO AND FOLLOWS       04/16/12         IN PROGRESS
                        INSTRUCTIONS FOR CORRECT
                        BREATHING AND COUGHING
                        TECHNIQUE, EVEN DURING
                        DYSPNEIC PERIODS
                      • VERBALIZES UNDERSTANDING OF   04/16/12         IN PROGRESS
                        CONDITION, TESTS, AND
                        TREATMENTS (BY 04/16/07,
                        2200).
                      • DECREASED REPORTS OF          04/16/12         IN PROGRESS
                        FEAR AND ANXIETY (NONE
                        WITHIN 12 HOURS).                              IN PROGRESS
                      • VOICE STEADY, NOT SHAKY.      04/16/12         IN PROGRESS
                      • RESP. RATE 12-22/MIN.         04/16/12         IN PROGRESS
                      • FREELY EXPRESSES CONCERNS     04/16/12         IN PROGRESS
                        ABOUT WORK AND PARENTING
                        ROLES, BUT PLACES THEM IN
                        PERSPECTIVE IN VIEW OF HER
                        ILLNESS.


   Nursing Orders:    • STAY WITH CLIENT WHEN SHE     04/16/12         IN PROGRESS
                        IS DYSPNEIC. REASSURE HER YOU
                        WILL STAY.
                      • REMAIN CALM; APPEAR           04/16/12         IN PROGRESS
                        CONFIDENT.
                      • ENCOURAGE SLOW, DEEP          04/16/12         IN PROGRESS
                        BREATHING WHEN CLIENT IS
                        DYSPNEIC.
                      • GIVE BRIEF EXPLANATIONS OF
                        TREATMENTS AND PROCEDURES.
                      • WHEN ACUTE EPISODE OVER,
                        GIVE DETAILED INFORMATION
                        ABOUT NATURE OF CONDITION,
                        TESTS, AND TREATMENTS.
```

FIGURE 10–13

(*continued*)

```
             DAILY CARE ACTIVITY SHEET                    PAGE 3

Patient: SANCHEZ, LUISA
Location: 221A      Sex: F   Age: 28    Birthdate: 1/25/79    Wt.: 125 lbs
Account #: 8-37838-1  MRN: 299333  Vst#: 00279 3    Admitted date: 04/16/12
```

NURSING PLAN OF CARE

		Start	Stop	Status
	• AS TOLERATED, ENCOURAGE TO EXPRESS AND EXPAND ON HER CONCERNS ABOUT HER CHILD AND HER WORK. EXPLORE ALTERNATIVES.	04/16/12		IN PROGRESS
	• NOTE WHETHER HUSBAND RETURNS AS EXPECTED. IF NOT, INSTITUTE CARE PLAN FOR ACTUAL ALTERED FAMILY PROCESSES.	04/16/12		IN PROGRESS
Prob. No.				
4. Nursing Diagnosis:	DISTURBED SLEEP PATTERN	04/16/12		IN PROGRESS
Related to:	COUGH, PAIN, ORTHOPNEA, FEVER, DIAPHORESIS	04/16/12		IN PROGRESS
Outcomes:	• OBSERVED SLEEPING AT NIGHT ROUNDS.	04/16/12		IN PROGRESS
	• REPORTS FEELING RESTED IN A.M.	04/16/12		IN PROGRESS
	• DOES NOT EXPERIENCE ORTHOPNEA (BY DAY 2).	04/16/12		IN PROGRESS
Nursing Orders:	• PROVIDE COMFORT MEASURES, SUCH AS BACK RUB, QUIET ENVIRONMENT, DIM LIGHTS, DRY LINEN WHEN DIAPHORETIC, AND MOUTH CARE.	04/16/12		IN PROGRESS
	• MONITOR AND INSTITUTE COLLABORATIVE MEASURES TO CONTROL PAIN, FEVER, AND DYSPNEA.	04/16/12		IN PROGRESS
	• USE FLASHLIGHT WHEN MAKING NIGHT ROUNDS.	04/16/12		IN PROGRESS
	• USE SEMI-FOWLER'S POSITION IF CLIENT CANNOT FALL ASLEEP IN FOWLER'S.	04/16/12		IN PROGRESS
	• INQUIRE DAILY IF CLIENT FEELS RESTED.	04/16/12		IN PROGRESS

FIGURE 10–13

(*continued*)

Evaluation

Step 10: Evaluate Results of Care, Revise Plan as Needed

During evaluation, you will compare patient progress with the predicted outcomes and revise the plan of care if necessary. Using an electronic patient care plan, such as in Figure 10–13, you would simply key in the changes and print out (or save to disk) a new plan. On this form, there is a column for problem "Status" and a "Start/Stop" column in which one can enter the date that a problem is discontinued. Of course, not all agencies have computerized plans of care. Table 10–1 indicates how changes might be made on a handwritten problem list; Table 10–2 shows how changes to Mrs. Sanchez's plan of care would look if it were not computerized. For brevity, only Problem 3 is shown in Table 10–2. The following scenario illustrates how the evaluation step might have been done for Mrs. Sanchez on the next morning after her admission.

> The IV fluids quickly restored Mrs. Sanchez's fluid balance, and by the next morning, she showed no signs of Fluid Volume Deficit (Problem 2). As you would expect, her ineffective airway clearance, along with Problems 4, 5, 6, and 9, did not improve as rapidly. These problems would resolve more slowly, as the antibiotics gradually controlled the pneumonia and her oxygenation improved. Therefore, Problems 1, 4, 5, 6, and 9 are unchanged in Table 10–1, the problem list.
>
> Improvement was noted in Problem 7. Because the oral ibuprofen was effective in lowering Mrs. Sanchez's temperature, she was no longer experiencing chills. Her husband returned as expected, removing the risk factor for interrupted family processes (Problem 8). Table 10–1 shows how these problems were redefined to reflect Mrs. Sanchez's changing condition.
>
> The evening and night nurses were able to effectively implement the nursing orders for Problem 3 (Anxiety). Resulting changes in the plan of care for anxiety are shown in Table 10–2. However, Anxiety remains on the problem list (Table 10–1) because not all the outcomes were achieved.

How to Mind Map a Plan of Care

As a student, you may wish (or your instructor may ask you) to make a care map as a part of your preparation for caring for a patient in the clinical setting. **Mind mapping** is a visual technique for showing graphic (picture) relationships among ideas and concepts. It is meant to stimulate critical thinking and is helpful for learners who are more visual than verbal. A mind-mapped plan of care uses shapes and pictures to represent the phases of the nursing process (i.e., assessment data, nursing diagnoses, patient goals, interventions, and evaluation), as well as the patient's pathophysiology, medications, and other relevant data. Because a care map must usually fit on one page, you must focus your thinking carefully and include only the most important points.

1. First place the main idea in the center or at the top of the page. This is the focus of your care plan. It is usually the patient rather than the disease or condition, although you must certainly consider the effect of the disease on the person.
2. As you think of them, connect other ideas to the main idea similar to the branches of a tree or the spokes of a wheel. For example, if your main idea is "Mrs. Sanchez," you might think, "difficulty breathing," "pain in chest," "anxious about her job," and

TABLE 10-2 Revised Plan of Care for Luisa Sanchez (Anxiety Only)

Nursing Diagnosis	Expected Outcomes	Evaluation Statements	Nursing Orders	Rationale
Anxiety r/t difficulty breathing and concerns about work and parenting roles (4/16/12 MM)	Demonstrates decreased anxiety, as evidenced by:		(a) When client is dyspneic, stay with her; reassure her you will stay.	(a) Presence of a competent caregiver reduces fear of being unable to breathe. Control of anxiety will help client to maintain effective breathing pattern.
	1. Listens and follows instructions for correct breathing and coughing technique, even during periods of dyspnea.	1. Outcome met. Performed coughing techniques as instructed during periods of dyspnea.	(b) Remain calm, appear confident.	(b) Reassures client the nurse can help her.
	2. Verbalizes understanding of condition, diagnostic tests, and treatments (by end of day 1).	2. Outcome met. See nurses' notes for 3–11 shift. Stated, "I know I need to try to breathe deeply even when it hurts." Demonstrated correct use of incentive spirometer and stated understanding of the need to use it. Understands IV is for hydration and antibiotics. (Evaluated 4/17/12 JW)	(c) Encourage slow, deep breathing to feel in control and decrease anxiety.	(c) Focusing on breathing may help client.
			(d) When dyspneic, give brief explanations of treatments and procedures.	(d) Anxiety and pain interfere with learning. Knowing what to expect reduces anxiety.
			(e) ~~When acute episode is over, give detailed information about nature of condition, treatments, and tests.~~ Reassess whether client needs any information about condition, etc. (4/17/12 JW)	(e) *Detailed information has been given. Because client shows understanding, there is no need to repeat information.*
	3. Reports of fear and anxiety decrease; none within 12 hrs.	3. Outcome met. States, "I know I can get enough air, but it still hurts to breathe."	(f) As client can tolerate, encourage her to express and expand on her concerns about her child and her work. Explore alternatives as needed.	(f) Awareness of source of anxiety enables client to gain control over it.
	4. Voice steady, not shaky.	4. Outcome met. Speaks in steady voice.		
	5. Respiratory rate of 12–22 per min.	5. Outcome not met. Rate 26–36 per minute.		
	6. Freely expresses concerns about work and parenting—places them in perspective in view of her illness.	6. Outcome partially met. Discussed only briefly on 3–11 shift. Not done on 11–7 shift because of client's need to rest. (Evaluated 4/17/12 JW)	(g) ~~Note whether husband returns as scheduled. If he does not, institute care plan for actual Interrupted Family Processes.~~ (4/17/12 Mr. Sanchez returned. JW)	(g) Husband's continued absence would constitute defining characteristic for this nursing diagnosis. It is important that this assessment be made right away so child care can be arranged if needed.

so on. It does not matter whether you begin creating branches with assessment data, nursing diagnoses, goals, interventions, or medical diagnoses and treatments.

3. Each of those branches may generate more ideas, which you also represent with pictures, shapes, or colors and cluster into groups. Notice that in Figure 10–14, there are two clusters of patient data, each connected to a different nursing diagnosis.

4. Draw arrows or lines to make connections between groups of ideas. For example, you might connect one of the data groups for Ms. Sanchez to a nursing diagnosis of "Ineffective Airway Clearance" and another to a nursing diagnosis of "Anxiety."

5. Write qualifying words on or beside the connecting lines to explain how the concepts or idea groups are related. In Figure 10–14, one such qualifier is "defining characteristics for."

Let your imagination roam freely. You can use pictures, drawings, shapes, and colors to represent your ideas and concepts. Use whatever is meaningful to you, whatever increases your understanding of the care of this patient, and whatever facilitates your learning.

Wellness in the Acute-Care Setting

Even in an acute-care setting, nurses do not focus entirely on problems and illness needs. You can increase your wellness focus by being sure to identify client strengths and to use those strengths in working to relieve the client's problems. Mrs. Sanchez's strengths are that she is able to communicate adequately, has a healthy lifestyle, is well educated, and understands and complies with treatment regimens. Realizing this, her nurse could use discussion, pamphlets, and diagrams as nursing interventions. Because Mrs. Sanchez has a stable family situation and finances, a special discharge plan is probably not needed.

Clients have health-promotion and illness-prevention needs beyond their admitting medical diagnoses. Sometime before discharge, the nurse might assess whether Mrs. Sanchez's health practices include regular exercise, eating balanced meals, and performing breast self-examinations. Notice, however, that the nurses must first focus on Mrs. Sanchez's more basic and immediate needs—adequate oxygenation, hydration, anxiety, and potential complications of pneumonia. This illustrates the difficulty of addressing wellness needs in an acute-care setting. Still, such an assessment could help Mrs. Sanchez to follow through on her own to improve her health after dismissal.

Ethical Considerations

Some say that because nursing affects people when they are most vulnerable, everything a nurse does has a moral aspect. Following this line of reasoning, the act of creating a patient plan of care has a moral dimension.

Conventional ethical principles are those that are widely held, expressed in practice, and enforced by sanctions. Two of the most basic conventional principles held by nurses are the following:

1. Nurses have an obligation to be competent in their work.
2. The good of the patient should be the nurse's primary concern.

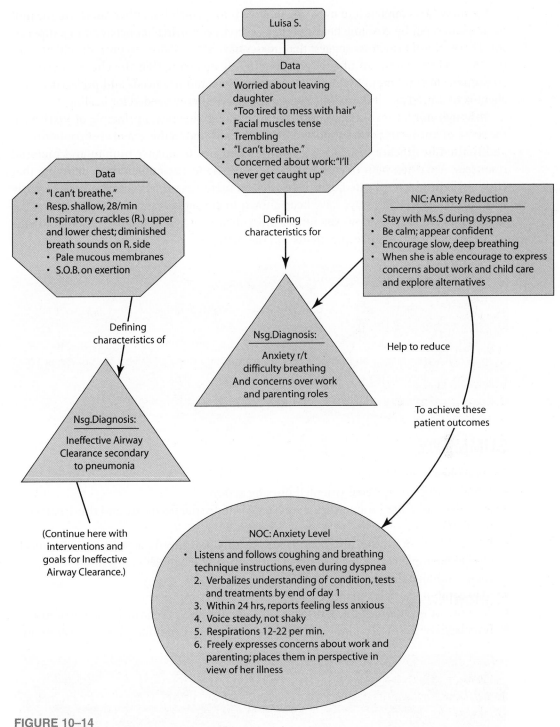

FIGURE 10–14

A mind-mapped plan of care for Luisa Sanchez

A nurse who is careless and uncaring violates both principles. Other nurses on the unit may sanction her by avoiding her or perhaps even by reporting her behavior to a supervisor. These ethical principles suggest that nurses have a moral duty to promote client healing. A good nursing plan of care aids healing by ensuring that the client's needs are communicated and met. When all caregivers understand her needs and preferences, the client is reassured and less anxious and can conserve energy needed for healing.

Although not a conventional principle of nursing, the moral principle of **justice** (in the sense of fairness) is also supported by good planning. In this era of cost containment and limited healthcare resources, it is important not to misuse human and material resources. A written plan of care makes efficient use of the nurse's time, ensuring that efforts will not be duplicated or time wasted in ineffective interventions. As previously mentioned, critical pathways have been shown to conserve resources by decreasing the length of hospital stays. However, nurses must always be careful not to overlook individual needs in their zeal to keep patients "on the pathway."

10-2 WHAT DO YOU KNOW?

1. List 10 steps in creating a patient plan of care (review Box 10–1 if you cannot remember all of them).
2. List as many guidelines for writing care plans as you can recall. For example, "For detailed treatments and procedures, refer to other sources" (if you cannot recall 10 more guidelines, review Box 10–2).

See answer to #10-2 What Do You Know? in Appendix A.

SUMMARY

A comprehensive care plan
- Is a written guide for goal-oriented nursing action.
- Provides the written framework necessary for individualized care and third-party reimbursement.
- Includes a client profile, instructions for meeting basic needs, aspects of the medical plan to be implemented by the nurse, and a nursing diagnosis care plan for the client's nursing diagnoses and collaborative problems.
- May combine both standardized and individualized approaches.
- Supports conventional ethical principles of nursing and the moral principle of justice.
- Is replaced by a critical pathway for frequently occurring conditions in some institutions.

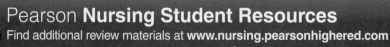

Pearson **Nursing Student Resources**
Find additional review materials at **www.nursing.pearsonhighered.com**
Prepare for success with additional NCLEX®-style practice questions,
interactive assignments and activities, Web links, animations and videos, and more!

Answer Keys to Questions Appearing in the Text

CHAPTER 1. OVERVIEW OF NURSING PROCESS

WHAT DO YOU KNOW? ANSWERS

#1-1

1. What is meant by describing nursing as an art?

   Answer: Art is more about your approach to what you do and less about what you know or what you do. Nursing art involves sensitivity, creativity, empathy, and the ability to adapt care—either to meet a patient's unique needs or in the face of uncertainty. It includes the ability to make connections, find meaning in client encounters, master nursing skills, use rational thinking, and practice ethically.

2. True or false? The ANA says that critical thinking is an essential feature of contemporary nursing practice.

   Answer: True. Nurses use critical thinking to apply scientific knowledge to diagnosis and treatment processes.

3. What are human responses?

   Answer: Reactions to an event or stressor.

4. How is nursing different from medicine?

   Answer: Physicians focus on diagnosis and treatment of disease; nurses focus on giving care during the cure. Physicians treat disease; nurses treat human responses.

#1-2

1. Nursing was first described as a process in:
   (a) The 1940s.
   (b) The 1950s.
   (c) The 1960s.
   (d) The 1970s.

   Answer: (b) Hall first described nursing as a process in 1955.

2. True or false? Using a systematic, logical process such as the nursing process interferes with the nurse's ability to focus on caring.

   Answer: False. Although the nursing process is systematic and logical, its use does not diminish the caring aspect of nursing. As you master the nursing process, it will become second nature to you and actually facilitate your caring.

#1-3

Define "intuition."

> **Answer:** Intuition is:
>
> - a problem-solving approach that relies on use of one's "inner sense" and "just a feeling" that something is wrong even though the person cannot say what prompted the feeling.
> - the "direct apprehension of a situation based upon a background of similar and dissimilar situations and embodied intelligence or skill" (Benner, 1984, p. 295).
> - the "immediate knowing of something without the conscious use of reason" (Schraeder & Fisher, 1987, p. 46).

#1-4

Give six examples of psychomotor skills a nurse might use.

> **Answer:** Some examples are changing a dressing, teaching CPR, giving injections, turning and positioning patients, attaching a heart monitor, and suctioning a tracheostomy. You may think of many others. If they require "doing" with the hands, they are psychomotor skills.

#1-5

1. In the wellness case study, the nurse provided teaching to help the client stop smoking. What kind of intervention was this?
   (a) Health promotion
   (b) Health protection
   (c) Disease prevention

   > **Answer:** (c) **Health promotion** activities (e.g., daily exercise) are directed toward achieving a higher level of wellness; they are not aimed at avoiding any particular disease. In health promotion, the client is seen as having more control and expertise, and the nurse serves as a facilitator. **Health protection** focuses on activities that decrease environmental threats to health (e.g., air pollution). **Disease prevention** involves actions that help prevent specific health problems or diseases (e.g., immunizations, prenatal care). Smoking cessation is intended to prevent lung cancer and other respiratory diseases, as well as heart disease.

2. In the parish nursing case study, the nurse conducted blood pressure screenings to identify those who might have an elevated blood pressure. What kind of intervention was this?
   (a) Health promotion
   (b) Health protection
   (c) Disease prevention

   > **Answer:** (c) **Health promotion** activities (e.g., daily exercise) are directed toward achieving a higher level of wellness; they are not aimed at avoiding any particular disease. In health promotion, the client is seen as having more control and expertise,

and the nurse serves as a facilitator. **Health protection** focuses on activities that decrease environmental threats to health (e.g., air pollution). **Disease prevention** involves actions that help to prevent specific health problems or diseases (e.g., immunizations, prenatal care). Blood pressure screening was intended to identify early those with elevated blood pressure so the condition could be treated to prevent complications associated with that condition.

THINK & REFLECT! SUGGESTED RESPONSES

There is usually no single, correct answer for these exercises because the intent is to have you practice thinking, not recall facts. The nature of a critical thinking problem is that it has more than one solution and that there may not be a "best" solution. You should compare your answers with those of your classmates—both your solutions and the thinking you used. Discussing your thinking processes is one way to help improve your thinking. Also, it is important for you to begin collaborating with your peers. During your nursing career, the thinking of other nurses will be an important resource to you, just as your thinking can be for them. You will usually not find answers here but ideas to help you think about the question.

#1-1

- Are all registered nurses professional nurses?
- Are all professional nurses registered nurses?
- The term "professional nurse" is used often. Who are the "nonprofessional" nurses, and what do they do?

    Suggested Response: This question is designed to help you discuss these issues with your peers. See what other people think and examine what you think.

#1-2

Why do you think the scientific method of problem solving would not work well in planning care for a patient?

    Hint: Look at Table 1–3. How are formal problem solving and the nursing process different? Could you use the first step of formal problem solving as the first step in the nursing process? Why not?

#1-3

1. Describe an incident in which you observed a nurse demonstrating cultural competence. What did the nurse do and say? (Or describe a nurse that was not culturally competent.)

    Suggested Response: Responses will differ based on each person's experiences. Listen to others to see how they practiced cultural competence.

2. Describe an incident in which you demonstrated either curiosity or creativity in patient care. If you have not yet given patient care, describe a different situation in which you showed those qualities.

   Suggested Response: Responses will differ based on each person's experiences. Listen to others to learn what curiosity and creativity mean to them.

CRITICAL THINKING AND CLINICAL REASONING: A CASE STUDY: SUGGESTED RESPONSES

1. I—settled her comfortably in bed
   A—interviewed her
   A—obtained a temperature
   A—examined Ms. Boiko's chart
   I—administered oxygen
   A—performed the physical examination
   D—wrote a diagnosis
   Po—chose an outcome

   Pi—wrote nursing orders for skin care
   I—bathing Ms. Boiko
   E—observed that her coccygeal area was still red (this could also be A, for ongoing assessment)
   E—concluded the outcome had not been achieved
   E—changed the order on the care plan

2. Client data are as follows: temp 101°F, pulse 120, resp. 32, B/P 100/68, reddened area over coccyx, unable to move about in bed, coccyx still red, a small area of skin was peeling off, there was some serous drainage. (Juan also obtained data that Ms. Boiko had been turned every 2 hours except for 6 hours each night. These data are about care that was given to Ms. Boiko but not data about her human responses.)

3. You should have circled the following as examples of reexamination of the nursing process phases (dynamic/cyclic):

   (1) . . . *concluded that the outcome had not been achieved.* This shows that Juan reexamined his original outcome.

   (2) *He was sure his data were adequate and that his nursing diagnosis was accurate.* This shows reexamination of the database and the original nursing diagnosis.

   (3) *The other staff members assured Juan that they had carried out the 2-hour turning schedule.* This shows that he checked to see if the nursing orders were properly implemented.

   (4) *He changed the order on the care plan.* This shows revision of the plan of care.

4. The nursing orders are:

   (1) to give skin care
   (2) a schedule for turning every 2 hours except at night
   (3) frequent, continued observation
   (4) to turn every 2 hrs around the clock

   Because the case states that Juan was bathing Ms. Boiko, you may have assumed that he wrote a nursing order for that; however, the case study does not say so, and you must use only the information provided. Juan did perform some other nursing activities, such as settling the client in bed; however, we do not know that they were written as nursing orders. Don't confuse nursing interventions or actions (carried out) with nursing orders (written).

5. This is the most obvious example of overlapping phases: "Two days later, when bathing Ms. Boiko, Juan observed that her coccygeal area was still red, a small area of skin was peeling off, and there was some serious drainage." In this example, Juan was implementing (bathing) at the same time he was assessing or evaluating (observing her coccygeal area).

   You might also have chosen: "Juan Apodaca, RN, settled her comfortably in bed and briefly interviewed her about her symptoms." *Settled* is implementation, but *interviewed* is assessment. As written, it isn't certain that these occurred at the same time; however, if you think they did, then this is also a case of overlapping phases.

6. Juan demonstrated creativity by not continuing to use the turning schedule that was routinely used on his unit. He was not content to do what was usually done but reasoned that in this case, something more was needed (he also used his cognitive skills here).

7. You should have chosen *planned* and *outcome oriented*: The nurse based interventions on the patient's needs, not on unit routines. You should also have chosen *flexible* because Juan did not adhere rigidly to his initial plan but changed it as needed.

CHAPTER 2. CRITICAL THINKING

WHAT DO YOU KNOW? ANSWERS

#2-1

Discuss four reasons why nurses need to think critically.

   Answer:
1. Nursing is an applied discipline. In an applied discipline (e.g., nursing), problems are messy and confusing. So the nurse must know how to identify knowledge and data gaps, find and use new information, and initiate and manage change. All of these skills require critical thinking.
2. Nursing draws on knowledge from other fields. Nurses use information and insights from other subject areas, such as physiology and psychology, in order to understand the meaning of patient data and to plan effective interventions. This, too, requires critical thinking.
3. Nurses deal with change in stressful environments. Therefore, routine behaviors and "the usual procedure" may not be adequate for the situation at hand. Treatments, medications, and technology change constantly, and a patient's condition may change from minute to minute. When anticipating or reacting to

changes, nurses must base their decisions on knowledge and rational thinking in order to respond appropriately under stress.

4. **Nurses make frequent, varied, and important decisions.** Nurses make many decisions. These are not trivial decisions; they often involve a client's well-being or even survival. Nurses use critical thinking to collect and interpret information and to make sound judgments and good decisions (e.g., to decide which of their many observations to report to physicians and which to handle on their own).

#2-2

List six characteristics of critical thinking.

Answer: Critical thinking:

- Is rational and reasonable.
- Involves conceptualization.
- Requires reflection.
- Involves both cognitive (thinking) skills and attitudes (feelings).
- Involves creative thinking.
- Requires knowledge.

#2-3

List and define at least five critical thinking attitudes.

Answer:

- *Independent thinking* means to think for yourself—to not passively accept the beliefs of others or just go along with the crowd.
- *Intellectual humility* means being aware of the limits of your knowledge, realizing that the mind can be self-deceptive, and admitting when you don't know something. It also includes rethinking conclusions when you have new knowledge
- *Intellectual courage* means being willing to consider and examine fairly your own beliefs and the views of others, especially those to which you may have a strongly negative reaction
- *Intellectual empathy* is the ability to imagine yourself in the place of others in order to understand them and their actions and beliefs.
- *Intellectual integrity* means being consistent in the thinking standards you apply (e.g., clarity, accuracy, completeness)—holding yourself to the same rigorous standards of proof to which you hold others.
- *Intellectual perseverance* is a sense of the need to struggle with confusion and unsettled questions over an extended period of time to achieve understanding and insight.
- *Intellectual curiosity* is an attitude of inquiry. It means having a mind filled with questions.
- *Faith in reason* implies that people can and should learn to think logically for themselves despite the natural tendencies of the mind to do otherwise.

Critical thinkers believe that well-reasoned thinking leads to trustworthy conclusions.

- *Fair-mindedness* involves making impartial judgments. It means treating all viewpoints alike without favoring one's own feelings or vested interests or those of one's friends, community, or nation. Fair-minded thinkers understand that their personal biases or social pressures and customs could unduly affect their thinking.
- *Interest in exploring thoughts and feelings* means to know that emotions can influence thinking and that all thought creates some level of feeling.

#2-4

List five guidelines to help you develop your critical thinking abilities.

Answer:

1. **Perform a self-assessment.**
2. **Tolerate dissonance and ambiguity.**
3. **Seek situations where good thinking is practiced.** *For example, attend conferences in clinical or educational settings that support open examination of all sides of issues and respect opposing viewpoints.*
4. **Create environments that support critical thinking.** *As leaders, nurses should encourage colleagues to examine evidence carefully before they come to conclusions and to avoid group think, the tendency to defer unthinkingly to the will of the group.*
5. **Practice critical thinking.**

THINK & REFLECT! SUGGESTED RESPONSES

There is usually no single, correct answer for these exercises because the intent is to have you practice thinking, not recall facts. The nature of a critical thinking problem is that it has more than one solution and that there may not be a "best" solution. You should compare your answers with those of your classmates—both your solutions and the thinking you used. Discussing your thinking processes is one way to help improve your thinking. Also, it is important for you to begin collaborating with your peers. During your nursing career, the thinking of other nurses will be an important resource to you, just as your thinking can be for them. You will usually not find answers here but ideas to help you think about the question.

#2-1

For each of the conventional moral principles above, write an example to illustrate how a nurse might demonstrate the principle. Compare your answers with those of a peer.

Suggested Responses: Responses will vary depending on each person's knowledge and past experiences. The following are some possibilities:

- **Be competent.** "I know a nurse who attends continuing education offerings even though they are not required by the employer or the state board of nursing."

- **Be loyal to each other.** "A nurse spoke up when someone was gossiping about another nurse."
- **Do not exploit patients.** "A patient offered this one nurse money for taking such good care of her. The nurse thanked the patient but refused the money."

#2-2

1. Which of the critical thinking attitudes do you believe to be your greatest strength? Explain your reasoning.

   Suggested Responses: Responses will vary depending on each person's knowledge and past experiences. Be certain that you explain your thinking on this point.

2. Which of the critical thinking attitudes do you most need to improve? Why do you think this?

   Suggested Responses: Responses will vary depending on each person's knowledge and past experiences. Be certain that you explain your thinking on this point.

#2-3

What do you think about the following definitions? Are they too broad, too narrow, or just right? Explain your answer.

1. A nurse is a professional.
2. A nurse is a professional woman who works in a hospital.

   Suggested Responses: The first definition is too broad and nonspecific; some might say it is incomplete. There are many professions other than nursing, so the definition doesn't help you to differentiate between nurses and other professionals. The second definition is more specific but is actually too specific. A nurse can be a woman or a man. Furthermore, nurses work in many settings other than hospitals. This definition would help you to identify *some* nurses, but it would cause you to fail to identify others.

#2-4

Recall an instance when you and a classmate heard a teacher's instructions differently (e.g., perhaps the teacher said to wear lab coats to orientation, but you thought you were supposed to wear your full uniform). Whose perception was inaccurate, and why?

   Suggested Responses: Everyone's answers will be different. Share your experiences with your classmates.

#2-5

Think about the nurses you have observed and about your own nursing experiences.

- What, exactly, is meant by "holistic" care?
- Do nurses always, or even usually, give holistic care?

- Is holistic care really a statement of what nurses are trying to achieve?
- What problems do nurses have in achieving this ideal?
- Is it realistic to try to achieve this ideal?

Suggested Responses: There are no single right answers to these questions. Discuss them with your classmates and compare the ideas you have about them. You will probably notice that some of the differences of opinion among you result from the different experiences each of you has had.

#2-6

1. What are some assumptions nurses commonly make about patients (e.g., patients are obligated to follow doctors' orders and to tell the truth when questioned about their symptoms)?
2. What are some assumptions you have about nurses (e.g., that they know what is best for patients; that they always chart accurate data)?
    Compare your assumptions with those of another student. How are they alike or different? Are they well-founded assumptions or are they in error?

Suggested Responses: Responses to these questions will differ on the basis of each person's knowledge and past experiences. The questions are meant for reflection and discussion and have no "best" answers.

#2-7

1. Write a paragraph describing a problem you have solved recently. Identify the problem-solving method you used.
2. Describe a decision you made in the clinical setting that was *not* made for the purpose of solving a problem.

Suggested Responses: Responses will vary among individuals. Discuss your experiences with your peers to determine whether you identified your problem-solving method accurately.

CRITICAL THINKING AND CLINICAL REASONING: A CASE STUDY: SUGGESTED RESPONSES

1. What factors does the nurse need to assess that might affect Mrs. Lutz's *ability* to consent?

    Suggested Responses: Examples of factors that may affect Mrs. Lutz's ability to consent: She is probably taking pain medications; the nurse needs to know what they are and how Mrs. Lutz responds to them. Mrs. Lutz may be depressed because of her illness. Her thinking may be affected by her weakened, malnourished state. She may be thinking of refusing treatment because it will present a financial burden to her family.

2. Before Mrs. Lutz signs the consent form, how can the nurse be certain that her consent was truly "informed"? (Informed consent means that the client has been informed about and understands the treatment, including its risks and benefits.)

   Suggested Responses: The nurse should ask Mrs. Lutz to verbalize the purpose of the treatment, its risks, and its benefits; what she can expect to feel during the treatment; and the advantages and disadvantages of the alternative treatments that are available.

3. Evaluate the nurse's approach to Mrs. Lutz in regard to this invasive procedure. (What do you think about it, and why?)

   Suggested Response: The nurse's approach was not appropriate. The nurse seems to be pressuring Mrs. Lutz into signing the form; she did not explain the risks of the procedure (she could have asked the physician if Mrs. Lutz had been informed about the risks); she did not explain what Mrs. Lutz would feel during the procedure, and she may even have been dishonest about that; she minimized the patient's fear by ignoring what she said.

4. Which phase of the nursing process is the nurse using in Items 1 and 2?

   Suggested Response: Assessment

5. In Items 1 and 2, which standard(s) of reasoning is/are involved (see Table 2–3).

   Suggested Response: Item 1 asks the nurse to apply the standard of accuracy: Will the data obtained from Mrs. Lutz be correct and accurate? Item 2 asks for the standards of breadth (Does she have the patient's true point of view?) and accuracy (Is that true? How could we check it?).

CHAPTER 3. ASSESSMENT

WHAT DO YOU KNOW? ANSWERS

#3-1

1. What is the difference between subjective and objective data?

   Answer: Subjective data are not measurable or observable. They can be obtained only from what the client tells you. Subjective data include the client's thoughts, beliefs, feelings, sensations, and perceptions of self and health (e.g., pain, dizziness, nausea, sadness, happiness). **Objective data** can be detected by someone other than the client. Examples of objective data include pulse rate, skin color, urine output, and results of diagnostic tests or radiographs.

2. What is the difference between primary and secondary data sources?

   Answer: The client is the **primary data** source; all other data sources are secondary. **Secondary data** are obtained from sources other than the client (e.g., other people, client records).

#3-2

1. Give three examples of data you could obtain from physical examination.

   Answers: Pulse rate, weight, heart sounds, palpation for abdominal masses or pain, bowel sounds

2. Give two examples of data you could obtain from observation.

   Answers: Pulse rate, body odor, condition of a dressing (e.g., drainage), safety hazards in the room, bed rails up (or down)

#3-3

1. State four conditions that require you to validate data.

   Answers:
   - Subjective and objective data do not agree.
   - Client statements differ at different times in the assessment.
   - The data seem very unusual or odd.
   - Factors are present that interfere with accurate measurement.

2. Define *validation.*

   Answer: Validation is the act of double checking or verifying data.

#3-4

List the phenomena to be assessed in a cultural assessment.

   Answers: Phenomena to assesss in a cultural assessment include the following:
   - Ethnicity, race, or cultural affiliation
   - Birthplace and place of residence
   - Communication
   - Food sanctions and restrictions
   - Religious beliefs and practices
   - Health beliefs
   - Folk practices
   - Family and social organization
   - Space orientation
   - Time orientation
   - Pain responses
   - Environmental control

#3-5

List six types of special-purpose assessment.

   Answers: Special-purpose assessments discussed in your text include home care and functional assessment, cultural assessment, spiritual assessment, wellness assessment, family assessment, and community assessment. You may have thought of others, such as nutritional assessment, neurological assessment, mental status examination, and so on.

THINK & REFLECT! SUGGESTED RESPONSES

There is usually no single, correct answer for these exercises because the intent is to have you practice thinking, not recall facts. The nature of a critical thinking problem is that it has more than one solution and that there may not be a "best" solution. You should compare your answers with those of your classmates—both your solutions and the thinking you used. Discussing your thinking processes is one way to help improve your thinking. Also, it is important for you to begin collaborating with your peers. During your nursing career, the thinking of other nurses will be an important resource to you, just as your thinking can be for them. You will usually not find answers here but ideas to help you think about the question.

#3-1

Think about the measurement criteria in Box 3–2 (ANA Standard I). Which of the standards of reasoning (in Table 3–1) are implied by each criterion? For example, Competency 1 implies "breadth" because comprehensive data collection helps ensure that data will be complete. What other standards are implied by Competency 1? By the other criteria?

Suggested Responses: The following are some examples of responses. This question is intended to encourage reflection and discussion, so not every possible answer is given:

- Criterion 2 implies breadth. Eliciting patient and family values helps ensure that you have all the data important to them, as well as those that are obvious to you.
- Criterion 3 implies accuracy, breadth, and significance. You always need to validate data with the patient for accuracy and to be certain the data are complete.
- Criterion 4 implies at least accuracy and precision because identifying barriers improves communication and allows you to obtain more information. More information can improve both accuracy and precision. For example, if the patient did not express herself clearly, communication enables you to clarify her statements.
- Criterion 5 implies accuracy. If you recognize the impact of the patient's personal attitudes, beliefs, and values, they may cue you to probe deeper into what the patient tells you.
- Criterion 6 implies accuracy because family dynamics can cause the patient or a family member to give inaccurate information. They may not be comfortable sharing some information in the presence of another family member.

#3-2

1. Observe a conversation between peers or family members. What nonverbal behaviors did you see? Did the speakers (a) put words in each other's mouth, (b) interrupt, or (c) make value judgments or give advice?

Suggested Responses: Responses will vary depending on students' experiences. Compare your experiences with those of your peers.

2. Recall a recent conversation between a nurse and a patient. Did the nurse do (a), (b), or (c)? Did the nurse make eye contact? Use silence as a technique?

    Suggested Responses: Responses will vary depending on students' experiences. Compare your experiences with those of your peers.

#3-3

Imagine you are a patient and the nurse says to you: "Lab will be here STAT to do a stick for gases, lytes, and enzymes. Then you'll go down for a CAT scan and an ECG. Meanwhile, I need to take your vitals. Also, do you take any OTC meds?"

- Would you understand what the nurse means?
- How would patients feel about these statements?
- Which terms are jargon that should be clarified?

    Suggested Responses: Whether you understand the nurse's meaning depends on your level of knowledge about medical terminology. Discuss these questions with your classmates. You might anticipate that patients would find the statements confusing. The following words are jargon: Lab, STAT, stick, gases, lytes, enzymes, CAT scan, ECG, vitals, OTC, meds.

#3-4

1. Does your school provide a nursing assessment form for you to use in clinical? What model(s) does it use to organize data? What are the major categories? How is it different from the forms used by the nurses on your clinical unit?

    Suggested Responses: Answers will vary according to the student's situation and experiences. Compare answers with your classmates and see if they agree with the conclusions you have drawn about your nursing assessment form.

#3-5

Scenario: You are making a focused assessment for Disturbed Sleep Pattern. Your patient says, "Well, of course, I'm tired! I didn't sleep a bit last night. My roommate snores like a freight train, and the night nurse was in here making noise all night long. If she'd get organized, she wouldn't have to disturb us so much."

1. In this case, what do you think of your text's directions to "record subjective data in the client's own words?"
2. What would you write when recording these data?

    Suggested Responses: Discuss your answers with your classmates. When the patient's words are too long or too negative, it is sometimes better to summarize rather than quote them exactly. You might, in this case, choose to write something like: "The patient states she didn't sleep last night because her roommate snored, and the nurse was in the room 'all night long.'" There is no need to include her solution that the nurse needs to "get organized."

CRITICAL THINKING AND CLINICAL REASONING: A CASE STUDY: SUGGESTED RESPONSES

1. What information do you need to gather when planning *safety* measures for Mr. Brown?
2. How is that information different from the information you'd need if everything in the case was the same except that instead of senile dementia, the medical diagnosis is fractured hip 1 week postoperatively?
3. Refer to Question 1. What data collection method will you use to get each piece of information? What data sources will you use?
4. What special techniques will you use to communicate with Mr. Brown? Write at least three questions (or statements) you would use when obtaining information from him.
5. What critical thinking attitudes or skills did you use in this exercise? Refer to Chapter 2, if necessary, to refresh your memory.

   Suggested Responses: Only a few suggestions are given. The best learning comes from discussion of the case.

   1. You may have listed: Is his disorientation continuous or just occasional? Is he just confused about where he is, or is his judgment poor about other things? Does he have a history of wandering about at night? What is his physical condition (e.g., strength, balance, ability to walk)? What is the facility's policy regarding patient safety and restraints?
   2. For a patient with a fractured hip, for example, you would need to know what pain medications he is taking (they may be causing the disorientation). You would do a focused pain assessment. You may not need as thorough a mental status assessment.
   3. To do a mental status examination, you must use primary source, subjective data obtained by interviewing Mr. Brown. You will use observation and physical examination. You will use secondary sources, such as the chart and the person bringing him to the hospital.
   4. For special techniques, refer to Chapter 3, "Interviewing Elderly Patients" and "Cognitive Deficits."
   5. For example, you used comparing and contrasting (data for senile dementia and fractured hip).

CHAPTER 4. DIAGNOSTIC REASONING

WHAT DO YOU KNOW? ANSWERS

#4-1

1. When did nursing diagnosis become incorporated into most nurse practice acts?

   Answer: In 1973, the American Nurses Association (ANA) Standards of Nursing Practice included nursing diagnosis as an important nursing activity, making it a legitimate function of professional nurses. During the 1970s and 1980s, the term *nursing diagnosis* was incorporated into nearly all state nurse practice acts, and diagnosis became a nursing obligation as well as a legal right. The term *nursing diagnosis* began to appear in the nursing literature in the 1950s to describe the functions of a professional nurse. In the 1960s, diagnosis was becoming an important part of the nursing process, but it was still necessary to establish that diagnosis was a thinking process that nurses could and should use and that they were not encroaching on medical territory.

2. State three reasons why nursing diagnosis is important.

    Answer: The following four reasons were given in the text:

    - Nursing diagnoses facilitate individualized care.
    - Nursing diagnoses promote professional accountability and autonomy by defining and describing the independent area of nursing practice.
    - Nursing diagnoses provide an effective vehicle for communication among nurses and other healthcare professionals.
    - Nursing diagnoses help determine assessment parameters.

#4-2

1. If there are no signs or symptoms present, is the problem an actual diagnosis, a potential diagnosis, or a possible diagnosis?

    Answer: It is a potential (risk) diagnosis. A possible diagnosis has at least one symptom present but not enough to allow you to identify the diagnosis.

2. A collaborative problem is a physiological complication of a disease or treatment that nurses can treat independently. True or false?

    Answer: False. Nurses cannot independently treat collaborative problems. Physician-prescribed interventions are also necessary. The nursing focus is on monitoring and prevention.

#4-3

1. What is a critical pathway?

    Answer: A critical pathway is a standardized care plan that indicates the patient and family care and outcomes that should occur within a specified time frame. It is a multidisciplinary plan that outlines the crucial care to be given for all patients of a certain type (e.g., all patients undergoing cardiac catheterization, all patients having a hysterectomy).

2. What is a variance?

    Answer: A **variance** occurs when the patient does not achieve a goal in the time predicted by the critical pathway.

#4-4

List the four main levels of data interpretation.

Answer:

- Identify significant cues.
- Cluster cues and identify data gaps.
- Draw conclusions about present health status.
- Determine etiologies and categorize problems.

THINK & REFLECT! SUGGESTED RESPONSES

There is usually no single, correct answer for these exercises because the intent is to have you practice thinking, not recall facts. The nature of a critical thinking problem is that it has more than one solution and that there may not be a "best" solution. You should compare your answers with those of your classmates—both your solutions and the thinking you used. Discussing your thinking processes is one way to help improve your thinking. Also, it is important for you to begin collaborating with your peers. During your nursing career, the thinking of other nurses will be an important resource to you, just as your thinking can be for them. You will usually not find answers here but ideas to help you think about the question.

#4-1

For each of the dimensions (physical dimension, psychological dimension, interpersonal/social dimension, or spiritual dimension), think of some ways a person might respond to the stressor of having a hysterectomy (removal of the uterus).

Suggested Responses: The following are only a few of the possible responses.

- Physical dimension: pain, bleeding, infection
- Psychological dimension: anxiety, fear, depression, crying, relief
- Interpersonal/social dimension: grief over loss of childbearing ability, fear that her significant other will not find her attractive, enhanced sexual satisfaction because there is no longer concern about becoming pregnant
- Spiritual dimension: praying, anger at God for allowing this to happen, gratitude to the Deity for allowing the surgery to go well

#4-2

Refer to Figure 4–4. Each of the following patients has undergone major abdominal surgery. Determine whether each set of cues represents a nursing diagnosis, a medical diagnosis, or a collaborative problem.

Patient A. Four days after surgery, incision is red, oozing pus, and not healing—symptoms of an infection.

Patient B. Two days after surgery, the patient's vital signs are normal, but he is breathing shallowly and not moving very much. These cues represent risk factors for postoperative pneumonia.

Patient C. The patient has just returned from surgery. The surgical dressing is dry but must be monitored to ensure that surgical hemostasis was obtained and that no excessive bleeding will occur.

Suggested Responses:

- Patient A has a medical diagnosis: infection. You cannot use the nursing diagnosis, Risk for Infection, because this is an actual rather than a potential problem.
- Patient B has a nursing diagnosis. Symptoms are present that identify Risk for Infection (Pneumonia) or perhaps Ineffective Breathing Pattern. If no symptoms were present, this would be a collaborative problem.
- Patient C has a collaborative problem. Bleeding is a potential physiological problem for all surgical patients. The nurse's main interventions are to monitor for and help prevent bleeding.

#4-3

Think about each of the following cue clusters. Do the cues fit together? Explain your reasoning.

Cluster 1—Osteoarthritis, difficulty getting out of bed, stiff joints, walks with walker

Cluster 2—Long-standing diabetes, legally blind, states feels lonely, wears glasses

Cluster 3—Incontinent of urine, wears incontinence pants, drinks adequate fluids, reddened area over coccyx

Cluster 4—Has bowel movement only every 3–4 days, sedentary lifestyle, history of urinary tract infections

Suggested Responses:

Cluster 1: All of these cues fit together. They all relate to a problem with mobility.

Cluster 2: These cues all fit together in that they may be related to diabetes. Diabetes can cause vision problems, and wearing glasses and being lonely may result from poor vision. These cues may indicate a problem with loneliness with an etiology of vision problems secondary to diabetes. More assessment would be needed to conclude that with certainty. You could make an argument that "states feels lonely" doesn't belong with this cluster; if so, you would be focusing on the vision problem. There are usually different possibilities for analyzing cue clusters.

Cluster 3: These cues fit together except that "drinks adequate fluids" is not an abnormal cue, and it not really relevant to identifying a skin problem related to urine incontinence.

Cluster 4: The sedentary lifestyle probably relates to the infrequent bowel movements. However, the history of urinary tract infections is irrelevant to those two cues.

#4-4

Your patient complains of abdominal cramping. He states that even though he takes a laxative every day, he must strain to have a bowel movement. What is your first hunch about the meaning of these data? Is there a problem? What is it? What data do you still need to feel more confident about your diagnosis? (Hint: Look up "Constipation" and "Perceived Constipation" in a nursing diagnosis handbook.)

> **Suggested Responses:** If you look up *Constipation* and *Perceived Constipation* in a nursing diagnosis handbook, you will see that these cues are associated with the nursing diagnosis of Constipation. That was probably your first hunch about the meaning of the data.

CRITICAL THINKING AND CLINICAL REASONING: A CASE STUDY: SUGGESTED RESPONSES

Only a few suggestions are given. Discuss the case with your peers.

1. Examples of feelings are fear, anger, and happiness
2. You may have thought, "He's doing this to himself" or many other things.
3. A value that "people should want to get well" or that "nurses should help people to get well" would certainly affect the way you see this situation.
4. What you say is highly individual and depends on Items 1 to 3.
5. He might be feeling anger, embarrassment, guilt, or . . . .
6. For example, many nurses may have already urged him to quit smoking, but maybe no one has ever focused on his feelings and how difficult it is to quit.
7. Noncompliance won't be a useful diagnosis unless you can find the reasons that the client continues to smoke. But the only etiology you can infer from these data is that he has an addiction to nicotine. You might speculate other reasons, such as "he doesn't care about his health," or "he is weak willed," but there are no data to suggest that.
8. There are no data to suggest that he smokes because of a lack of knowledge.
9. Based just on the data provided, you might consider Activity Intolerance r/t inadequate oxygenation. Or perhaps Self-Care Deficit (Bathing/Hygiene, Feeding) r/t Activity Intolerance. Based on his outburst, you might consider a "possible" diagnosis of Ineffective Denial or Ineffective Coping—but there are not enough data to confirm these as actual diagnoses.

CHAPTER 5. DIAGNOSTIC LANGUAGE

WHAT DO YOU KNOW? ANSWERS

#5-1

1. List four reasons standardized nursing languages are needed.

Answer:

1. They help to expand nursing knowledge.
2. They support computerized records.
3. They define and communicate unique nursing knowledge to nurses and others.
4. They can improve nursing care quality by providing researchable data.
5. They can influence health policy decisions—again, by generating data that represents nursing practice more accurately.

2. (True or false) Taxonomies classify ideas and objects on the basis of their similarities.

   Answer: True

#5-2

1. What are the four components of a NANDA-I diagnosis?

   Answer: Label (title or name), definition, defining characteristics, and related or risk factors

2. Define the term *NANDA-I label.*

   Answer: A label (also called *title* or *name*) is a concise word or phrase describing the client's health. Labels can be used as either the problem or the etiology in a diagnostic statement.

3. What is the difference between related factors and risk factors?

   Answer: Defining characteristics are subjective and objective data (cues, signs, and symptoms) that indicate the presence of the diagnostic label for an actual problem. Risk factors are the defining characteristics for potential problems—problems that don't exist at the time but that can be expected to occur if the nurse does not intervene to control or remove the risk factors.

#5-3

Why do nurses use "r/t" instead of "due to" to join the problem and etiology of a nursing diagnosis?

   Answer: Because the phrase *due to* implies a direct cause-and-effect relationship, which is hard to prove in a nursing diagnosis. Usually, there are multiple factors that interact to "cause" a problem, and it is possible that even if those factors were eliminated, the problem response might still exist. At best, you can say that it is highly likely that the factors are influencing, creating, or contributing to the problem.

#5-4

1. Which part of the diagnostic statement determines the patient outcomes needed to measure change in the problem status?

   Answer: The first part of the diagnostic statement (the problem) states what needs to change; thus, it determines the patient outcomes needed to measure this change.

2. (True or false) Interventions are sometimes suggested by the problem label instead of the etiology.

   Answer: True. Nursing interventions can be suggested by either part of the diagnostic statement. A few problem labels suggest particular nursing interventions regardless of the cause of the problem (e.g., Decisional Conflict; Fear; Hopelessness; Ineffective Denial; and Risk for Self-Directed, or Other-Directed, Violence). As the NANDA-I labels become more specific, you will probably discover more instances in which the etiology cannot be treated by independent nursing actions, and both the goals and nursing orders will be determined by the problem. For example, the nurse cannot treat a spinal cord lesion. Both the outcome and nursing orders are suggested by the problem label "Reflex Incontinence."

#5-5

1. Using preservation of life as a criterion, state whether the following are high, medium, or low priority diagnoses. Those that:
   a. Are life threatening
   b. Are concerned with developmental needs and need minimal nurse support
   c. Would bring about destructive physical or emotional changes

   Answers:

   a: high
   b: low
   c: medium

2. List the Maslow/Kalish needs in order from lowest (survival) to highest.

   Answers:

   > Physiologic (survival, then stimulation)
   > Safety and security
   > Social
   > Esteem
   > Self-actualization

THINK & REFLECT! SUGGESTED RESPONSES

There is usually no single, correct answer for these exercises because the intent is to have you practice thinking, not recall facts. The nature of a critical thinking problem is that it has more than one solution and that there may not be a "best" solution. You should compare your answers with those of your classmates—both your solutions and the thinking you used. Discussing your thinking processes is one way to help improve your thinking. Also, it is important for you to begin collaborating with your peers. During your nursing career, the thinking of other nurses will be an important resource to you, just as your thinking can be for them. You will usually not find answers here but ideas to help you think about the question.

#5-1

Use the Taxonomy II (Table 5–2) axes to write a problem statement for the following data: An elderly client with left-sided paralysis has a red area of abraded ("broken") skin over his sacrum. (The concept, Axis 1, is Skin Integrity.)

Suggested Responses: The following are possible responses. You may have thought of others.

From Axis 1: Skin Integrity

From Axis 2: Individual (but not necessary to include in the diagnostic statement)

From Axis 3: Impaired

From Axis 4: Skin (but not necessary in the diagnostic statement because it is a part of the concept from Axis 1)

From Axis 7: Actual (the patient has symptoms/defining characteristics).

So the diagnosis label would be Actual Impaired Skin Integrity

#5-2

Think of a problem, other than Decisional Conflict and Chronic Low Self-Esteem, that could be caused by a complex etiology.

Suggested Responses: Some possible problems might include Ineffective Health Maintenance, Sedentary Lifestyle, Deficient Knowledge, and Ineffective Activity Planning. You may have thought of others.

#5-3

In Culture A, pain is considered a punishment for sins, so the person is expected to tolerate pain without complaint in order to make atonement. In Culture B, expressions of pain elicit attention and sympathy. Suppose you are caring for a client with a fractured arm. He is holding his arm, pacing the floor, cursing, and complaining loudly of unbearable pain.

- If you are from Culture A, what would be your most likely interpretation of these cues?
- If you are from Culture B, what would be your most likely interpretation?
- If you and the client are both from Culture A, would your interpretation be accurate?
- If you are from Culture A and the client is from Culture B, would your interpretation be accurate?

Suggested Responses: Responses will depend on your knowledge and personal experiences. Compare your answers with those of your peers and then discuss with them how their knowledge and experience differ from yours. You may have said that if you are from Culture A, you'd interpret that the patient must have sinned and is being punished for it. You might not be very sympathetic to his complaints, but perhaps he is angry because he thinks he is being unjustly punished. If you were from Culture B., you might feel sorry for the person and spend time trying to make him comfortable. If both you and the client are from Culture A, your interpretation that he ought to be more stoic or that he has been punished unjustly might be accurate. If the two of you are from different cultures, you are more likely to misinterpret his behaviors unless you take his culture into account.

CRITICAL THINKING AND CLINICAL REASONING: A CASE STUDY: SUGGESTED RESPONSES

Only a few suggestions are given. Discuss the case with your peers.

1. Correct. The data do not explain why Mr. Gomez is in denial (if he actually is).
2. Incorrect. There are no data to suggest that Mr. Gomez lacks knowledge about anything, although that could be the case. It would be correct to say *possibly* r/t lack of knowledge.
3. Incorrect. Failure to change lifestyle is a defining characteristic for that NANDA-I label, not a related factor. It is a symptom of the problem, not a cause.
4. Probably Ineffective Individual Therapeutic Regimen Management. Mr. Gomez has the defining characteristics for Noncompliance; however, that NANDA-I definition requires "an *agreed-upon* . . . treatment plan." This situation does not say whether Mr. Gomez ever actually agreed to his prescribed treatment plan. This question is certainly open to discussion.
5. You may have written something like: Ineffective Therapeutic Regimen Management (diet, smoking, work pattern) possibly r/t denial of seriousness of illness A.M.B. working 60 hours/week, high-fat diet, smoking, exacerbation of physical symptoms, and statement ". . . working too hard . . . just need pills." Mr. Gomez's statement is the strongest cue that he is in denial but by itself is not proof. His behaviors may be caused by something other than denial. The most important issue in this question is it is probably most useful to use denial in the etiology rather than as a problem.
6. This would depend on the framework you use. In a preservation of life framework, the collaborative problem would have highest priority.
7. Your perspective will affect your speculations about Mr. Gomez's priority. However, it appears from the data that he is probably most concerned about fatigue.
8. Answers are completely individual.

CHAPTER 6. PLANNING: OVERVIEW AND OUTCOMES

WHAT DO YOU KNOW? ANSWERS

#6-1

Give an example of each of the following: informal planning, formal planning, time-sequenced planning, initial planning, ongoing planning.

Answer: The following are examples. You may have thought of others.

1. Informal planning: The nurse assesses a patient's skin while performing a bath.
2. Formal planning: The nurse writes a plan for a patient's care.
3. Time-sequenced planning: The nurse plans to help the patient ambulate before visiting hours so the patient can receive visitors.
4. Initial planning: After receiving a patient from surgery, the nurse plans care for the remainder of the shift.
5. Ongoing planning: On a patient's second hospital day, the nurse revises the care plan to reflect improvements in the patient's mobility.

#6-2

1. List the components of a goal statement.

   Answer: Subject, action verb, performance criteria, target time, and special conditions.

2. (True or false) Special conditions should be a component of all goals.

   Answer: False. Not all goals need special conditions; they are included only if they are important. If the performance criteria clearly specify the expected performance, then special conditions are not necessary.

#6-3

List as many guidelines as you can recall for judging the quality of outcome statements.

Answer: The following are the guidelines presented in your textbook:

1. *Standards: Accuracy, Logic:* The outcome is appropriate to and derived from the nursing diagnosis.
2. *Standard: Logic:* Each outcome is derived from only one nursing diagnosis.
3. *Standard: Logic:* The outcome is stated in terms of patient responses rather than nurse activities.
4. *Standard: Accuracy:* The desired outcomes are revised to reflect changes in patient status.
5. *Standard: Clarity:* Desired outcomes are phrased in positive terms.
6. *Standard: Clarity:* The outcome statement is concise.
7. *Standard: Precision:* The goal or outcome is directly observable or measurable.
8. *Standard: Precision:* The goal or outcome is specific and concrete.
9. *Standard: Depth:* Each goal or outcome statement has all the necessary components.
10. *Standard: Depth:* Desired outcomes are adequate (e.g., in number) to address each nursing diagnosis.
11. *Standard: Breadth:* The goal or outcome is valued by the client, family, or community.
12. *Standard: Breadth:* The goal or outcome is congruent with the total treatment plan.

13. *Standard: Breadth:* Remember that goals or outcomes can be written for families and communities as well as individuals.
14. *Standards: Breadth and Depth:* The desired outcomes are realistic and achievable in terms of the client's internal and external resources.

THINK & REFLECT! SUGGESTED RESPONSES

There is usually no single, correct answer for these exercises because the intent is to have you practice thinking, not recall facts. The nature of a critical thinking problem is that it has more than one solution and that there may not be a "best" solution. You should compare your answers with those of your classmates—both your solutions and the thinking you used. Discussing your thinking processes is one way to help improve your thinking. Also, it is important for you to begin collaborating with your peers. During your nursing career, the thinking of other nurses will be an important resource to you, just as your thinking can be for them. You will usually not find answers here but ideas to help you think about the question.

#6-1

Write as many examples of action verbs as you can think of (not more than 50).

Suggested Responses: The following are some action verbs. You may have thought of others.

Apply	List
Breathe	Move
Choose	Prepare
Communicate	Report
Define	Share
Demonstrate	Sit
Describe	Sleep
Design	Talk
Drink	Transfer
Explain	Turn
Express	Use
Identify	Verbalize
Inject	Walk

CRITICAL THINKING AND CLINICAL REASONING: A CASE STUDY: SUGGESTED RESPONSES

Only a few suggestions are given. Remember that answers will vary based on knowledge, experience, and values. The most meaningful learning comes from discussing the case with others.

1. Items *a to e* should have helped you work through this question. If not, read more about diabetes and insulin. If you are still having trouble, see your instructor for help.
2. Poor peripheral circulation is one risk factor that supports a nursing diagnosis of Risk for Delayed Wound Healing.
3. A general goal would be that the foot would heal at an optimum rate; evidence of that would be approximation of edges and a clean, dry incision, for example.
4. To answer this question, ask: (a) Can the nurse provide most of the care to prevent delayed wound healing? (b) Are there factors that put this patient at higher risk for delayed wound healing than the "norm"? If so, you may want to write a nursing diagnosis. This is a difficult question, because *a* is probably No, and *b* is Yes.
5. Example of an outcome for the patient: Will state the signs and symptoms of infection.
6. Answers will vary, depending on your perspective. Is it possible to give culturally competent care to someone of a different race, culture, or sex than the nurse? Are there situations in which someone of the same race, culture, or sex might be more effective or increase the patient's comfort in some way?
7. The patient will probably not be able to care for his nutritional and self-care needs. For example, his nutritional needs are different because of the surgery, and he is probably less able to shop and cook; his appetite may not be good because of the antibiotic side effects or because of his probable decreased activity.
8. Examples of outcomes that would demonstrate nutritional and self-care needs are being met: Will maintain present weight. Will state that he cooks and eats at least three meals per day.
9. The highest priority is to determine how his care needs can be managed at home and make those arrangements. Second to that, the priority is to assure that he knows the signs and symptoms of infection and antibiotic reactions.
10. Perhaps the home health nurse's highest priority would be to monitor the diabetes to be sure it remains stable because of the effect diabetes can have on wound healing. Or perhaps the nurse will teach and give care to prevent infection of the wound. It depends on the framework you are using to prioritize. For example, the *most likely* problem is that he will fall; the *most serious* is either that his diabetes will not be controlled or his wound will become infected. Because the diabetes is controlled at present, the main focus should probably be wound care to prevent infection. However, none of these is an actual problem. If you identified an actual problem (e.g., inability to buy and prepare food), that might receive a higher priority.

CHAPTER 7. PLANNING: INTERVENTIONS

WHAT DO YOU KNOW? ANSWERS

#7-1

1. Which type of nursing intervention is ordered by the primary care provider: independent, dependent, or collaborative?

2. Which type of nursing intervention is an autonomous action based on scientific rationale: independent, dependent, or collaborative?

   Answers:

   1. Dependent
   2. Independent

#7-2

List the four steps to follow in generating and selecting nursing interventions.

   Answer:

   1. Review the nursing diagnosis.
   2. Review the patient goals/outcomes.
   3. Identify alternative interventions or actions.
   4. Select the best options.

#7-3

List the six components of a nursing order.

   Answer:

   1. Date the order was written
   2. Subject
   3. Action verb
   4. Descriptive qualifiers
   5. Specific times
   6. Signature

#7-4

1. (True or false) The nurse should choose the NIC intervention labels and activities best suited to your patient's needs.

   Answer: True. The NIC will have several interventions appropriate for a single nursing diagnosis. Different interventions will be required depending on the etiology of the diagnosis. In addition, NIC lists many *activities,* specific actions a nurse might take in performing an intervention. Not all activities will be needed for a particular client, so the nurse chooses them to fit the supplies, equipment, and other resources available in the agency, as well as the client's needs.

2. Which classification system was developed specifically for community health: NIC, Omaha, or CCC?

   Answer: The Omaha System was developed specifically for community health; CCC was developed for home health; and NIC is a broad classification for use in all settings.

THINK & REFLECT! SUGGESTED RESPONSES

There is usually no single, correct answer for these exercises because the intent is to have you practice thinking, not recall facts. The nature of a critical thinking problem is that it has more than one solution and that there may not be a "best" solution. You should compare your answers with those of your classmates—both your solutions and the thinking you used. Discussing your thinking processes is one way to help improve your thinking. Also, it is important for you to begin collaborating with your peers. During your nursing career, the thinking of other nurses will be an important resource to you, just as your thinking can be for them. You will usually not find answers here but ideas to help you think about the question.

#7-1

Describe one activity you have performed (or have seen another nurse perform) in clinical in each of the following categories: observation, treatment, prevention, and health promotion.

Suggested Responses: Examples will vary depending on each person's clinical experience. Use Table 7–1 to evaluate your examples.

#7-2

When deciding whether to make a referral or deal with a patient's problem yourself, ask (1) What are my knowledge and experience in this area? (2) Does this require in-depth or specialized knowledge that I lack? (3) Do I have any values, beliefs, or biases that could interfere with the quality of care I give for this problem? Which of the following situations would you refer? Why?

Suggested Responses: Responses will vary, depending on each person's experience, knowledge, and personal values.

1. Mary has come to the clinic for a prenatal visit. When you comment on some bruises, she tells you that her husband beats her. She says, "I'm even afraid for my kids. We need to get out of there, but I don't know where to go or how I'd support the kids."

   Suggested Responses: As a nurse, you would probably refer Mary unless you have had special training in counseling abuse victims. Another reason is that legal assistance may be needed to protect the patient and her children.

2. Elaine has just given birth and plans to breastfeed her baby. She is about 25 lb overweight now, and she asks you how she can lose the weight and still maintain her milk supply.

   Suggested Responses: You would probably refer Elaine if you think you lack adequate knowledge of the nutritional needs of and interventions for infants and lactating women.

3. A patient's care plan has a nursing diagnosis of "Impaired Gas Exchange r/t changes in alveolar-capillary membranes secondary to chronic lung disease."

Suggested Responses: You would probably refer this patient if you do not know enough about chronic lung disease and Impaired Gas Exchange to manage Impaired Gas Exchange on your own. In any event, you would probably need to seek medical prescriptions to help treat the Impaired Gas Exchange.

4. Would an experienced community health nurse or psychiatric nurse practitioner have addressed the first situation the same way as you did?

Suggested Responses: Probably both nurses would address the first situation differently than you did because their knowledge and experience would be vastly different from yours.

CRITICAL THINKING AND CLINICAL REASONING: A CASE STUDY: SUGGESTED RESPONSES

Note: Answers do not contain comprehensive information. Only a few suggestions are given.

1. Respiratory complications such as pneumonia and atelectasis
2. Anesthesia, incisional pain, obesity, fatigue. Obese persons may have decreased alveolar expansion related to a sedentary lifestyle. She may be taking shallow breaths to decrease the pain—also because she is tired.
3. Has she recently received medication for pain? If so, is it adequately relieving her pain? These answers would be obtained by looking at the medication record (in the chart) to see if any medication has been administered and by asking the patient (a) whether she has recently had medication and (b) how she would rate her pain on a scale of 1 to 10.
4. To prevent respiratory complications
5. First, be sure pain relief is optimal. Then you may, for example, teach her to splint her incision with a pillow while doing the exercises to minimize tension on the incision. Explain that consistent performance of the exercises will actually decrease her fatigue (by increasing the availability of oxygenated blood).
6. One action would be to demonstrate the exercises and then breathe along with her while she performs them. Verbal feedback (e.g., saying, "Well done") would support her efforts. Communicate the plan to other caregivers; check often to see if she is complying.
7. She will have no respiratory complications. Assess vital signs (especially temperature and respirations), lung sounds, skin color, and so on.

CHAPTER 8. IMPLEMENTATION

WHAT DO YOU KNOW? ANSWERS

#8-1

List at least three ways you can encourage patients to adhere to treatment regimens.

Answer:

1. Accept the patient as he is.
2. Ask the patient what *he* wants to know and what *his* concerns are.
3. Be realistic. Patients are more likely to make behavioural and lifestyle changes gradually.
4. Do not assume. Every patient's situation is different.
5. Promote patient confidence.
6. Remind the patient that change takes time. Refer him to a support or self-help group for encouragement.

#8-2

1. List four functions of client records.

   Answer:

   - Communication (among health professionals)
   - Planning care
   - Evaluating and improving patient care
   - Providing information to regulating agencies (e.g., The Joint Commission)
   - Reimbursement from Medicare, Medicaid, and private insurance companies
   - Serving as a legal document
   - Research, education, and statistics

2. What do the letters S-O-A-P stand for in SOAP charting?

   Answer: Subjective data, objective data, assessment, and planning

3. What do the letters P-I-E stand for in PIE charting?

   Answer: Problems, Interventions, Evaluation (or patient responses to care)

4. (True or false) CBE organizes the progress notes by using the key words *data, action,* and *response.*

   Answer: False. Focus® charting organizes progress notes by using the key words, *data, action,* and *response.* CBE is a system in which only significant findings or exceptions to stated norms are recorded.

#8-3

1. State two rules relating to *when* to chart.

   Answer:

   - Date and time each entry.
   - Indicate both the time the entry was made and the time the observation or intervention occurred, if different.
   - Record the nursing action or client response as soon as possible after it occurs.
   - Never leave the unit for an extended time unless all important information has been charted.
   - Do not document interventions before carrying them out.

- Document in chronological order. If you forget to chart something, record it as soon as possible, marking it "Late Entry."

2. State three rules relating to *what* to chart.

Answer:

- As a rule, do not chart actions performed by someone else.
- Progress notes must be accurate and correct.
- Go beyond flowsheet data. Chart judgments about the data to indicate whether the patient is doing better or worse. Compare current patient status with previous data.
- Progress notes should be factual. Chart what you see, hear, smell, or observe.
- Progress notes should be clear and specific. Do not use vague generalities, such as *good*, *normal*, or *sufficient*.
- Do not use negative, prejudicial terms.
- To organize a narrative entry, include D–I–E (data, intervention, and evaluation).
- Record only appropriate and relevant data.
- Progress notes should be complete.
- Be brief. Omit unnecessary words, such as *patient*.
- Balance conciseness with completeness.

3. State one thing you should *not chart*.

Answer: Any one of the following:

- Words suggesting errors (e.g., *accidentally, unintentionally, by mistake*)
- That an incident report has been filed
- Staff conflicts or critical comments about the behaviors or care given by other team members
- Staffing problems or staff shortages (use a confidential memo or incident report instead)

4. State two rules about *how* to chart.

Answer:

- Use dark ink. Most agencies specify black ink. Erasable ink is not acceptable.
- Write legibly or print.
- Use correct grammar, spelling, and punctuation.
- Use standard symbols, terminology, and abbreviations carefully.
- Do not use abbreviations from The Joint Commission's "do not use" list ("U" or "u" for unit; "IU" for International Unit; Q.D., QD, q.d., qd.; Q.O.D., QOD, q.o.d., qod).

5. List three items of *essential data* to chart (from Box 8–8).

Answer:

- A physical symptom that:
      Is severe (e.g., extreme shortness of breath)
      Recurs or persists (e.g., vomiting after every meal)
      Is not normal (e.g., elevated temperature)
      Becomes worse (e.g., fever increases from 102° to 104°F)

Is not relieved by prescribed actions (e.g., patient unable to sleep after taking sleeping pill)

Is a symptom of a complication (e.g., inability to void after surgery)

Is a known danger signal (e.g., a lump in the breast)

- Changes in physical function
- Behavior changes and relationship changes
- Nursing interventions, especially those performed in response to symptoms and changes in patient status
- Patient responses to nursing interventions; evaluation of outcomes or goal achievement
- Inability to carry out prescribed treatments or patient's refusal of treatments or interventions
- Teaching about the need for treatment and the possible consequences of nonadherence
- Patient's ability to manage care after discharge
- All medical visits and consultations
- Discussions with the primary provider about your concerns with medical orders

#8-4

1. What do the letters in the mnemonic SBAR stand for?

   Answer: Situation, background, assessment, and recommendation

2. What do the letters in the mnemonic PACE stand for?

   Answer: Patient or problem, assessment or actions, continuing or changes, and evaluation

THINK & REFLECT! SUGGESTED RESPONSES

There is usually no single, correct answer for these exercises because the intent is to have you practice thinking, not recall facts. The nature of a critical thinking problem is that it has more than one solution and that there may not be a "best" solution. You should compare your answers with those of your classmates—both your solutions and the thinking you used. Discussing your thinking processes is one way to help improve your thinking. Also, it is important for you to begin collaborating with your peers. During your nursing career, the thinking of other nurses will be an important resource to you, just as your thinking can be for them. You will usually not find answers here but ideas to help you think about the question.

#8-1

Write a scenario illustrating overlapping between implementation and each of the following steps: Assessment, diagnosis, and evaluation. Do not use examples given in your textbook.

Suggested Responses: Examples will vary depending on each student's clinical experience and imagination. Some possibilities are the following:

- Implementation overlaps with assessment: While bathing a client, the nurse observes a rash on the patient's back.
- Implementation overlaps with diagnosis: While teaching a client about a diet modification, the nurse observes that the client often asks her to repeat instructions. She diagnoses Disturbed Sensory Perception (Auditory).
- Implementation overlaps with evaluation: The nurse administers an oral pain medication before teaching a client about diet modifications. During the teaching session, the nurse observes that the client is restless, grimaces occasionally, and does not seem to be listening closely. The nurse inquires further and discovers that the client's pain has not been relieved by the medication.

#8-2

On the critical pathway for Ms. Fischer, one of the nursing orders for today (postoperative day 2) is "Discontinue IV fluids." However, Ms. Fischer's bowel sounds are infrequent, and she is taking only scant amounts of oral fluids. As her nurse, what would you do?

Suggested Responses: Discuss your response with other students. The nurse should notify the primary care provider of these findings before discontinuing the IV fluids. If you did not know to do that, don't be too concerned. As you gain clinical experience and theoretical knowledge, such questions will be easier to answer. For now, and in this text, they are meant to get you started thinking like a nurse even if you don't always have the best answer.

#8-3

Recall a time when you did not follow a doctor's or other health professional's advice. For example, you may have not taken all of the antibiotic capsules, even though the instructions clearly said to do so.

1. List all the reasons you had for not complying.
2. What, if anything, could a nurse have done that would have changed what you did in that situation?

Suggested Responses: Responses will vary depending on individual experiences. Discuss responses with other students.

CRITICAL THINKING AND CLINICAL REASONING: A CASE STUDY: SUGGESTED RESPONSES

Note: Other answers may be possible. Only a few suggestions are given.

1. *Actual Diagnoses*: Functional Urinary Incontinence; Bathing/Hygiene Self-Care Deficit, Toileting S-CD, Dressing/Grooming S-CD (You could write Total Self-Care Deficit instead of these.)

   Potential Diagnoses: Risk for Disturbed Body Image or Situational Low Self-Esteem; Risk for Disuse Syndrome (a complication of immobility that includes Risk for Constipation, Impaired Urinary Elimination, disorientation, Disturbed Body Image, and Powerlessness), Risk for Disturbed Thought Processes.

2. (a) No; not based on the information given. (b) He does have risk factors: decreased self-care abilities, incontinence, body changes, and inability to communicate all may be damaging to his self-esteem.

3. Add urinary incontinence as an etiology because the dampness increases the risk for skin breakdown. There is also a possibility of inadequate nutrition related to his illness and his inability to feed himself. Inadequate nutrition is a risk factor for impaired skin integrity. It is important to add these etiological factors because they suggest nursing interventions.

4. Monitor for redness, breakdown, edema, excessive dryness or moistness, color and temperature, and hydration.

5. Refer to Box 2–9 in Chapter 2.

6. (a) All activities are appropriate, except for "provide trapeze . . " Mr. W. is probably not yet able to use the trapeze; this may be appropriate later. You might have drawn a line through "fecal" in the first activity because he has not been incontinent of stool. In the second activity, draw a line through "as appropriate." In the third activity, draw a line through "at least daily"—that is not often enough. In the last activity, draw a line through "as appropriate." (b) The last activity should specify the type of "specialty" bed or mattress (e.g., foam, air, sheepskin).

7. Bleeding or hemorrhage

8. Use a soft bristle toothbrush. Use an electric razor only. Bathe gently. Tell the nurse if you see any bleeding (e.g., nose, mouth, or urine) or bruises.

9. Keep linens dry, taut, and wrinkle free. Because he is immobile, wrinkled or damp linens will contribute to skin breakdown.

10. Example: Will be able to feed himself with his right hand within 3 weeks.

11. (a) Because of his Impaired Verbal Communication, he cannot call for help. Also, he cannot tell the nurse of any subjective symptoms that are developing.
    (b) Place the call light or bell where he can reach it with his right hand. Ask "yes/no" questions about any symptoms of complications that you may be concerned about (e.g., dizziness, disorientation).

12. The nurse might refer Mr. Williams to the following professionals:
    - Speech therapist to practice speech-therapy activities and find alternative methods of communication
    - Nutritionist to suggest high-protein menus to promote healthy skin, and high-fiber menus to prevent constipation; also, foods that he can feed himself
    - Physical therapist for range-of-motion and muscle-strengthening exercises
    - Occupational therapist for assistive devices for eating and other self-care and for training in self-care

13. One nursing order might be: Provide passive range-of-motion exercises for left arm and leg and active range-of-motion exercises for right arm and leg every 4 hours while awake.

CHAPTER 9. EVALUATION

#9-1

What are three important evaluations nurses make?

Answer: As a nurse, you will make frequent and varied evaluations. Because the client is your primary concern, the most important evaluations involve the following:

1. The client's progress toward health goals
2. The success of the nursing plan of care in helping the client to achieve desired outcomes
3. The overall quality of care given to defined groups of clients

#9-2

List the five-step process for evaluating client progress.

Answer:

1. Review the desired outcomes (indicators).
2. Collect evaluation data.
3. Compare patient status with desired outcomes and draw a conclusion.
4. Write the evaluative statement.
5. Relate nursing interventions to outcomes.

THINK & REFLECT! SUGGESTED RESPONSES

There is usually no single, correct answer for these exercises because the intent is to have you practice thinking, not recall facts. The nature of a critical thinking problem is that it has more than one solution and that there may not be a "best" solution. You should compare your answers with those of your classmates—both your solutions and the thinking you used. Discussing your thinking processes is one way to help improve your thinking. Also, it is important for you to begin collaborating with your peers. During your nursing career, the thinking of other nurses will be an important resource to you, just as your thinking can be for them. You will usually not find answers here but ideas to help you think about the question.

#9-1

Mrs. Adams needed to lose 60 lb (28 kg). With her input, the nurse included in the care plan a goal to "Lose 6 lb (2.8 kg) by 5/2/12." A nursing order in the care plan was to

"Explain how to plan and prepare a 1,000-calorie diet." When Mrs. Adams weighed herself on May 2, she had lost 10 lb. The goal had been met.

1. Does this mean that the nursing order was effective?
2. What do you need to know in order to decide if that nursing action led to the weight loss?
3. What other factors might have caused Mrs. Adams to lose weight?
4. If Mrs. Adams says, "I forgot what you said about the diet, so I just ate out a lot," what conclusion would you draw about the nursing strategy?

Suggested Responses:

1. No, meeting the goal does not necessarily mean it was the nursing order that caused goal achievement, although that may be so. Recall that a number of variables can affect outcome achievement, for example:
   - Actions and treatments performed by other healthcare professionals
   - Influence of family members and significant others
   - Client's attitudes, desire, and motivation
   - Client's failure to give accurate or sufficient information during data collection
   - Client's prior experiences and knowledge
   - Other variables are possible; nurses cannot control all the variables that might influence the outcome of care. Therefore, in determining the effect of a nursing action, you should try to identify other factors that might have promoted or interfered with its effectiveness.

2. In order to decide if that nursing action led to the weight loss, you need to know a variety of things. For example, to know if the nursing order was responsible for the weight loss, and you need to know whether Mrs. Adams did indeed plan and prepare a 1,000-calorie diet. You also need to know whether she actually limited her food intake to 1,000 calories per day.

3. Other factors might have caused Mrs. Adams to lose weight, including the following: Other professional treatments may have been given, such as medications that caused a loss of appetite or promoted weight loss by increasing her metabolic rate. Or perhaps Mrs. Adams started a new exercise program that helped her burn calories. Or perhaps Mrs. Adams was ill during the period before 5/2/12 and had no appetite. You may think of many others.

4. If Mrs. Adams says, "I forgot what you said about the diet, so I just ate out a lot," you would probably conclude that the nursing strategy had very little to do with her weight loss.

#9-2

Explain the difference between relevance and significance when evaluating the plan of care.

Suggested Responses: *Relevance* pertains to how well the data related to the stated goals, for example. Whether you are talking about data, goals, or

interventions, in simple terms it means: What does this have to do with the matter at hand—with the problem or with the patient. *Significance* refers to the importance of the data, goals, or interventions. For instance, certain data might be related to the problem but not be very important.

#9-3

In the past 3 months, several medication errors have been made on your nursing unit. The unit has instituted some policies and procedures to improve the safety of this task. Develop criteria to use to evaluate whether this practice problem has been solved. Include criteria to measure structure, process, and outcomes. To begin, answer these questions:

- What is the purpose of the evaluation?
- What is being evaluated; what is the function of the "thing" being evaluated?
- What different points of view may exist?

Suggested Responses: The purpose of this exercise is to encourage you to think about what you have learned. Discuss and compare your answers with those of other students. To help you get started, in this sample case, the purpose of the evaluation is to determine whether the new policies have had any effect on the number of medications being made on your nursing unit. Answer the other two guiding questions above and then write your structure, process, and outcomes criteria. Review structure, process, and outcomes evaluation in your textbook, as needed.

CRITICAL THINKING AND CLINICAL REASONING: A CASE STUDY: SUGGESTED RESPONSES

1. Probably not. Ms. Jackson doesn't have the necessary defining characteristics to diagnose either Dysfunctional Grieving (duration too short) or Ineffective Coping. She appears to be experiencing a normal grief process, for which there is no NANDA diagnosis. However, because her grief seems to be affecting her nutrition, the nurse should find a way to include it in the description of her health status.
2. Do the defining characteristics fit Ms. Jackson? Is the etiology specific or descriptive enough to provide direction for the nursing interventions?
3. For example, you might add "as manifested by . . " or "secondary to grief over loss of husband."
4. Item #1 is vague and not observable. What is "optimal" daily caloric intake? For example, you might write, "Will decrease calorie intake by 500 calories/day." You need to add a fourth goal that would indicate resolution of the problem–that she will lose weight. State specifically how much weight and by when (e.g., "Will lose 1 lb/week.")
5. *c.* You need to know how many calories it takes to produce a 1-lb weight loss; otherwise, you might set an impossible goal (e.g., 10 lb/week would mean she has to reduce her intake by 5,000 calories/day—probably more than her total intake has

been). Principle *a* is the only one that does not apply. Principle *b* explains the reason for dietary changes (to lose weight); *c* also explains relationship between calories and weight; *d* explains the concern for a "well-balanced" diet.

6. Refer her to support groups (e.g., a grieving support group).
7. *Outcome #1*—This goal is impossible to evaluate because it is stated in broad, non-specific terms. Her dietary log indicates she is eating well-balanced meals, but is that "optimal" intake? It is impossible to judge by her weight loss because there was no goal to specify what that was to be. She lost less than 1 lb/week, however, so she is probably still consuming too many calories.

   Outcome #2—Not met. She is only walking 20 minutes/day, not 30.

   Outcome #3—Partially met. She realizes that she eats when she is bored and depressed, but there are probably other, more specific activities that are associated with her eating (e.g., watching TV).
8. 2b—Because there is no evidence that this has been done.

   3a—Because there is no evidence that this has been done except for verbalizing that she eats when she is bored.

   3b—Because there is no evidence that this has been done; it is important as motivation. The nurse should do all of these things at this clinic visit.
9. **a.** For example, when she watches TV, she might start doing something that requires her to use her hands (e.g., sewing, ironing, working on a photo album). "Stop watching TV" doesn't apply this principle nor would "Stop snacking."
   b. She has not stopped smoking, but she has substituted better quality, healthier (and we assume lower calorie) foods.
10. No suggestions. Answers will be unique to each person.

CHAPTER 10. CREATING A PLAN OF CARE

WHAT DO YOU KNOW? ANSWERS

#10-1

1. List the five components of a comprehensive plan of care.
2. In which component of the care plan would you expect to find a patient's religious preferences listed?
3. Where would you look to find the plan of care for a patient with special teaching needs?

Answer:

1. The five components of a comprehensive plan of care are:
   - Client profile
   - Instructions for meeting basic needs
   - Aspects of the medical plan to be implemented by the nurse
   - Nursing diagnoses and collaborative problems
   - Addendum care plans

2. In the client profile
3. Addendum care plans

#10-2

1. List 10 steps in creating a patient plan of care (review Box 10–1 if you cannot remember all of them).

   Answers:

   a. Collect data.
   b. Analyze and synthesize data.
   c. List all problems (working problem list).
   d. Make formal list of labelled problems.
   e. Determine which problems can be addressed by critical pathways, standards of care, model care plans, protocols, and policies and procedures.
   f. Individualize model plans of care, protocols, and so forth, as needed.
   g. Transcribe medical, collaborative, activities of daily living, and basic care needs to the Kardex or electronic plan.
   h. Develop an individualized plan of care for remaining nursing diagnoses and collaborative problems.
   i. Implement the care plan (do or delegate; document).
   j. Evaluate the results of care.

2. List as many guidelines for writing care plans as you can recall. For example, "For detailed treatments and procedures, refer to other sources" (if you cannot recall 10 more guidelines, review Box 10–2).

   Answer:

   a. Include each of these components: client profile, basic needs, aspects of medical plan, nursing diagnoses and collaborative problems, special or complex teaching, and discharge needs.
   b. Date and sign the initial plan and any revisions.
   c. List or number the nursing diagnoses in order or priority.
   d. Write the plan in clear, concise terms.
   e. Write legibly in ink.
   f. For detailed treatments and procedures, refer to other sources (e.g., standards of care).
   g. Be sure the plan is holistic.
   h. Include the collaborative and coordination aspects of the client's care.
   i. Include discharge plans

THINK & REFLECT! SUGGESTED RESPONSES

There is usually no single, correct answer for these exercises because the intent is to have you practice thinking, not recall facts. The nature of a critical thinking problem is that it has more than one solution and that there may not be a "best" solution. You should compare your answers with those of your classmates—both your solutions and the thinking you used. Discussing your thinking processes is one way to help improve your thinking. Also, it is important for you to begin collaborating with your peers. During your nursing career, the thinking of other nurses will be an important resource to you, just as your thinking can be for them. You will usually not find answers here but ideas to help you think about the question.

#10-1

You have the following standardized documents:

a. Critical pathway
b. Protocol
c. Agency policy

1. Which one would you probably use to find out how long a patient's friend may visit him in the intensive care unit?
2. Which one would you probably use when a physician is coming to your unit to insert chest tubes in a patient for whom you are providing nursing care?
3. A patient is being admitted for a hip replacement, and you need a map of the collaborative care to be provided during the patient's stay. Which one would you use?

Suggested Responses:

1. (c) agency policy
2. (b) protocol
3. (a) critical pathway

ANA Code of Ethics for Nurses: Provisions

Provision 1. The nurse, in all professional relationships, practices with compassion and respect for the inherent dignity, worth, and uniqueness of every individual, unrestricted by considerations of social or economic status, personal attributes, or the nature of health problems.

Provision 2. The nurse's primary commitment is to the patient, whether an individual, family, group, or community.

Provision 3. The nurse promotes, advocates for, and strives to protect the health, safety, and rights of the patient.

Provision 4. The nurse is responsible and accountable for individual nursing practice and determines the appropriate delegation of tasks consistent with the nurse's obligation to provide optimum patient care.

Provision 5. The nurse owes the same duties to self as to others, including the responsibility to preserve integrity and safety, to maintain competence, and to continue personal and professional growth.

Provision 6. The nurse participates in establishing, maintaining, and improving healthcare environments and conditions of employment conducive to the provision of quality health care and consistent with the values of the profession through individual and collective action.

Provision 7. The nurse participates in the advancement of the profession through contributions to practice, education, administration, and knowledge development.

Provision 8. The nurse collaborates with other health professionals and the public in promoting community, national, and international efforts to meet health needs.

Provision 9. The profession of nursing, as represented by associations and their members, is responsible for articulating nursing values, for maintaining the integrity of the profession and its practice, and for shaping social policy.

Source: Reprinted with permission from American Nurses Association, *Code of Ethics for Nurses with Interpretive Statements,* © 2001. American Nurses Publishing, American Nurses Association, Washington, DC.

Multidisciplinary (Collaborative) Problems Associated with Diseases and Other Physiological Disorders

Source: Wilkinson, J. M., & Ahern, N. R. (2009). *Prentice Hall nursing diagnosis handbook* (9th ed.). Upper Saddle River, NJ: Prentice Hall Health.

PC = potential complications

CANCER
PC of Cancer*

Anemia
Bowel obstruction
Cachexia
Clotting disorders
Electrolyte imbalance
Fractures, pathological
Hemorrhage
Obstructive uropathy
Metastasis to vital organs (e.g., brain, lungs)
Pericardial effusions, tamponade
Sepsis→septic shock
Spinal cord compression
Superior vena cava syndrome
Tissue anoxia→necrosis

PC of Antineoplastic Medications
Specify for each drug (e.g., anemia, bone marrow depression, cardiac toxicity, CNS toxicity, congestive heart failure, electrolyte imbalance, enteritis, leukopenia, necrosis at IV site, pneumonitis, renal failure, thrombocytopenia)

PC of Narcotic Medications
Depressed respirations, consciousness, and blood
  pressure
Cardiovascular collapse
Biliary spasm

PC of Radiation Therapy
Increased intracranial pressure
Myelosuppression
Inflammation
Fluid/electrolyte imbalances

CARDIAC FUNCTION DISORDERS
PC of Angina/Coronary Artery Disease
Myocardial infarction

PC of Congestive Heart Failure

Ascites
Cardiac decompensation, severe
Cardiogenic shock
Deep vein thrombosis
Gastrointestinal congestion→malabsorption
Hepatic failure
Pulmonary edema, acute
Renal failure

PC of Digitalis Administration
Toxicity

PC of Dysrhythmias

Decreased cardiac output→Decreased myocardial
  perfusion→Heart failure
Severe atrioventricular conduction blocks
Thromboemboli formation→Stroke
Ventricular fibrillation

*Also see specific disorders, such as Gastrointestinal Function Disorders, for effects of cancer on those patterns

PC of Myocardial Infarction

Cardiogenic shock
Dysrhythmia
Infarct extension or expansion
Myocardial rupture
Pulmonary edema
Pulmonary embolism
Pericarditis
Thromboembolism
Ventricular aneurysm

PC of Pericarditis/Endocarditis

Cardiac tamponade
Congestive heart failure
Emboli (pulmonary, cerebral, renal, spleen, heart)
Valvular stenosis

PC of Rheumatic Fever/Rheumatic Heart Disease

Congestive heart failure
Decreased ventricular function
Endocarditis
Pericardial effusion
Valvular changes

ENDOCRINE FUNCTION DISORDERS

PC of Adrenal Gland Disorders

PC of Addison's Disease
Addisonian crisis (shock, coma)
Diabetes mellitus
Thyroid disease

PC of Cushing's Disease
Congestive heart failure
Hyperglycemia
Hypertension
Pancreatic tumors
Potassium and sodium imbalance
Psychosis

PC of Diabetes Mellitus

Coma
Coronary artery disease
Hypoglycemia
Infections
Ketoacidosis
Nephropathy
Peripheral vascular disease
Retinopathy

PC of Parathyroid Gland Disorders

PC of Hyperparathyroidism
Hypercalcemia→Cardiac arrhythmias
Hypertension
Metabolic acidosis
Pathologic fractures
Peptic ulcers
Psychosis
Renal calculi, renal failure

PC of Hypoparathyroidism
Hypocalcemia→Cardiac arrhythmias
Convulsions
Malabsorption
Psychosis
Tetany

PC of Pituitary Gland Disorders

PC of Anterior Pituitary Disorders
Acromegaly
Congestive heart failure
Seizures

PC of Posterior Pituitary Disorders
Loss of consciousness
Hypernatremia
Seizures

PC of Thyroid Gland Disorders

PC of Hyperthyroidism
Exophthalmos
Heart disease
Negative nitrogen balance
Thyroid crisis

PC of Hypothyroidism
Adrenal insufficiency
Cardiovascular disorders
Myxedema coma
Psychosis

GASTROINTESTINAL (GI) FUNCTION DISORDERS

PC of Esophageal Disorders

PC of Esophageal Diverticula
Obstruction
Pulmonary aspiration of regurgitated food

PC of Esophageal Surgery
Reflux esophagitis
Stricture formation

PC of Hiatal Hernia
Incarceration
Necrosis→Hemorrhage

PC of Gallbladder, Liver, and Pancreatic Disorders

PC of Cholelithiasis and Cholecystitis
Fistula
Gallbladder perforation
Intestinal ileus/obstruction
Obstruction of common bile duct→liver
    damage
Pancreatitis
Peritonitis

PC of Cirrhosis
Anemia
Ascites
Diabetes
Disseminated intravascular coagulation (DIC)
Esophageal varices
GI bleeding/hemorrhage
Hepatic encephalopathy
Hyperbilirubinemia
Hypokalemia
Splenomegaly
Peritonitis
Renal failure

PC of Hepatic Abscess
Fluid/electrolyte imbalance
Hyperbilirubinemia

PC of Hepatitis
Cirrhosis
Hepatic encephalopathy
Hepatic necrosis

PC of Metronidazole or Iodoquinol Administration
Bone marrow suppression

PC of Pancreatitis
Ascites
Cardiac failure

Coma
Delirium tremens
Diabetes mellitus
Hemorrhage
Hyper/hypoglycemia
Hypocalcemia
Hypovolemic shock
Pancreatic abscess
Pancreatic pseudocyst
Pleural effusion/respiratory failure
Psychosis
Renal failure
Tetany

PC of GI Infections

PC of Appendicitis
Abscess
Gangrenous appendicitis
Perforated appendix
Peritonitis
Pylephlebitis

PC of Bacterial or Viral Infections (e.g., Food Poisoning)
Bowel perforation
Dehydration
Hemolytic uremic syndrome
Hypokalemia
Hypovolemic shock
Metabolic acidosis
Metabolic alkalosis
Peritonitis
Respiratory muscle paralysis
Thrombotic thrombocytopenic
    purpura

PC of Helminthic Infections
Anemia
Bowel, biliary, or pancreatic
    duct obstruction
Migration to liver or lungs

PC of Peritonitis
Hypovolemic shock
Septicemia
Septic shock

PC of GI Inflammatory Diseases (e.g., diverticulitis, gastritis, peptic ulcer, ulcerative colitis)

Abscess
Anal fissure
Anemia
Colorectal carcinoma
Fistula
Fluid/electrolyte imbalances
GI bleeding/hemorrhage
Intestinal obstruction
Intestinal perforation
Peritonitis
Pyloric obstruction
Toxic megacolon

PC of Gastrectomy, Pyloroplasty
Dumping syndrome

PC of Structural and Obstructive GI Disorders

PC of Hemorrhoids and
Anorectal Lesions
Anemia
Infection
Thrombosed hemorrhoid
Sepsis

PC of Hernias
Bowel infarction
Bowel perforation
Hernia incarceration and strangulation
Peritonitis

PC of Intestinal Obstruction
Bowel wall necrosis
Gangrene
Fluid and electrolyte imbalance
Hypovolemic or septic shock
Intestinal perforation
Peritonitis

PC of Malabsorption Syndromes
Anemia
Bleeding
Delayed maturity
Lack of growth
Muscle wasting

Rickets (and other nutrient deficiencies)
Tetany

HEMATOLOGIC DISORDERS
PC of Aplastic Anemia

Congestive heart failure
Hemorrhage
Infections

PC of Coagulation Disorders

Hemorrhage (Specific effects are determined by
  site of bleeding, e.g., increased intracranial
  pressure in the brain, adult respiratory distress
  syndrome in the cardiovascular system.)
Joint deformity/disability

PC of Leukemias

Anemia
Bleeding difficulties/internal hemorrhage
Bone infarctions
Coma
Hepatomegaly
Infections
Renal failure
Seizures
Splenomegaly
Tachycardia

PC of Nutritional Anemias

Impaired cardiac functioning
Impaired neurologic functioning
  (e.g., problems with proprioception)

PC of Cyanocobalamin Therapy
Hypersensitivity
Hypokalemia
Peripheral vascular thrombosis
Pulmonary edema

PC of Iron Therapy
Hypersensitivity
Toxicity (cardiovascular collapse, liver necrosis,
  metabolic acidosis)

PC of Polycythemia

Bone marrow fibrosis
Gastrointestinal bleeding and ulcers
Splenomegaly
Thrombosis (various organs)

PC of Sickle Cell Anemia

Multisystem organ failure (e.g., congestive heart
    failure, hyperuricemia, hepatomegaly, hepatic
    abscesses/fibrosis, hyperbilirubinemia,
    gallstones, bone marrow aplasia, osteomyelitis
    aseptic bone necrosis, skin ulcers, vitreous
    hemorrhage, retinal detachment)
Sickle cell crisis

PC of Sickle Cell Crisis

Aplastic crisis
Cerebrovascular accident
Hemosiderosis (from repeated transfusions)
Infections (e.g., pneumonia)
Seizures
Splenic sequestration→circulatory collapse

IMMUNE FUNCTION DISORDERS

PC of Altered Immune Function

Allergic reactions→Anaphylaxis
Autoimmune disorders (e.g., systemic lupus
    erythematosus)
Delayed wound healing
Infections (e.g., nosocomial, opportunistic)
Spesis→septicemia
Tissue inflammation, acute/chronic
    (e.g., granulomas)
Transplant/graft rejection

PC of Autoimmune Deficiency Syndrome (AIDS)

HIV wasting syndrome
Malignancies: Cervical cancer, Kaposi's sarcoma,
    lymphomas
Neurologic: Dementia complex, meningitis
Opportunistic infections (e.g., candida,
    cytomegalovirus, herpes, *Mycobacterium
    avium, Pneumocystis carinii* pneumonia,
    toxoplasmosis, tuberculosis)

IMMOBILIZED PATIENT

PC of Immobility

Contractures
Decreased cardiac output
Decubitus ulcers
Embolus
Hypostatic pneumonia
Joint ankylosis
Orthostatic hypotension
Osteoporosis
Renal calculi
Thrombophlebitis

MUSCULOSKELETAL DISORDERS AND TRAUMA

PC of Amputation

Contracture
Delayed healing
Edema of the stump
Infection

PC of Fractures

Compartment syndrome
Deep vein thrombosis
Delayed union
Fat embolism
Infection
Necrosis
Reflex sympathetic dystrophy
Shock

PC of Gout

Nephropathy
Uric acid stones→renal failure

PC of Osteoarthritis

Contractures
Herniated disk

PC of Osteomyelitis

Cutaneous sinus tract formation
Necrosis
Soft tissue abscesses

PC of Osteoporosis, Osteomalacia

Fractures
Neuropathies
Posttraumatic arthritis

PC of Paget's Disease

Bone tumors
Cardiovascular complications
   (e.g., arteriosclerosis, hypertension, CHF)
Degenerative osteoarthritis
Dementia
Fractures
Renal calculi

PC of Rheumatoid Arthritis

Anemia
Bony and/or fibrous ankylosis
Carpal tunnel syndrome
Contractures
Episcleritis or scleritis of the eye
Felty's syndrome
Muscle atrophy
Neuropathy
Pericarditis
Pleural disease
Vasculitis

PC of Corticosteroid Intraarticular Injections

Intraarticular infection
Joint degeneration

PC of Corticosteroid Systemic Administration

Atherosclerosis
Cataract formation
Congestive heart failure
Cushing's syndrome
Delayed wound healing
Depressed immune response
Edema
Growth retardation (children)
Hyperglycemia
Hypertension
Hypokalemia
Muscle wasting
Osteoporosis
Peptic ulcers
Psychotic reactions

Renal failure
Thrombophlebitis

PC of Nonsteroidal Anti-inflammatory Medications

Gastric ulcers/bleeding, nephropathy

NEUROLOGIC DISORDERS

PC of Brain Injury and Intracranial Hemorrhage

Brain ischemia
Herniation
Increased intracranial pressure

PC of Brain Tumor

Hyperthermia
Increased intracranial pressure
Paralysis
Sensorimotor changes

PC of Cerebrovascular Accident (CVA)

(NOTE: The manifestations and complications of a CVA vary according to the area of the brain affected. Also, it is difficult to determine which effects are manifestations or symptoms and which are actually complications. Furthermore, many of the complications of CVA are caused by the resulting immobility rather than to the pathophysiology of the CVA itself. Refer to "Immobilized Patient.")

Behavioral changes
Brain stem failure
Cardiac dysrhythmias
Coma
Elimination disorders
Increased intracranial pressure
Language disorders
Motor deficits
Respiratory infection
Seizures
Sensory-perceptual deficits

PC of Increased Intracranial Pressure (e.g., Cerebral Edema, Hydrocephalus)

CNS ischemic response (increased mean arterial pressure, increased pulse pressure, and bradycardia)

Coma
Failure of autoregulation of cerebral blood
    flow
Hyperthermia resulting from impaired
    hypothalamic function
Motor impairment (decorticate or decerebrate
    posturing)

PC of Intracranial Aneurysm

Hydrocephalus
Hypothalamic dysfunction
Rebleeding
Seizures
Vasospasm

PC of Meningitis and Encephalitis

Arthritis
Brain infarction
Coma
Cranial nerve damage
Hydrocephalus
Increased intracranial pressure
Seizures

PC of Multiple Sclerosis

Dementia
Pneumonia
Sudden progression of neurological symptoms:
    convulsions, coma
Urinary tract infection

PC of Myasthenia Gravis

Aspiration
Cholinergic crisis
Dehydration
Myasthenic crisis
Pneumonia

PC of Organic Brain Diseases
(e.g., Alzheimer's)

Aspiration pneumonia
Dehydration
Delusions
Depression
Falls
Malnutrition

Paranoid reactions
Pneumonia

PC of Parkinson's Disease

Depression and social isolation
Falls
Infections related to immobility (e.g., pneumonia)
Malnutrition related to dysphagia and immobility
Oculogyric crisis
Paranoia and hallucinations
Pressure ulcers

PC of Seizure Disorder

Accidental trauma (e.g., burns, falls)
Aspiration
Head injury
Status epilepticus→Acidosis, hyperthermia,
    hypoglycemia, hypoxia

PC of Spinal Cord Injury

Autonomic dysreflexia
Cardiac dysrhythmias
Complications due to immobility (See
    "Immobilized Patient.")
Hypercalcemia
Necrosis of spinal cord tissue
Paralytic ileus
Respiratory infection secondary to decreased
    cough reflex
Spinal shock

PERIPHERAL VASCULAR AND LYMPHATIC DISORDERS
PC of Aneurysms

PC of Aortic Aneurysm
Dissection
Hemiplegia and lower extremity paralysis
    (with dissection)
Rupture→hypovolemic shock

PC of Femoral and Popliteal Aneurysms
Embolism
Gangrene
Rupture
Thrombosis

PC of Hypertension

Aortic dissection
Cerebrovascular accident
Congestive heart failure
Hypertensive crisis
Malignant hypertension
Myocardial ischemia
Papilledema
Renal insufficiency
Retinal damage

PC of Lymphedema

Cellulitis
Lymphangitis

PC of Peripheral Arterial Disease

Arterial thrombosis
Cellulitis
Cerebrovascular accident
Hypertension
Ischemic ulcers
Tissue necrosis→gangrene

PC of Thrombophlebitis

Chronic leg edema
Pulmonary embolism
Stasis ulcers

PC of Varicose Veins

Cellulitis
Hemorrhage
Vascular rupture
Venous stasis ulcers

RESPIRATORY FUNCTION DISORDERS
PC of Asthma

Atelectasis
Cor pulmonale
Dehydration
Pneumothorax
Respiratory infection
Status asthmaticus

PC Corticosteroid Therapy

Hypertension, hypokalemia, hypoglycemia,
    immunosuppression, osteoporosis, ulcers

PC of Methylxanthine Therapy

Toxicity (seizures, circulatory failure, respiratory
arrest)

PC of Chronic Obstructive Pulmonary Disease (COPD)

Hypoxemia
Respiratory acidosis
Respiratory failure
Respiratory infection
Right-sided heart failure
Spontaneous pneumothorax

PC of Pneumonia

Bacteremia→Endocarditis, meningitis, peritonitis
Lung abscess and empyema
Lung tissue necrosis
Pleuritis

PC of Pulmonary Edema

Cerebral hypoxia
Multisystem organ failure
Right-sided heart failure

PC of Pulmonary Embolism

Pulmonary infarction with necrosis
Right ventricular heart failure
Sudden death

PC of Tuberculosis

Bacteremia—extrapulmonary tuberculosis (e.g.,
    genitourinary tuberculosis, meningitis,
    peritonitis, pericarditis)
Bronchopleural fistula
Empyema

PC of Medications for Tuberculosis

Hepatotoxicity, hypersensitivity, nephrotoxicity,
    peripheral neuropathy (isoniazid), optic neuritis
    (ethambutol)

SEXUALLY TRANSMITTED DISEASES
PC of Chlamydial Infections

Females: Abortion, infertility, pelvic abscesses, pelvic inflammatory disease, postpartum endometritis, spontaneous abortion, stillbirth
Males: Epididymitis, prostatitis, urethritis
Neonates: Ophthalmia neonatorum, pneumonia

PC of Genital Herpes

All: Herpes keratitis
Females: Cervical cancer
Males: Ascending myelitis, lymphatic suppuration, meningitis, neuralgia, urethral strictures
Neonates: Potentially fatal infections; infections of eyes, skin, mucous membranes, and central nervous system

PC of Genital Warts

All: Urinary obstruction and bleeding
Females: Increased risk of cancer of the cervix, vagina, vulva, and anus; obstruction of the birth canal during labor; transmission to neonate
Neonates: Respiratory papillomatosis

PC of Gonorrhea

All: Secondary infection of lesions, fistulas, chronic ulcers, sterility
Females: Abdominal adhesions, ectopic pregnancy, pelvic inflammatory disease
Males: Epididymitis, nephritis, prostatitis, urethritis
Neonates: Ophthalmia neonatorum

PC of Syphilis

Blindness, paralysis, heart failure, liver failure, mental illness

SHOCK
PC of Shock

Cerebral hypoxia→coma
Multiple-organ system failure
Paralytic ileus
Pulmonary emboli
Renal failure

SKIN INTEGRITY DISORDERS
PC of Burns

Airway obstruction (inhalation injury)
Curling's ulcer
Hypervolemia
Hypothermia
Hypovolemic shock
Infection secondary to suppression of immune system
Negative nitrogen balance
Paralytic ileus
Renal failure
Sepsis
Stress ulcers

PC of Skin Lesions/Dermatitis/Acne

Cyst formation
Infection
Malignancy

PC of Herpes Zoster

Dissemination→Visceral lesions
Encephalitis
Loss of vision

PC of Pressure Ulcer

Necrotic damage to muscle, bone, tendons, joint capsule
Infection
Sepsis

URINARY ELIMINATION DISORDERS
PC of Cystitis

Bladder ulceration
Bladder wall necrosis
Renal infection

PC of Polycystic Kidney Disease

Renal calculi
Renal failure
Urinary tract infection

PC of Pyelonephritis

Bacteremia
Chronic pyelonephritis
Renal failure
Renal insufficiency

PC of Renal Failure, Acute

Electrolyte imbalance
Fluid overload
Metabolic acidosis
Pericarditis
Platelet dysfunction
Secondary infections

PC of Renal Failure, Chronic

Anemia
Cardiac tamponade, pericarditis

Congestive heart failure
Fluid and electrolyte imbalance
Gastrointestinal bleeding
Hyperparathyroidism
Infections
Medication toxicity
Metabolic acidosis
Pleural effusion
Pulmonary edema
Uremia

PC of Urolithiasis

Hydronephrosis
Hydroureter
Infection
Pyelonephritis
Renal insufficiency

Multidisciplinary (Collaborative) Problems Associated with Surgical Treatments

Source: Wilkinson, J. M., & Ahern, N. R. (2009). *Prentice Hall nursing diagnosis handbook* (9th ed.). Upper Saddle River, NJ: Prentice Hall Health.

Type of Surgery	Potential Complications (Multidisciplinary Problems)
Potential Complications of General Surgery	
(Complications that can occur regardless of type of surgery)	Atelectasis
	Bronchospasm or laryngospasm on extubation (with general anesthesia)
	Electrolyte imbalance
	Excessive bleeding→Shock
	Fluid imbalance
	Headache from leakage of cerebrospinal fluid (with regional anesthesia)
	Hypotension (with regional anesthesia)
	Ileus
	Infection
	Stasis pneumonia
	Urinary retention→Bladder distention
	Venous thrombosis→Pulmonary embolism
	Wound dehiscence→Evisceration

Instructions: Choose complications from "General Surgery" above; then choose those that apply to patient's particular type of surgery, following. These complications are in addition to the complications for "General Surgery."

Potential Complications of:	
Abdominal surgery	Dehiscence
	Fistula formation
	Paralytic ileus
	Peritonitis
	Renal failure
	Surgical trauma (e.g., to ureter, bladder, or rectum)
Breast surgery	Cellulitis
	Hematoma
	Lymphedema
	Seroma
Chest surgery: Coronary artery bypass graft	Cardiovascular insufficiency
	Renal insufficiency
	Respiratory insufficiency
Chest surgery: Thoracotomy	Adult respiratory distress syndrome
	Bronchopleural fistula
	Cardiac dysrhythmias
	Empyema of the chest cavity

Type of Surgery	Potential Complications (Multidisciplinary Problems)
Chest surgery: Thoracotomy	Hemothorax Infection at chest tube sites Mediastinal shift Myocardial infarction Pneumothorax Pulmonary edema Subcutaneous emphysema
Craniotomy	Cardiac dysrhythmias Cerebral or cerebellar dysfunction Cerebrospinal fluid leaks Cranial nerve impairment Gastrointestinal bleeding Hematomas Hydrocephalus Hygromas Hyperthermia or hypothermia Hypoxemia Increased intracranial pressure Meningitis or encephalitis Residual neurological defects Seizures
Eye surgery	Enophthalmus Hyphema Increased intraocular pressure Lens implant dislocation Macular edema Retinal detachment Secondary glaucoma
Musculoskeletal surgeries	Bone necrosis Fat embolus Flexion contractures Hematoma Joint dislocation or displacement of prosthesis Nerve damage Sepsis Synovial herniation
Neck surgeries	Airway obstruction Aspiration Cerebral infarction Cranial nerve damage Fistula formation (e.g., between hypopharynx and skin) Flap rejection (in radical neck dissection) Hypertension or hypotension Hypoparathyroidism (in thyroidectomy or parathyroidectomy)

Type of Surgery	Potential Complications (Multidisciplinary Problems)
Neck surgeries	Local nerve damage (e.g., laryngeal nerve) Respiratory distress Tetany (in thyroidectomy) Thyroid storm Tracheal stenosis Vocal cord paralysis
Rectal surgery	Fistula formation Stricture formation
Skin grafts	Edema Flap necrosis Graft rejection Hematoma
Spinal surgery	Bladder or bowel dysfunction Cerebrospinal fistula Displacement of bone graft (in laminectomy or spinal fusion) Hematoma Nerve root injury Paralytic ileus Sensorineural impairments Spinal cord edema or injury
Urologic surgery	Bladder neck constriction Bladder perforation (intraoperative) Epididymitis Paralytic ileus Retrograde ejaculation (in prostate resection or prostatectomy) Stomal necrosis, stenosis, obstruction (in urostomy or nephrostomy) Urethral stricture Urinary tract infection
Vascular surgery: Aortic aneurysm resection	Congestive heart failure Myocardial infarction Renal failure Rupture of the suture line→Hemorrhage Spinal cord ischemia
Vascular surgery: Other	Cardiac dysrhythmia Compartmental syndrome Failure of anastomosis Lymphocele Occlusion of graft

Selected References

Chapter 1

American Nurses Association. (1980). *Nursing: A social policy statement.* Kansas City, MO: Author.

American Nurses Association. (1992). *House of Delegates report: 1992 convention, Las Vegas, NV* (pp. 104–120). Kansas City, MO: Author.

American Nurses Association. (2001). *Code of ethics for nurses with interpretive statements.* Washington, DC: American Nurses Publishing. Retrieved September 10, 2009, from http://nursingworld.org/ethics/code/protected_nwcoe813.htm.

American Nurses Association. (2003). *Nursing's policy statement.* Washington, DC: Author.

American Nurses Association. (2004). *Nursing: Scope and standards of practice* (3rd ed.). Washington, DC: Author.

American Nurses Association. (in press). *Nursing: Scope and standards of practice* (2nd ed.). (Public Comment draft, January). Silver Spring, MD: Author. Available at http://nursebooks.org.

Anderson, C. A. (1998). Nursing: A thinking profession. *Nursing Outlook, 46,* 197–198.

Anthony, M. K. (2004). Shared governance models: The theory, practice, and evidence. *Online Journal of Issues in Nursing, 9*(1). Retrieved May, 2010, from http://www.nursingworld.org/MainMenuCategories/ANAMarketplace/ANAPeriodicals/OJIN/TableofContents/Volume92004/No1Jan04/SharedGovernanceModels.aspx.

Association for Registered Nurses in Newfoundland and Labrador. (2007). *Standards for nursing practice.* St. John's, Newfoundland, Canada: Author.

Baggs, J. G. (January 31, 2005). Overview and summary: Partnerships and collaboration: What skills are needed? *Online Journal of Issues in Nursing, 10*(1). Retrieved December 10, 2005, from http://www.nursingworld.org/ojin/topic26/tpc26ntr.htm.

Benner, P. (1984) *From novice to expert.* Menlo Park, CA: Addison-Wesley Publishing Co.

Benner, P., & Tanner, C. (1987). How expert nurses use intuition. *American Journal of Nursing, 87,* 23–31.

Benner, P., & Wrubel, J. (1989). *The primacy of caring: Stress and coping in health and illness.* Menlo Park, CA: Addison-Wesley.

Bulechek, G. M., Butcher, H. K., & Dochterman, J. M. (Eds.) (2008). *Nursing Interventions Classification (NIC)* (5th ed.). St. Louis: C. V. Mosby.

Canadian Nurses Association. (1987). *A definition of nursing practice. Standards for nursing practice.* Ottawa, Ontario, Canada: Author.

Cleak, H., & Williamson, D. (2007). Preparing health science students for interdisciplinary professional practice. *Journal of Allied Health, 36*(3), 141–149.

College & Association of Registered Nurses of Alberta (2005). *Nursing Practice Standards.* Edmonton, Alberta, Canada: Author. Retrieved January 23, 2010, from https://www.nurses.ab.ca/Carna-Admin/Uploads/Nursing%20Practice%20Standards_1.pdf.

College of Nurses of Ontario. (1996). *Professional standards for registered nurses and registered practical nurses in Ontario.* Toronto, Ontario, Canada: Author.

College of Registered Nurses of Nova Scotia. (2004). *Standards for nursing practice.* Halifax, Nova Scotia, Canada: Author.

Dawson, D. (2006). The art of nursing: A hidden science? *Intensive and Critical Care Nursing, 22*(6), 313–314.

Finfgeld-Connett, D. (2008). Concept synthesis of the art of nursing. *Journal of Advanced Nursing, 62*(3), 381–388.

Frauman, A. C., & Skelly, A. H. (1999). Evolution of the nursing process. *Clinical Excellence for Nurse Practitioners, 3*(4), 238–244.

Gardner, D. (2005). Ten lessons in collaboration. *Online Journal of Issues in Nursing, 10*(1). Retrieved May, 2010, from http://www.nursingworld.org/MainMenuCategories/ANAMarketplace/ANAPeriodicals/OJIN/TableofContents/Volume102005/No1Jan05/tpc26_116008.aspx.

Gramling, K. L. (2004). A narrative study of nursing art in critical care. *Journal of Holistic Nursing, 22*(4), 379–398.

Hall, L. (June 1955). Quality of nursing care. *Public Health News.* New Jersey State Department of Health.

Hicks, D. (2007). Are we losing the art of nursing? *Journal of Diabetes Nursing, 11*(10).

Johnson, D. (1959). A philosophy for nursing diagnosis. *Nursing Outlook, 7,* 198–200.

Johnson, J. (1994). A dialectical examination of nursing art. *Advances in Nursing Science, 17*(1), 1–14.

The Joint Commission (2008). *Hospital Accreditation Standards.* Oakbrook Terrace, IL: The Joint Commission.

Leininger, M. (1978). *Transcultural nursing: Concepts, theories, and practice.* New York: Wiley.

Mason, G. M., & Attree, M. (1997). The relationship between research and the nursing process in clinical practice. *Journal of Advanced Nursing, 26*(5), 1045–1049.

Miskelly, S. (1995). A parish nursing model: Applying the community health nursing process in a church community. *Journal of Community Health Nursing, 12*(1), 1–14.

Moorhead, S., Johnson, M., Maas, M., & Swanson, E. (Eds.). (2008). *Nursing Outcomes Classification (NOC)* (4th ed.). St. Louis: C. V. Mosby.

Musk, A. (2004). Proficiency with technology and the expression of caring: Can we reconcile these polarized views? *International Journal of Human Caring, 8*(2), 13–20.

NANDA International. (2009). *NANDA nursing diagnoses: Definitions & classification 2009–2011.* Ames, IA: Wiley-Blackwell.

Neuman, B. (1972). The Betty Neuman model: A total person approach to viewing patient problems. *Nursing Research, 21*(3), 264–269.

Neuman, B. (1980). The Betty Neuman health-care systems model: A total person approach to patient problems. In J. Riehl & C. Roy (Eds.), *Conceptual models for nursing practice.* New York: Appleton-Century-Crofts.

Nightingale, F. (1969). *Notes on nursing. What it is, what it is not.* New York: Dover Publications (Original work published in 1859).

Nuñez, D. E., Armbruster, C., Phillips, W. T., & Gale, B. J. (2003). Community-based senior health promotion program using a collaborative practice model: The Escalante Health Partnerships. *Public Health Nursing, 20*(1), 25–32.

Nurses Association of New Brunswick. (2005). *Standards of practice for registered nurses.* Fredericton, New Brunswick, Canada: Author.

Orem, D. (1971). *Nursing: Concepts of practice.* New York: McGraw-Hill.

Orlando, I. (1961). *The dynamic nurse-patient relationship.* New York: GP Putnam's Sons.

Parse, R. (1974). *Nursing fundamentals.* Flushing, NY: Medical Examination Publishing.

Parse, R. (1981). *Man-living-health: A theory of nursing.* New York: John Wiley & Sons.

Parse, R. (1987). *Nursing science: Major paradigms, theories, and critiques.* Philadelphia: W. B. Saunders.

Patterson, E., & McMurray, A. (2003). Collaborative practice between registered nurses and medical practitioners in Australian general practice: Moving from rhetoric to reality. *Australian Journal of Advanced Nursing, 20*(4), 43–48.

Pavlovich-Danis, S., Forman, H., Simek, P. P., et al. (1998, July/August). The nurse-physician relationship. Can it be saved? *Journal of Nursing Administration, 28*(7–8), 17–20.

Pender, N. J., Murdaugh, C. L., & Parsons, M. A. (2006). *Health promotion in nursing practice.* (5th ed.). Upper Saddle River, NJ: Prentice Hall.

Peplau, H. (1952). *Interpersonal relations in nursing.* New York: GP Putnam's Sons.

Price, S., Arbuthnot, E., Benoit, R., Landry, D., Landry, M., & Butlere, L. (2007). The art of nursing: Communication and self-expression. *Nursing Science Quarterly, 20*(2), 155–160.

Registered Nurses Association of British Columbia. (2003). *Standards for registered nursing practice in British Columbia.* Vancouver: Author.

Registered Nurses Association of the Northwest Territories and Nunavut. (2006). *Standards of nursing practice for registered nurses.* Yellowknife, NT: Author.

Rogers, M. E. (1970). *The theoretical basis of nursing.* Philadelphia: F. A. Davis.

Rogers, M. E. (1980). Nursing: A science of unitary man. In J. P. Riehl & S. C. Roy (Eds.), *Conceptual models for nursing practice* (2nd ed, pp. 329–337.). New York: Appleton-Century-Crofts.

Roy, C. (1970). A conceptual framework for nursing. *Nursing Outlook, 18*(3), 42–45.

Roy, C. (1976*). Introduction to nursing: An adaptation model.* Englewood Cliffs: NJ: Prentice Hall.

Roy, C. (1980). The Roy adaptation model. In J. Riehl & C. Roy (Eds.), *Conceptual models for nursing practice* (2nd ed.). New York: Appleton-Century-Crofts.

Schraeder, B., & Fischer, D. (1987). Using intuitive knowledge in the neonatal intensive care nursery. *Holistic Nursing Practice, 1*(3), 45–51.

U.S. Department of Health and Human Services, Public Health Service. (2010a). *Healthy People 2020.* Washington, DC: U.S. Government Printing Office.

U.S. Department of Health and Human Services, Public Health Service. (2010b). *Healthy People 2020 objectives—List for public comment.* Washington, DC: U.S. Government Printing Office. Retrieved January 18, 2010, from http://www.healthypeople.gov/hp2020/Objectives/TopicAreas.aspx.

Vitale, B., Schultz, N., & Nugent, P. (1974). *A problem-solving approach to nursing care plans: A program.* St. Louis: C. V. Mosby.

Watson, J. (1988). *Nursing: Human science and human care. A theory of nursing.* New York: National League for Nursing.

Wiedenbach, E. (1963). The helping art of nursing. *American Journal of Nursing, 63*(11), 54–57.

Chapter 2

Adams, B. L. (1999). Nursing education for critical thinking: An integrative review. *Journal of Nursing Education, 38*(3), 111–119.

Alfaro-LeFevre, R. (2008). *Critical thinking indicators: 2007–2008 evidence-based version.* Retrieved November 29, 2009, from http://www.alfaroteachsmart.com/2008_2009CTI.pdf.

Alfaro-LeFevre, R. (2009). *Critical thinking and clinical judgment: A practical approach to outcome-focused thinking* (4th ed.). Philadelphia: Saunders-Elsevier.

American Nurses Association. (2001). *Code of ethics for nurses with interpretive statements.* Washington, DC: American Nurses Publishing.

American Nurses Association. (2004). *Nursing: Scope and standards of practice* (3rd ed.). Washington, DC: Author.

American Nurses Association. (in press). *Nursing: Scope and standards of practice* (2nd ed.). (Public Comment draft, January). Silver Spring, MD: Author. Available at http://nursebooks.org.

Assessment Technologies Institute. (2003). Critical thinking assessment developmental and statistical manual. Overland Park, KS: Assessment Technologies Institute.

Benner, P. (1984). *From novice to expert.* Menlo Park, CA: Addison-Wesley Publishing Co.

Berman, A., Snyder, S., Kozier, B., & Erb, G. (2008). *Fundamentals of nursing: Concepts, process, and practice* (8th ed.). Upper Saddle River, NJ: Prentice-Hall.

Brookfield, S. D. (1991). *Developing critical thinkers.* San Francisco: Jossey-Bass.

Brunt, B. A. (2005). Critical thinking in nursing: An integrated review. *Journal of Continuing Education in Nursing, 36*(2), 60–67.

Carper, B. (1978). Fundamental patterns of knowing in nursing. *Advances in Nursing Science, 1*(October), 13–23.

Chaffee, J. (1990). *Thinking critically* (3rd ed.). Boston: Houghton Mifflin.

Chinn, P., & Kramer, M. (1991). *Theory and nursing.* St. Louis: Mosby Year Book.

DiVito, T. P. (2005). Nursing student stories on learning how to think like a nurse. *Nurse Educator, 30*(3), 133–136.

Ennis, R. H. (n.d.) Definition of critical thinking. Retrieved December 1, 2009, from http://www.critical thinking.net.

Ennis, R. H. (1962). A concept of critical thinking. *Harvard Educational Review, 32,* 81–111.

Ennis, R. H. (1996). *Critical thinking.* Upper Saddle River, NJ: Prentice-Hall.

Ennis, R. H. (2006). *A super-streamlined conception of critical thinking.* Retrieved January 13, 2008, from http://faculty.ed.uluc.edu/rhennis.

Facione, P. A., & N. C. (2007). *Thinking and reasoning in human decision making: The method of argument and heuristic analysis.* Millbrae, CA: The California Academic Press LLC.

Fesler-Birch, D. M. (2005). Critical thinking and patient outcomes: A review. *Nursing Outlook, 53*(2), 59–65.

Foundation for Critical Thinking (1996). *Critical thinking workshop handbook.* Rohnert Park, CA: Author.

Gaberson, K., & Oermann, M. (1999). *Clinical teaching strategies in nursing.* New York: Springer.

Giddens J., & Gloeckner, G.W. (2005). The relationship of critical thinking to performance on the NCLEX-RN. *Journal of Nursing Education, 44*(2), 85–89.

Green, C. (2000). *Critical thinking in nursing. Case studies across the curriculum.* Upper Saddle River, NJ: Prentice Hall Health.

Hatcher, D., & Spencer. L. A. (2000). *Reasoning and writing: From critical thinking to composition.* Boston: American Press.

Jameton, A. (1984). *Nursing practice. The ethical issues.* Englewood Cliffs, NJ: Prentice-Hall.

Johns, C., & Freshwater, D. (2005). *Transforming nursing through reflective practice.* Malden, MA: Blackwell Publishing.

Jones, S. A., & Brown, L. N. (1993). Alternative views on defining critical thinking through the nursing process. *Holistic Nursing Practice, 7*(3), 71–76.

Kurfiss, J. G. (1988). *Critical thinking: Theory, research, practice, and possibilities: ASHE-ERIC/Higher Education Research Report,* 17(2) (2nd printing). San Francisco: Jossey-Bass Wiley.

Lipman, M. (1988). The concept of critical thinking. *Teaching Thinking and Problem Solving, 10*(3).

Ludwick, R., & Sedlak, C. A. (1998). Ethical perspectives. Ethical issues and critical thinking: Students' stories. *Nursing Connections, 11*(3), 12–18.

Matthews, C. A., & Gaul, A. L. (1979). Nursing diagnosis from the perspective of concept attainment and critical thinking. *Advances in Nursing Science, 2*(1), 17–26.

McPeck, J. (1981). *Critical thinking and education.* New York: St. Martin's.

Parker, M. (1993). *Patterns of nursing theories in practice.* New York: National League for Nursing Press.

Parker, R. (2005). *Critical thinking* (8th ed.). Columbus, OH: McGraw-Hill.

Paul, R. (1988). What, then, is critical thinking? *The Eighth Annual and Sixth International Conference on Critical Thinking and Educational Reform.* Rohnert Park, CA: The Center for Critical Thinking and Moral Critique, Sonoma State University.

Paul, R. (1990). *Critical thinking.* Rohnert Park, CA: The Center for Critical Thinking and Moral Critique, Sonoma State University.

Paul, R. W. (1993). *Critical thinking: What every person needs to survive in a rapidly changing world* (3rd ed.). Santa Rosa, CA: Foundation for Critical Thinking.

Paul, R., & Elder, L. (2001). *The miniature guide to critical thinking: Concepts and tools* (p. 1). Dillon Beach, CA: The Foundation for Critical Thinking.

Paul, R. W., Ennis, R. H., & Norris, S. (1996). In B. Fowler (Ed.), *Critical thinking definitions. (Critical Thinking Across The Curriculum Project).* Lee's Summit, MO: Longview Community College.

Profetto-McGrath, J., Hesketh, K. L., Lang, S., & Estabrooks, C. A. (2003). A study of critical thinking and research utilization among nurses. *Western Journal of Nursing Research, 25*(3), 322–337.

Reilly, D. E., & Oermann, M. H. (1992). *Clinical teaching in nursing education.* New York: National League for Nursing.

The Roy Adaptation Model (n.d.), Boston College. Retrieved March 3, 2010, from http://www2.bc.edu/~royca/htm/ram.htm.

Roy, C. (1970). A conceptual framework for nursing. *Nursing Outlook, 18*(3), 42–45.

Roy, C. (1980). The Roy adaptation model. In J. Riehl & C. Roy (Eds.), *Conceptual models for nursing practice* (2nd ed.). New York: Appleton-Century-Crofts.

Scriven, M., & Paul, R. (1987). *Defining critical thinking. Critical thinking as defined by the National Council for Excellence in Critical Thinking.* A statement presented at the 8th Annual International Conference on Critical Thinking and Education Reform, Summer 1987. The Critical Thinking Community website. Retrieved December 1, 2009, from http://www.criticalthinking.org/aboutct/define_critical_thinking.cfm.

Tanner, C. A. (2000). Critical thinking: Beyond nursing process. *Journal of Nursing Education 39*(8), 338–339.

Tanner, C. A. (2005). What have we learned about critical thinking in nursing? *Journal of Nursing Education, 44*(2), 47–48.

Warnick, B., & Inch, E. (1994). *Critical thinking and communication* (2nd ed., p. 11). New York: Macmillan.

Wilkinson, J., & Treas, L. (2011). Critical thinking and nursing process. In *Fundamentals of nursing: Theory, concepts, and applications* (Vol. 1, 2nd ed.). Philadelphia: F. A. Davis.

Ziegler, S., Vaughan-Wrobel, B., & Erlen, J. (1986). *Nursing process, nursing diagnosis, nursing knowledge: Avenues to autonomy.* Norwalk, CT: Appleton-Century-Crofts.

Chapter 3

Acute Pain Management Guideline Panel. (1992). *Acute pain management in adults: Operative procedures, quick reference guide for clinicians.* (AHCPR Publication No. 92-0019). Rockdale, MD: Author.

Alfaro-LeFevre, R. (2010). *Applying nursing process: A tool for critical thinking* (7th ed.). Philadelphia: Lippincott Williams & Wilkins.

American Nurses Association. (1991). *Position statement on cultural diversity in nursing practice.* Kansas City, MO: Author.

American Nurses Association. (2001). *Code of ethics for nurses with interpretive statements.* Washington, DC: American Nurses Publishing. Retrieved January 10, 2010, from http://nursingworld.org/ethics/code/protected_nwcoe813.htm.

American Nurses Association. (2004). *Nursing: Scope and standards of practice* (3rd ed.). Washington, DC: American Nurses Publishing.

American Nurses Association. (2007). *Public health nursing: Scope and standards of practice.* Silver Spring, MD: Author.

American Nurses Association. (in press). *Nursing: Scope and standards of practice* (2nd ed.). (Public Comment draft, January). Silver Spring, MD: Author. Available at http://nursebooks.org.

Andrews, H., & Roy, C. (1986). *Essentials of the Roy adaptation model.* Norwalk, CT: Appleton-Century-Crofts.

Andrews, M. M., & Boyle, J. S. (2007). *Transcultural concepts in nursing care* (5th ed.). Philadelphia: Lippincott.

Barry, C. (1998). Assessing the older adult in the home. *Home Health Nurse, 16*(8), 519–530.

Cathell, D. (1991). A spiritual assessment without asking spiritual questions [lecture]. Merriam, KS: Shawnee Mission Medical Center.

Centers for Medicare and Medicaid Services (2009). *OASIS C. Home Health Quality Initiatives.* Baltimore, MD: U.S. Department of Health and Human Services. Available at http://www.cms.hhs.gov/HomeHealthQualityInits/06_OASISC.asp#TopOfPage.

College & Association of Registered Nurses of Alberta. (2005). *Nursing practice standards.* Retrieved January 23, 2010, from https://www.nurses.ab.ca/Carna-Admin/Uploads/Nursing%20Practice%20Standards_1.pdf.

Danter, J. H. (2003). Put a realistic spin on geriatric assessment. *Nursing 2003, 33*(12), 52–55.

Eskreis, T. R. (1998). Seven common legal pitfalls in nursing. *American Journal of Nursing, 98*(4), 34–40.

Galanti, G. A. (2004). *Caring for patients from different cultures* (3rd ed.). Philadelphia: University of Pennsylvania Press.

Giger, J. N., & Davidhizar, R. (2008). *Transcultural nursing: Assessment and intervention* (5th ed.). St. Louis: Mosby.

Gordon, M. (1994). *Nursing diagnosis: Process and application* (3rd ed.). St. Louis: Mosby.

Gorman, L. M., Raines, M. L., & Sultan, D. F. (2008). *Psychosocial nursing for general patient care* (3rd ed.) Philadelphia, F. A. Davis.

Gowri, A., & Hight, E. (2001). Spirituality and medical practice: Using the HOPE questions as a practical tool for spiritual assessment. *American Family Physician, 63,* 81–88.

Grainger, M. (2004). What about accountability? *British Journal of Nursing, 13*(21), 1241.

Joint Commission on Accreditation of Healthcare Organizations. (2008). *Hospital accreditation standards.* Oakbrook Terrace, IL: The Joint Commission.

Leininger, M. M., & McFarland, M. R. (2002). *Transcultural nursing: Concepts, theories, research and practices.* (3rd ed.). New York: McGraw-Hill.

Mahoney, F., & Barthel, D. (1965). Functional evaluation: The Barthel Index. *Maryland Medical Journal, 14*(2), 61–65.

Maslow, A. H. (1970). *Motivation and personality* (2nd ed.). New York: Harper & Row.

Maslow, A., & Lowery, R. (Eds.). (1998). *Toward a psychology of being* (3rd ed.). New York: Wiley & Sons.

McCaffery, M., & Pasero, C. (1999). *Pain clinical manual* (2nd ed.). St. Louis: C. V. Mosby.

McDowell, I. (2006). Measuring health: A guide to rating scales and questionnaires. New York: Oxford University Press.

Moskowitz, E., & McCann, C. (1957). Classification of disability in the chronically ill and aging. *Journal of Chronic Disease, 5,* 342–346.

NANDA International. (2009) *Nursing diagnoses: definitions & classification 2009–2010*. Philadelphia: NANDA International.

Neal, L. J. (1998). Current functional assessment tools. *Home Healthcare Nurse, 16*(11), 766–772.

Orem, D. E. (1991). *Nursing: Concepts of practice* (4th ed.). St. Louis: Mosby-Year Book.

Pender, N. J., Murdaugh, C. L., & Parsons, M. A. (2006). *Health promotion in nursing practice* (5th ed.). Upper Saddle River, NJ: Prentice Hall.

Pope, A. M., Snyder, M. A., & Mood, L. H. (Eds.). (1995). *Nursing, health and environment.* Washington, DC: Institute of Medicine, National Academy Press [classic].

Purnell, L. D., & Paulanka, B. J. (2008). *Transcultural health nursing: A culturally competent approach* (3rd ed.). Philadelphia: F. A. Davis.

Roy, C., & Andrews, H. A. (1991). *The Roy adaptation model: The definitive statement.* Norwalk, CT: Appleton & Lange.

Spector, R. E. (2004). *Cultural diversity in health and illness* (6th ed.). Upper Saddle River, NJ: Prentice-Hall.

Stewart, M. J. (1993). *Integrating social support in nursing.* Newbury Park, CA: Sage.

Stoll, R. (1979). Guidelines for spiritual assessment. *American Journal of Nursing, 79,* 1574–77.

Sumner, C. H. (1998). Recognizing and responding to spiritual distress. *American Journal of Nursing, 98*(1), 26–30.

Suzuki, L. A., & Ponterotto, J. G. (2007). *Handbook of multicultural assessment* (3rd ed.). New York: Jossey-Bass, Inc.

Todd, R. (2007). Place-based learning in teacher education: A windshield survey. *Social Studies Research and Practice, 2*(3), 390–402.

Townsend, M. (2009). *Psychiatric mental health nursing* (6th ed.). Philadelphia: F. A. Davis.

U.S. Census Bureau. (2005). *Race and Hispanic Origin in 2005*. Available at http://www.census.gov/population/pop-profile/dynamic/RACEHO.pdf.

U.S. Census Bureau. (2010). *2010 Census questionnaire reference book*. Available at http://2010.census.gov/partners/pdf/langfiles/qrb_English.pdf.

Wilkinson, J., & Treas, L. (2011). Culture & ethnicity. In *Fundamentals of nursing: Theory, concepts, and applications* (Vol. 1, 2nd ed.). Philadelphia: F. A. Davis.

Wilkinson, J., & Treas, L. (2011). Nursing process: Assessment. In *Fundamentals of nursing: Theory, concepts, and applications* (Vol. 1, 2nd ed.). Philadelphia: F. A. Davis.

Williams, S. R., & Schlenker, E. D. (2003). *Essentials of nutrition and diet therapy* (8th ed.). St. Louis: Mosby.

Young, T. (2009). Towards a code of practice for effective communication with people with dementing illnesses. *Journal of Language and Social Psychology, 28*(2), 174–189.

Zimmerman, P. G. (1998). Effective communication with patients with dementia. *Journal of Emergency Nursing, 24*(5), 412–415.

Chapter 4

Abdellah, F. (1957). Methods of identifying covert aspects of nursing problems. *Nursing Research, 6*(1), 4–23.

American Medical Association. (2008). *Current procedural terminology: CPT 2008.* Chicago: Author.

American Nurses Association. (1955). *Model nurse practice act,* Washington, DC: Author.

American Nurses Association. (1973). *Standards of nursing practice.* Kansas City, MO: Author.

American Nurses Association. (1980). *Nursing: A social policy statement.* Washington, DC: Author.

American Nurses Association. (2006). ANA recognized terminologies and data element sets. Nursing Practice Information Infrastructure. Retrieved March 14, 2008, from http://nursingworld.org/npii/terminologies.htm.

American Nurses Association. (in press). *Nursing: Scope and standards of practice* (2nd ed.). (Public Comment draft, January). Silver Spring, MD: Author. Available at http://nursebooks.org.

American Psychiatric Association. (2000). *Diagnostic and statistical manual of mental disorders.* Arlington, VA: American Psychiatric Publishing.

Benner, P., & Tanner, C. (1987). How expert nurses use intuition. *American Journal of Nursing, 87*(1), 23–31.

Carpenito-Moyet, L. J. (2006). *Nursing diagnosis: Application to clinical practice* (11th ed.). Philadelphia: Lippincott.

Carpenito, L. (1997). *Nursing diagnosis* (7th ed.). Philadelphia: J. B. Lippincott.

College & Association of Registered Nurses of Alberta (2005). *Nursing practice standards.* Edmonton, Alberta, Canada: Author. Retrieved January 23, 2010, from https://www.nurses.ab.ca/Carna-Admin/Uploads/Nursing%20Practice%20Standards_1.pdf.

Cronenwett, L., Sherwood, G., Barnsteiner, J., Disch, J., Johnson, J., Mitchell, P., Taylor-Sullivan, D., & Warren, J. (2007). Quality and safety education for nurses. *Nursing Outlook, 55*(3), 122–131.

da Cruz, D., & Peres, R. (2003). Accuracy of nursing diagnosis: Interrater agreement. *International Journal of Nursing Terminologies and Classifications, 14*(4) (Supplement), 47.

Dossey, B. M. (1998). Holistic modalities and healing moments. *American Journal of Nursing, 98*(6): 44–47.

Florin, J., Ehrenberg, A., & Ehnfors, M. (2005). Quality of nursing diagnoses: Evaluation of an educational intervention. *International Journal of Nursing Terminologies and Classifications, 15*(2), 33–43.

Fry, V. (1953). The creative approach to nursing. *American Journal of Nursing, 53*(3), 301–302.

Gambrill, E. (2005). *Critical thinking in clinical practice: Improving the quality of judgments and decisions* (2nd ed.). Hoboken, NJ: John Wiley & Sons.

Gordon, M. (1994). *Nursing diagnosis: Process and application* (3rd ed.). St. Louis: Mosby.

Gordon, M., Murphy, C., Candee, D., et al. (1994). Clinical judgment: An integrated model. *Advances in Nursing Science, 16*(4), 55–70.

Jaco, M. K., Gordon, M. D., & Marvin, J. A. (2003). Nursing rounds link nursing diagnoses to clinical practice. *International Journal of Nursing Terminologies and Classifications, 14*(4) (Supplement), 53.

Keenan, G., Falan, S., Heath, C., & Treder, M. (2003). Establishing competency in the use of North American Nursing Diagnosis Association, Nursing Outcomes Classification, and Nursing Interventions Classification terminology. *Journal of Nursing Measurement, 11*, 183–198.

Lavin, M. A., Meyer, G., & Carlson, J. H. (1999). A review of the use of nursing diagnosis in U.S. nurse practice acts. *Nursing Diagnosis, 10*(2), 57–64.

Levin, R., Lunney, M., & Krainovich-Miller, B. (2004). Improving diagnostic accuracy using an evidence-based nursing model. *International Journal of Nursing Language and Classification, 15*(4), 114–122.

London, S. (1998). DXplain: A web-based diagnostic decision support system for medical students. *Medical Reference Services Quarterly, 17*(2), 17–28.

Lunney, M. (2003). Critical thinking and accuracy of nurses' diagnoses. *International Journal of Nursing Terminologies and Classifications, 14*(3), 96–107.

Lunney, M. (2008). Critical need to address accuracy of nurses' diagnoses. *Online Journal of Issues in Nursing* (January 31).

McManus, L. (1951). Assumption of functions of nursing. In *Regional planning for nursing and nursing education.* New York: Teachers College Press.

Mrayyan, M. T. (2005). The influence of standardized languages on nurses' autonomy. *Journal of Nursing Management, 13*(3), 238–241.

Müller-Staub, M., Lavin, M. A., Needham, I., & Van Achterberg, T. (2006). Nursing diagnoses, interventions and outcomes—Application and impact on nursing practice: Systematic review. *Journal of Advanced Nursing, 56*(5j), 514–531.

NANDA International. (2009). *NANDA International nursing diagnoses: Definitions & classification, 2009–2011.* Philadelphia: Author.

O'Neill, J. A. (1997). The consequences of meeting "Mrs. Wisdom": Teaching the nursing diagnostic process with case studies (pp. 131–138). In M. A. Rantz & P. LeMone (Eds.), *Classification of nursing diagnoses: Proceedings of the Twelfth Conference, North American Nursing Diagnosis Association.* Philadelphia: NANDA.

Parris, K. M., Place, P. J., Orellana, E., Calder, J., Jackson, K., Karolys, A., Meza, M., Middough, C., Nguyen, V., Shim, N. W., & Smith, D. (1999). Integrating nursing diagnoses, interventions, and outcomes in public health nursing practice. *Nursing Diagnosis, 10*(2), 49–56.

Powers, P. (2003). A discourse analysis of nursing diagnosis. *Quality Health Research, 12*(7), 945–965.

Ramnarayan, P., Tomlinson, A., Rao, A., Coren, M., Winrow, A., & Britto, J. (2003). ISABEL: A web-based differential diagnostic aid for paediatrics: Results from an initial performance evaluation. *Archives of Diseases in Childhood, 88,* 408–413.

Robichaud, A. L. (2003). Healing and feeling: The clinical ontology of emotion. *Bioethics, 17*(1), 59–68.

Roy, Sr. C. (1984). *Introduction to nursing: An adaptation model.* Englewood Cliffs, NJ: Prentice Hall.

Smith, H. K., & Donald, J. G. (2002, April). Thinking processes used by nurses in clinical decision making. *Journal Nursing Education, 41*(4), 145–153.

Wang, J., Lo, C. K., & Ku, Y. (2004). Problem solving strategies integrated into nursing process to promote clinical problem solving abilities of RN-BSN students. *Nurse Educator Today, 24*(8), 589–595.

Wilbraham, A., et al. (1990). *Critical thinking worksheets.* A supplement of *Addison-Wesley chemistry.* Menlo Park, CA: Addison-Wesley.

Wilkinson, J. M., & Ahern, N. R. (2009). *Prentice Hall nursing diagnosis handbook* (9th ed.). Upper Saddle River, NJ: Prentice Hall Health.

Wilkinson, J. M., & Treas, L. S. (2011). *Fundamentals of nursing* (2nd ed.). Philadelphia: F. A. Davis.

Chapter 5

Abdellah, F. (1957). Methods of identifying covert aspects of nursing problems. *Nursing Research, 6*(1), 4–23.

American Medical Association. (2010). *Current procedural terminology: CPT 2010.* Chicago: Author.

American Nurses Association. (1973). *Standards of nursing practice.* Kansas City, MO: Author.

American Nurses Association. (1980). *ANA social policy statement.* Washington, DC: Author.

American Nurses Association. (2003). *Nursing's social policy statement.* (2nd ed.). Washington, DC: Author.

American Nurses Association. (2006). ANA recognized terminologies and data element sets. *Nursing practice information infrastructure.* Retrieved March 14, 2008, from http://nursingworld.org/npii/terminologies.htm.

American Nurses Association. (in press). *Nursing: Scope and standards of practice* (2nd ed.). (Public Comment draft, January). Silver Spring, MD: Author. Available at http://nursebooks.org.

American Psychiatric Association. (2000). *Diagnostic and statistical manual of mental disorders.* Arlington, VA: American Psychiatric Publishing.

Barton, A., Gilbert, L., Erickson, V., Baramee, J., Sowers, D., & Robertson, K. (2003, May-June). A guide to assist nurse practitioners with standardized nursing language. *CIN: Computers, Informatics, Nursing, 21*(3), 128–133.

Bates, D. W., Ebell, M., Gotlieb, E., Zapp, J., & Mullins, H. C. (2003). A proposal for electronic medical records in U.S. primary care. *Journal of the American Medical Informatics Association, 10*(1), 1–10.

Beyea, S. (1999, November). Standardized language-making nursing practice count. *AORN Journal, 70*(5), 831–832, 834, 837, 838.

Beyea, S. (2000, May). Standardized nursing vocabularies and the perioperative nursing data set: Making clinical practice count. *CIN Plus, 3*(2), 1, 5, 6.

Blegen, M. A., & Tripp-Reimer, T. (1997). Implications of nursing taxonomies for middle-range theory development. *Advances in Nursing Science, 19*(3), 37–49.

Brokel, J., & Heath, C. (2009). The value of nursing diagnoses in electronic health records (pp. 28–31). In *Nursing diagnoses definitions and classification 2009–2011.* Ames, IA: John Wiley & Sons.

Carpenito, L. J. (2006). *Nursing diagnosis: Application to clinical practice* (11th ed.). Philadelphia: Lippincott.

Conrick, M. (2005). The International Classification for Nursing Practice: A tool to support nursing practice? *Collegian, 12*(3), 9–13.

Cosgrove, L. (2006). When labels mask oppression: Implications for teaching psychiatric taxonomy to mental health counselors. *Journal of Mental Health Counseling, 27*(4), 283–296.

Craft-Rosenberg, M. (1999). NDEC guidelines for development and evaluation of diagnoses. *Nursing Diagnosis, 10*(2), 84–85.

Delaney, C., Herr, K., Maas, M., & Specht, J. (2000). Reliability of nursing diagnoses documented in a computerized nursing information system. *Nursing Diagnosis, 11*(3), 121–134.

Engebretson, J. (1996). Considerations in diagnosing in the spiritual domain. *Nursing Diagnosis, 7*(3), 100–107.

Fry, V. (1953). The creative approach to nursing. *American Journal of Nursing, 98*(6), 44–47.

Gebbie, K. (1976). Development of a taxonomy of nursing diagnosis. In J. Walter (Ed.), *Dynamics of problem-oriented approaches: Patient care and documentation.* Philadelphia: J. B. Lippincott.

Geissler, E. (1992). Nursing diagnoses: A study of cultural relevance. *Journal of Professional Nursing, 8*(5), 301–307.

Gordon, M. (1998). Nursing nomenclature and classification system development. *Online Journal of Issues in Nursing, 2*(2). Retrieved May 27, 1999, from http://www.nursingworld.org/ojin/tpc7/tpc7_1.htm.

Gordon, M., & Butler-Schmidt, B. (1997). High frequency–high treatment priority nursing diagnoses in home health care nursing. In M. J. Rantz & P. LeMone (Eds.), *Classification of nursing diagnoses: Proceedings of the Twelfth Conference, North American Nursing Diagnosis Association.* Glendale, CA: CINAHL Information Systems.

Green, P. M., & Slade, D. S. (2001). Environmental nursing diagnoses for aggregates and community. *Nursing Diagnosis, 12*(1), 5–13.

Henderson, V. (1964). The nature of nursing. *American Journal of Nursing, 64*(8), 62–68.

International Council of Nurses (2009). ICNP® *Version 2. International Classification for Nursing Practice.* Retrieved January 30, 2010, from http://www.icn.ch/icnp.htm.

Johnson, M. (2002, January/March). Criteria for standardized nursing language. *Outcomes Management. 6*(1), 1–3.

Johnson, M., Bulechek, G., Dochterman, J. M., Maas, M., Moorhead, S., Swanson, E., & Butcher, H. (2006). *Nursing diagnoses, outcomes, and interventions: NANDA, NOC, and NIC linkage,* (2nd ed.). St. Louis: Mosby.

Johnson, M., & Maas, M., Eds. (1997). *Nursing outcomes classification.* St. Louis: C. V. Mosby.

Kalish, R. (1983). *The psychology of human behavior* (5th ed.). Monterey, CA: Brooks/Cole.

Keeling, A., Utz, S., Shuster, G. III, & Boyle, A. (1993). Noncompliance revisited: A disciplinary perspective of a nursing diagnosis. *Nursing Diagnosis, 4*(3), 91–98.

Kim, M., McFarland, G., & McLane, A. (1984). *Proceedings of the Fifth National Conference, North American Nursing Diagnosis Association.* St. Louis: C. V. Mosby.

Kritek, P. (1985). Nursing diagnosis: Theoretical foundations. *Occupational Health Nursing* (August), 393–396.

Leininger, M. (1990). Issues, questions, and concerns related to the nursing diagnosis cultural movement from a transcultural nursing perspective. *Journal of Transcultural Nursing, 2,* 23–32.

Lesh, K. (1997). Use of nursing diagnosis in public health nursing. In M. J. Rantz & P. LeMone (Eds.), *Classification of nursing diagnoses: Proceedings of the Twelfth Conference, North American Nursing Diagnosis Association.* Glendale, CA: CINAHL Information Systems.

Lunney, M. (2008). Critical need to address accuracy of nurses' diagnoses. *Online Journal of Issues in Nursing* (January 31).

Lunney, M. (2009). Nursing diagnosis and research. In *Nursing diagnoses definitions and classification 2009–2011* (pp. 32–36). Ames, IA: John Wiley & Sons.

Martin, K. S. (2005). *The Omaha System: A key to practice, documentation, and management* (2nd ed.). New York: Elsevier.

Martin, K. S., & Norris, J. (1996). The Omaha system: A model for describing practice. *Holistic Nursing Practice, 11*(1), 75–83.

Martin, K. S., & Scheet, N. J. (1992). *The Omaha system: Applications for community health nursing.* Philadelphia: W. B. Saunders.

Maslow, A. (1970). *Motivation and personality.* (2nd ed.). New York: Harper & Row.

Maslow, A. (1971). *The farther reaches of human nature.* New York: The Viking Press.

Maslow, A., & Lowery, R. (Ed.). (1998). *Toward a psychology of being* (3rd ed.). New York: Wiley & Sons.

McCloskey, J. C., & Bulechek, G. M. (Eds.). (1992). *Nursing interventions classification (NIC).* St. Louis: Mosby.

Müller-Staub, M., Lavin, M. A., Needham, I., & Van Achterberg, T. (2006). Nursing diagnoses, interventions and outcomes—Application and impact on nursing practice: Systematic review. *Journal of Advanced Nursing, 56*(5j), 514–531.

NANDA International. (2009). *NANDA nursing diagnoses: Definitions & classification 2009–2011.* Ames, IA: Wiley-Blackwell.

Nursing Information and Data Set Evaluation Center. (2006). Retrieved February 5, 2010, from http://www.nursingworld.org/npii/terminologies.htm.

O'Brien, M. (1982). The need for spiritual integrity (pp. 81–115). In H. Yura & M. Welsh (Eds.), *Human needs and the nursing process.* Norwalk, CT: Appleton-Century-Crofts.

Ollson, P. T., & Gardulf, A. (2006). Nurses and head nurses views of nursing diagnoses at a geriatric clinic. *Journal of Clinical Nursing, 15*(10), 1338–1339.

The Omaha System (2009, updated). Problem classification scheme. Domains and problems of the problem classification system. Retrieved February 1, 2010, from http://www.omahasystem.org/problemclassification scheme.html.

Parris, K. M., Place, P. J., Orellana, E., Calder, J., Jackson, K., Karolys, A., Meza, M., Middough, C., Nguyen, V., Shim, N. W., & Smith, D. (1999). Integrating nursing diagnoses, interventions, and outcomes in public health nursing practice. *Nursing Diagnosis, 10*(2), 49–56.

Pesut, D. J., & Herman, J. (1999). *Clinical reasoning: The art and science of critical & creative thinking.* Albany, NY: Delmar.

Rutherford, M. A. (2008, January 31). Standardized nursing language: What does it mean for nursing practice? *Online Journal of Issues in Nursing, 13*(1). Retrieved January 29, 2010, from http://www.nursing world.org/MainMenuCategories/ANAMarketplace/ANAPeriodicals/OJIN/TableofContents/vol132008/No1Jan08/ArticlePreviousTopic/StandardizedNursingLanguage.aspx.

Saba, V. (2006). *Clinical Care Classification (CCC) system manual. A guide to nursing documentation.* New York: Springer Publishing Company.

Saba, V. K. (1995). Home health care classifications (HHCCs): Nursing diagnoses and nursing interventions. In *An emerging framework: Data system advances for clinical nursing practice.* ANA Publication #NP-94. Washington, DC: American Nurses Publishing.

Saba, V. K. (1997). Why the home health care classification is a recognized nursing nomenclature. *Computers in Nursing, 15*(2), 69–76.

Shelly, B., & Hawks, J. (2005). Proper terminology enhances collaboration. *Urology Nursing, 25i*(4), 285.

Smith, H. K., & Donald, J. G. (2002, April). Thinking processes used by nurses in clinical decision making. *Journal of Nursing Education, 41*(4), 145–153.

Sumner, C. H. (1998). Recognizing and responding to spiritual distress. *American Journal of Nursing, 98*(1), 26, 28–30.

Wilkinson, J. M., & Ahern, N. R. (2009). *Prentice Hall nursing diagnosis handbook* (9th ed.). Upper Saddle River, NJ: Prentice Hall Health.

Wilkinson, J. M., & Treas, L. S. (2011). *Fundamentals of nursing* (2nd ed.). Philadelphia, F. A. Davis.

World Health Organization. (2007). *International statistical classification of diseases and related health problems* (10th rev.). Geneva, Switzerland: Author. Retrieved January 29, 2010, from http://apps.who.int/classifications/apps/icd/icd10online.

Chapter 6

Agency for Health Care Policy and Research. (1993). *Clinical practice guideline development, AHCPR program note,* AHCPR Publication Number 93-0023. Last modified July 31, 1995.

Agency for Health Care Policy and Research. (1998). Invitation to submit guidelines to the National Guideline Clearinghouse™, *Federal Register, 63*(70), 18027. Retrieved March 12, 2008, from http://www.ahrq.gov/fund/ngcguidl.htm.

American Medical Association. (2008). *CPT® 2008 professional edition.* Chicago: Author.

American Nurses Association. (2001). *Code of ethics for nurses with interpretive statements.* Washington, DC: American Nurses Publishing. Retrieved February 10, 2010, from http://nursingworld.org/ethics/code/protected_nwcoe813.htm.

American Nurses Association. (2006). *ANA recognized terminologies and data element sets.* Retrieved March 13, 2008, from http://www.nursingworld.org/npli/terminologies.htm.

American Nurses Association. (in press). *Nursing: Scope and standards of practice* (2nd ed.). (Public Comment draft, January). Silver Spring, MD: Author. Available at http://nursebooks.org.

American Nurses Association/Nursing Information & Data Set Evaluation Center. (2008). *Nursing Information & Data Set Evaluation Center,* American Nurses Association, NursingWorld. Retrieved March 12, 2008, from http://www.nursingworld.org/MainMenuCategories/ThePracticeofProfessionalNursing/DocInfo/NIDSEC.aspx.

Anthony, M., & Hudson-Barr, D. (2004). A patient-centered model of care for hospital discharge. *Clinical Nursing Research, 13*(2), 117–136.

Aroskar, M. A. (1995). Managed care and nursing values: A reflection. *Journal of Nursing Law, 24*(4), 63–70.

Berman, A, Snyder, S., Kozier, B., & Erb, G. (2008). *Kozier & Erb's fundamentals of nursing* (8th ed.). Upper Saddle River, NJ: Pearson/Prentice Hall.

Beyea, S. (2000, May). Standardized nursing vocabularies and the perioperative nursing data set: Making clinical practice count. *CIN Plus, 3*(2), 1, 5, 6.

Bonaiuto, M. M. (2007). School nurse case management: Achieving health and educational outcomes. *Journal of School Nursing, 23*(4), 202–209.

Bulechek, G., Butcher, H., & Dochterman, J. M. (2008). *Nursing Intervention Classification (NIC)* (5th ed.). St. Louis: Mosby.

Bull, M. J., Hansen, H. E., & Gross, C. R. (2000). Differences in family caregiver outcomes by their level of involvement in discharge planning. *Applied Nursing Research, 13*(2), 76–82.

Carr, P. (1990). Two halves don't make a whole. *RN, 53*(7), 96.

College & Association of Registered Nurses of Alberta. (2005). *Nursing practice standards.* Edmonton, Alberta, Canada, Author.

College of Registered Nurses of Nova Scotia. (2003). *Standards for nursing practice.* Halifax, Nova Scotia, Canada: Author.

Damiani, G. (2009). Hospital discharge planning and continuity of care for aged people in an Italian local health unit: Does the care-home model reduce hospital readmission and mortality rates [abstract]? *BMC Health Serv Res, 9,* 22.

Dedhia, P. (2009). A quality improvement intervention to facilitate the transition of older adults from three hospitals back to their homes. *Journal of the American Geriatrics Society, 57*(9), 1540–1546.

Ellis-Hill, C., Robison, J., Wiles, R., McPherson, K., Hyndman, D., & Ashburn, A., on Behalf of the Stroke Association Rehabilitation Research Centre Team. (2009). Going home to get on with life: Patients and carers experiences of being discharged from hospital following a stroke. *Disability & Rehabilitation, 31*(2), 61–72.

Frenn, M., & Malin, S. (1998). Health promotion: Theoretical perspectives and clinical applications. *Holistic Nursing Practice, 12*(2), 1–7.

Given, B., & Sherwood, P. (2005). Nursing-sensitive patient outcomes—a white paper. *Oncology Nursing Forum 32*(4), 773–784.

Gordon, M., Murphy, C., & Candee, D. (1994). Clinical judgment: An integrated model. *ANS, 16*(4), 55–70.

Greenwald, J. L., Denham, C. R., & Jack, B. W. (2007). The hospital discharge: A review of a high risk care transition with highlights of a reengineered discharge process. *Journal of Patient Safety, 3*(2), 97–106.

Harris, B. L. (1990). Becoming deprofessionalized: One aspect of the staff nurse's perspective on computer-mediated nursing care plans, *ANS, 13*(2), 63–74.

Head, B., Maas, M., & Johnson, M. (1997). Outcomes for home and community nursing in integrated delivery systems. *Caring, 16*(1), 50–56.

Hinck, S., Webb, P., Simms-Giddens, S., Helton, C., Hope, K., Utley, R., et al. (2006). Student learning with concept mapping of care plans in community-based education. *Journal of Professional Nursing, 22,* 23–29.

Hunt, S. (2008). Data management in home care: Using data to drive acute care hospitalization. *Home Health Care Management & Practice, 20*(2), 175–179.

Johnson, M., Bulechek, G., Butcher, H., Dochterman, J.M., Maas, M. Moorhead, S., Swanson, E. (2006). *Nursing diagnoses, outcomes, and interventions: NANDA, NOC, and NIC linkage* (2nd ed.). St. Louis: Mosby.

Kay, D., Blue, A., Pye, P., Lacy, A., Gray, C., & Moore, S. (2006). Heart failure: Improving the continuum of care. *Care Management Journals, 7*(2), 58–63.

Maas, M., & Delaney, C. (2004). Nursing process outcome linkage research: Issues, current status, and health policy implications. *Medical Care, 42*(2) (Supplement), II-40–48.

Maas, M., Johnson, M., Moorhead, S., Reed, D., & Sweeney, S. (2003). Evaluation of the reliability and validity of Nursing Outcomes Classification patient outcomes and measures. *Journal of Nursing Measurement, 11*(2), 97–117.

Martin, K. (2005). *The Omaha System: A key to practice, documentation, and information management.* (2nd ed.). Philadelphia: Saunders.

McCloskey, J. C., & Bulechek, G. M. (Eds.). (1992). *Nursing interventions classification (NIC).* St. Louis: Mosby.

McGinty, J. (1997). Issues and interventions. Look at cost savings and care paths with an ethical eye. *Nursing Case Management, 2*(6), 267–268.

Meyer, J., & Sturdy, D. (2004). Exploring the future of gerontological nursing outcomes. *Journal of Clinical Nursing, 13*(6b): *(International Journal of Older People Nursing),* 128–134.

Moorhead, S. (1999). *Health care terminology: Nursing Outcomes Classification (NOC). NCVHS Hearings on Medical Terminology and Code Development.* Rockville, MD. Retrieved November 18, 2010 from http://www.ncvhs.hhs.gov/990518t4.htm.

Moorhead, S., Johnson, M., Maas, M., & Swanson, E. (2008). *Nursing Outcomes Classification (NOC)* (4th ed.). St. Louis: Mosby.

Nazarko, L. (1998). Improving discharge: the role of the discharge coordinator. *Nursing Standard, 12*(49), 35–37.

Nelson, R. (2004). Measuring outcomes in home health care: Beyond the OASIS data set. *Home Health Care Management Practice, 16*(3), 200–205.

Nolan, S. (2008). Nursing M&M reviews: Learning from our outcomes. *RN, 71*(1), 36–40.

NSW Department of Health (2007). Policy directive. Discharge planning: Responsive standards (rev. November 2007). Retrieved March 10, 2008, from http://www.health.nsw.gov.qu/policies.

Parkes, S., McClaren, J., & Phillips, C., Lannin, N., Clemson, L., McCluskey, A., Cameron, I., & Barras, S. (January 20, 2010). Discharge planning from hospital to home. *Cochrane Database Systematic Reviews* (1):CD00313. Retrieved February 8, 2010, from http://www.ncbi.nlm.nih.gov/pubmed/20091507?ordinalpos=1&itool=EntrezSystem2.PEntrez.Pubmed.Pubmed_ResultsPanel.Pubmed_SingleItemSupl.Pubmed_Discovery_RA&linkpos=2&log$=relatedreviews&logdbfrom=pubmed.

Parlocha, P. K., & Henry, S. B. (1998). The usefulness of the Georgetown Home Health Care Classification system for coding patient problems and nursing interventions in psychiatric home care. *Computers in Nursing, 16*(1), 45–52.

Rivera, J., & Parris, K. (2003). Use of NANDA- and NIC-based nursing care plans in public health nursing practice. *International Journal of Nursing Terminologies and Classifications,14*(4) (Supplement), 55.

Rutherford, M. A. (1998). Standardized nursing language: What does it mean for nursing practice? *Online Journal of Issues in Nursing, 3*(2). Retrieved March 13, 2008, from http://www.nursingworld.org/SpecialPages/Search.aspx?SearchMode=1&SearchPhrase=nidsec.

Saba, V. (2006). *Clinical Care Classification (CCC) system manual. A guide to nursing documentation.* New York: Springer Publishing Company.

Schneider, J., Barkaauskas, V., & Keenan, G. (2008). Evaluating home health care nursing outcomes with OASIS and NOC. *Journal of Nursing Scholarship, 40*(1), 76–82.

Schneider, J., Hornberger, S. Booker, J., et al. (1993). A medication discharge planning program. Measuring the effect on readmissions. *Clinical Nursing Research, 2*(1), 41–53.

Simpson, R. (1998). Setting the informatics standards: An overview of NDISEC's information systems evaluation criteria. *Nursing Economics (September–October).*

Smith, K., Smith, V., Krugman, M., & Oman, K. (2005). Evaluating the impact of computerized clinical documentation. *CIN: Computers, Informatics, Nursing, 23*(3), 132–138.

Stephens, N. (2005). Complex care packages: Supporting seamless discharge for child and family. *Paediatric Nursing, 17*(7), 30–32.

Tirk, J. (1992). Determining discharge priorities. *Nursing, 22*(7), 55.

Tuazon, N. (1992). Discharge teaching: Use this MODEL. *RN, 55*(4), 19–22.

U.S. Department of Health and Human Services. (2010). *Healthy people 2020.* Washington, DC: U.S. Government Printing Office.

Walker, C., Hogstel, M., & Curry, L. (2007). Hospital discharge of older adults. *American Journal of Nursing, 107*(6), 60–71.

Walsh, S. (2004). Formulation of a plan of care for culturally diverse patients. *International Journal of Nursing Terminologies and Classifications, 15*(1), 17–26.

Weissman, M. A., & Jasovsky, D. A. (1998). Discharge teaching for today's times. *RN, 61*(6), 38–40.

Wilkinson, J., & Treas, L. (2011). *Fundamentals of nursing* (2nd ed.). Philadelphia: F. A. Davis.

Zander, K. (1998). Historical development of outcomes-based care delivery. *Critical Care Nursing Clinics of North America, 10*(1), 1–11.

Chapter 7

American Medical Association. (2008). *CPT® 2008 Professional Edition.* Chicago: Author.

American Nurses Association. (2001). *Code of ethics for nurses with interpretive statements.* Washington, DC: ANA.

American Nurses Association. (in press). *Nursing: Scope and standards of practice* (2nd ed.). (Public Comment draft, January). Silver Spring, MD: Author. Available at http://nursebooks.org.

American Nurses Association/Nursing Information & Data Set Evaluation Center. (2002, January 23). *Recognized languages for nursing.* Retrieved September 1, 2002, from http://nursingworld.org/nidsec/classlst.htm.

Aranda, S. (2008). Designing nursing interventions. *Collegian, 15*(1), 19–25.

Benner, P. (2004). Designing formal classification systems to better articulate knowledge, skills, and meanings in nursing practice. *American Journal of Critical Care, 13,* 426–430.

Berlin, E. A., & Fowkes, W. C. (1983). A teaching framework for cross-cultural health care. *Western Journal of Medicine, 139*(b), 934–938.

Bolton, L., Donaldson, N., Rutledge, D., et al. (2007). The impact of nursing interventions: Overview of effective interventions, outcomes, measures, and priorities for future research. *Medical Care Research & Review, 64*(2) (Supplement), 123S–143S.

Bowker, G. C., Star, S. L., & Spasser, M. A. (2001, March). Classifying nursing work. *Online Journal of Issues in Nursing.* Retrieved September 9, 2002, from http://www.nursingworld.org/ojin/tpc7/tpc7_6.htm.

Bulechek, G., Butcher, H., & Dochterman, J. (2008). *Nursing Interventions Classification (NIC)* (5th ed.). St. Louis: Mosby.

Burkhart, L., Konicek, D., Moorhead, S., & Androwich, I. (2005). Mapping parish nurse documentation into the Nursing Interventions Classification: A research method. *CIN: Computers, Informatics, Nursing, 23*(4), 220–229.

Button, P. S. (1997). Computers in practice: Challenges and uses—using standardized nursing nomenclature in an automated careplanning and documentation system. In M. J. Rantz & P. LeMone (Eds.), *Classification of nursing diagnoses: Proceedings of the Twelfth Conference, North American Nursing Diagnosis Association* Glendale, CA: CINAHL, 327–331.

Carpenito-Moyet, L. (2005). *Nursing diagnosis: Application to clinical practice* (11th ed.). Philadelphia: Lippincott, Williams & Wilkins.

College and Association of Registered Nurses of Alberta (CARNA). (2003). *Nursing practice standards.* Available at http://www.nursingworld.org/DocumentVault/NursingPractice/Draft-Nursing-Scope-Standards-2nd-Ed.aspx.

deCordova, P., Lucero, R., Hyun, S., et al. (2010). Using the Nursing Interventions Classification as a potential measure of nurse workload. *Journal of Nursing Care Quality, 25*(1), 39–45.

DeVliegher, K., Paquay, L., Grypdonck, M., Wouters, R., Debaillie, R., & Geys, L. (2005). A study of core interventions in home nursing. *International Journal of Nursing Studies, 42*(5), 513–520.

Dicenso, A., Guyatt, G., & Ciliska, D. (2005). *Evidence-based nursing: A guide to clinical practice.* St. Louis: Elsevier Mosby.

DiJoseph, J., & Cavendish, R. (2005). Expanding the dialogue on prayer relevant to holistic care. *Holistic Nursing Practice, 19,* 147–155.

Dochterman, J. C., & Bulechek, G. M. (Eds.). (2004). *Nursing Interventions Classification (NIC)* (4th ed.). St. Louis: Mosby.

Dochterman, J., Titler, M., Wang, J., Reed, D., Pettit, D., Mathew-Wilson, M., Budreau, G., Bulechek, G., Kraus, V., & Kanak, M. (2005). Describing use of nursing interventions for three groups of patients. *Journal of Nursing Scholarship, 37*(1), 57–66.

Doran, D., Harrison, M., Laschinger, H., et al. (2006). Relation between nursing interventions and outcome achievement in acute care settings. *Research in Nursing & Health, 29*(1), 61–70.

Giger, J., & Davidhizar, R. (2007). Promoting culturally appropriate interventions among vulnerable populations. (2007). *Annual Review of Nursing Research, 25,* 293–316.

Grant, D. (2004). Spiritual interventions: How, when, and why nurses use them. *Holistic Nursing Practice, 18,* 36–41.

Hendry, C., & Walker, A. (2004). Priority setting in clinical nursing practice: Literature review. *Journal of Advanced Nursing, 47,* 427–436.

International Council of Nurses (ICN). (2005). *ICNP Version 1.0.* Geneva, Switzerland: Author. Retrieved March 23, 2008, from http://www.icn.ch/icnp_v1.htm.

Iowa Intervention Project. (1997). Proposal to bring nursing into the information age. *Journal of Nursing Scholarship, 29*(3), 275–281.

Johnson, M., Bulechek, G., Dochterman, J.M., Maas, M. Moorhead, S., Swanson, E. & Butcher, H. (2006). *Nursing diagnoses, outcomes, and interventions: NANDA, NOC, and NIC linkages* (2nd ed.). St. Louis: Mosby.

Laukhuf, G., & Werner, H. (1998). Spirituality: The missing link. *Journal of Neuroscience Nursing, 30*(1), 60–67.

Lunney, M. (2006). NANDA diagnoses, NIC interventions, and NOC outcomes used in an electronic health record with elementary school children. *Journal of School Nursing, 22*(2), 94–101.

Lunney, M. (2006). Staff development. Helping nurses use NANDA, NOC, and NIC: Novice to expert. *Journal of Nursing Administration, 36*(3), 118–125.

Lustria, M., Cortese, J., Noar, S., et al. (2009). Computer-tailored health interventions delivered over the Web: Review and analysis of key components. *Patient Education & Counseling, 74*(2), 156–173.

Martin, K. S. (2005). *The Omaha system: A key to practice, documentation, and information management* (2nd ed.). St. Louis: Elsevier.

Martin, K. S., & Scheet, N. J. (1992). *The Omaha system: Applications for community health nursing.* Retrieved September 1, 2002, from http://www.omahasystem.org/shminter.htm.

Müller-Staub, M., Needham, I., Odenbreit, M., et al. (2007). Improved quality of nursing documentation: Results of a nursing diagnoses, interventions, and outcomes implementation study. *International Journal of Nursing Terminologies & Classifications, 18*(1), 5–17.

Mundinger, M. O. (1980). *Autonomy in nursing.* Gaithersburg, MD: Aspen Systems.

Nursing Practice Information Infrastructure. (2007). ANA recognized terminologies and data element sets (last updated May 11, 2006). Retrieved March 23, 2008, from http://nursingworld.org/npii/terminologies.htm.

Parris, K. M., Place, P. J., & Orellana, E. (1999). Integrating nursing diagnoses, interventions, and outcomes in public health nursing practice. *Nursing Diagnosis, 10*(2), 49–56.

Pender, N. J., Murdaugh, C. L., & Parsons, M. A. (2006). *Health promotion in nursing practice* (5th ed.). Upper Saddle River, NJ: Prentice Hall.

Reed, D., Titler, M. G., Dochterman, J. M., Shever, L. L., & Kanak, M. (2007). Measuring the dose of nursing interventions. *International Journal of Nursing Terminologies and Classifications, 18*(4), 121–130.

Rivera, J. C., & Parris, K. M. (2003). Use of NANDA- and NIC-based nursing care plans in public health nursing practice. *International Journal of Nursing Terminologies and Classifications, 14*(4) (Supplement), 55.

Russell, C. (2006). Culturally responsive interventions to enhance immunosuppressive medication adherence in older African American kidney transplant recipients. *Progress in Transplantation, 16*(3), 187–196.

Saba, V. K. (1997). Why the Home Health Care Classification is a recognized nursing nomenclature. *Computers in Nursing, 15*(2), S69–S76.

Saba, V. K. (2003). *CCC Sabacare. Clinical Care Classification (CCC) System.* Retrieved January 23, 2006, from http://www.sabacare.com.

Saba, V. K. (2006). *Clinical care classification system manual: A guide to nursing documentation.* New York: Springer.

Sakano, L., & Yoshitome, A. (2007). Diagnosis and nursing interventions on elderly inpatients. *Acta Paulista de Enfermagem, 20*(4), 495–498.

Sellers, S. C., & Haag, B. A. (1998). Spiritual nursing interventions. *Journal of Holistic Nursing, 16*(3), 338–354.

Shever, L., Titler, M., Dochterman, J., et al. (2007). Patterns of nursing intervention use across 6 days of acute care hospitalization for three older patient populations. *International Journal of Nursing Terminologies & Classifications, 18*(1), 18–29.

Thoroddsen, A. (2005). Applicability of the Nursing Interventions Classification to describe nursing. *Scandinavian Journal of Caring Sciences, 19*(2), 128–139.

Wilkinson, J. M. & Ahern, N. R. (2009). *Prentice Hall's nursing diagnosis handbook* (9th ed.). Upper Saddle River, NJ: Pearson/Prentice Hall.

Wong, E. (2008). Novel nursing terminologies for the rapid response system. *International Journal of Nursing Terminologies & Classifications, 20*(2), 53–63.

Wong, E. (2009). Coining and defining novel nursing terminology. Part 2: Critical incident nursing intervention. *International Journal of Nursing Terminologies & Classifications, 20*(2), 53–63.

Ziegler, S. M. (1993). *Theory-directed nursing practice.* New York: Springer Publishing.

Chapter 8

American Nurses Association. (1992). *Position statements. Registered nurse education relating to the utilization of unlicensed assistive personnel.* Washington, DC: Author. Retrieved January 24, 2008, from http://nursingworld.org/readroom/position/uap/uapuse.htm.

American Nurses Association. (1996). *Registered professional nurses and unlicensed assistive personnel* (2nd ed.). Washington, DC: Author.

American Nurses Association. (2001). *Code of ethics for nurses with interpretive statements.* Washington, DC: ANA.

American Nurses Association. (2005). Safe staffing saves lives. *ANA principles for delegation.* Retrieved August 3, 2010, from http://www.safestaffingsaveslives.org//WhatisSafeStaffing/SafeStaffingPrinciples/PrinciplesforDelegationhtml.aspx.

American Nurses Association. (2007). *Revised position statement: Registered nurses utilization of nursing assistive personnel in all settings.* Retrieved March 1, 2008, from http://www.nursingworld.org/MainMenuCategories/HealthcareandPolicyIssues/ANAPositionStatements/uap/UnlicensedAssistivePersonnel.aspx.

American Nurses Association. (in press). *Nursing: Scope and standards of practice* (2nd ed.). (Public Comment draft, January). Silver Spring, MD: Author. Available at http://nursebooks.org.

American Nurses Association (ANA) and the National Council of State Boards of Nursing (NCSBN). (2006). *Joint statement on delegation.* Retrieved February 1, 2008, from https://www.ncsbn.org/joint_statement.pdf.

Ayers, D. M. M., & Montgomery, M. (2008). Delegating the "right" way. *Nursing2008, 38*(4), 57–58.

Anonymous. (2001). Baldridge criteria spur ongoing change. *QI/TQM. 11*(8), 89.

Anonymous. (2002). Baldridge National Quality Program. *Health care criteria for performance excellence.* Retrieved January 24, 2008, from http://www.quality.nist.gov.

Barter, M. (1999). Delegation and supervision outside the hospital. *American Journal of Nursing, 99*(2), 24.

Barter, M. (1999). Delegation and supervision outside the hospital. *American Journal of Nursing, 99*(7), 24A–24B, 24D.

Basco, M. (2008). Overcoming the myths surrounding adherence. *The Clinical Advisor, 11*(10), 74, 76–78.

Batsie, C. (1999). Patient call system provides efficient delegation. *Nursing Management, 30*(1), 50.

Bentley, J. (2001). Promoting patient partnership in wound care. *British Journal of Community Nursing, 6*(10), 493–494, 496, 498, 500.

Bulechek, G., Butcher, H., & Dochterman, J. (2008). *Nursing interventions classification (NIC)*. (5th ed.). St. Louis: Mosby.

Catanzano, F. (1994). Nursing information/documentation system increases quality care, shortens stay at Desert Samaritan Medical Center. *Computers in Nursing, 12*(4), 184–185.

Chapman, G. F. (1999). Charting tips. Documenting an adverse incident. *Nursing 99, 29*(2), 17.

Chase, S. K. (1997). Charting critical thinking: Nursing judgments and patient outcomes. *Dimensions of Critical Care Nursing, 16*(2), 102–111.

Cronenwett, L., Sherwood, G., Barnsteiner, J., Disch, J., Johnson, J., Mitchell, P., Sullivan, D. T., & Warren, J. (2006). Quality and safety education for nurses. *Nursing Outlook, 55*(3), 122–131.

Cummins, K. M., & Hill, M. T. (1999). Charting by exception: A timely format for you? *American Journal of Nursing, 99*(3), 24G.

Davidson, S. G., & Scott, R. (1999). Professional practice: Thinking critically about delegation. *American Journal of Nursing, 99*(6), 61–62.

Dickens, G., Stubbs, J., & Haw, C. (2008). Delegation of medication administration: An exploratory study. *Nursing Standard, 22*(22), 35–40.

Dowding, D. (2001). Examining the effects that manipulating information given in the change of shift report has on nurses' care planning ability. *Journal of Advanced Nursing, 33*(6), 836–846.

Eggland, E. T., & Heinemann, D. S. (1994). *Nursing documentation. Charting, recording, and reporting*. Philadelphia: J. B. Lippincott.

Eskreis, T. R. (1998). Seven common legal pitfalls in nursing. *American Journal of Nursing 98*(4), 34–40.

Fisher, M. (2000). Do you have delegation savvy? *Nursing 2000, 30*(12), 58–59.

Groah, L., & Reed, E. (1983). Your responsibility in documenting care. *AORN Journal, 37*, 1174–1185.

Gropper, E. I., & Dicapo, R. (1995). The P.A.R.T. system. *Nursing Management, 26*(4), 46, 48.

Haig, K., Sutton, S., & Whittington, J. (2006). SBAR: A shared mental model for improving communication between clinicians. *Joint Commission Journal of Quality and Patient Safety, 32*(3), 167–175.

Hill, M., Labik, M., & Vanderbilt, D. (1997). Managing skin care with the CareMap system. *Journal of Wound Ostomy and Continence Nursing, 24*(1), 26–37.

Hopkins, D. L. (2002). Evaluating the knowledge deficits of registered nurses responsible for supervising nursing assistants. A learning needs assessment tool. *Journal of Nursing Staff Development, 18*(3), 152–156.

Institute for Healthcare Improvement (n.d.). Reducing harm from falls. Retrieved October 31, 2010, from http://www.ihi.org/IHI/Topics/PatientSafety/ReducingHarmfromFalls.

The Joint Commission. (2008). *Hospital accreditation standards: Accreditation policies, standards, and intent statements*. Oakbrook Terrace, IL: Author.

Kaiser Permanente of Colorado. (n.d.). *SBAR technique for communication*. Institute for Healthcare Improvement. Retrieved August 16, 2008, from http://www.ihi.org/IHI/Topics/PatientSafety/SafetyGeneral/Tools/SBARTechniqueforCommunicationASituationalBriefingModel.htm.

Kennedy, J. (1999). An evaluation of non-verbal handover. *Professional Nurse, 14*(6), 391–394.

Kleinman, C. S., & Saccomano, S. J. (2006). Registered nurses and unlicensed assistive personnel: An uneasy alliance. *The Journal of Continuing Education in Nursing, 37*(4), 162–170.

Kozier B., Erb, G., & Berman, A. (2008). *Kozier & Erb's Fundamentals of nursing: Concepts, process, and practice* (8th ed.). Upper Saddle River, NJ: Prentice-Hall.

Kummeth, P., de Ruiter, H., & Capelle, S. (2001). Developing a nursing assistant model: Having the right person perform the right job. *Medsurgical Nursing, 10*(5), 255–263.

Lampe, S. (1985). Focus charting: Streamlining documentation. *Nursing Management, 16*(7), 43–46.

London, F. (1998). Improving compliance. What you can do. *RN, 61*(1), 43–46.

McKenna, L. G. (1997). Improving the nursing handover report. *Professional Nurse, 12*(9), 637–639.

Murphy, J., & Burke, L. J. (1990). Charting by exception: A more efficient way to document. *Nursing 1990, 20,* 65–69.

National Council of State Boards of Nursing. (1995). *Delegation: Concepts and decision-making process.* Chicago: National Council of State Boards of Nursing.

National Council of State Boards of Nursing, Inc. (1997). Delegation decision-making grid (based on a concept developed by the American Association of Critical Care Nurses). Retrieved December 20, 1999, from http://www.ncsbn.org/files/uap/delegationgrid.pdf.

National Council of State Boards of Nursing, Inc. (1997). Delegation decision-making tree. Retrieved December 20, 1999, from http://www.ncsbn.org/files/uap/delegationtree.pdf.

National Council of State Boards of Nursing, Inc. (1997). The five rights of delegation. Retrieved December 20, 1999, from http://www.ncsbn.org/files/uap/fiverights.pdf.

National Council of State Boards of Nursing, Inc. (1998). *The continuum of care framework: Roles of the licensed nurse and assistive personnel (AP) in relation to the client.* Retrieved January 24, 2004, from http://www.ncsbn.org/public/res/uap/contcaregrid.pdf.

Parkman, C. A. (1996). Delegation. Are you doing it right? *American Journal of Nursing, 96*(9), 43–47.

Parsons, L. C. (1999). Building RN confidence for delegation decision-making skills in practice. *Journal of Nursing Staff Development, 15*(6), 263–269.

Phillips, E. (1998). Directing UAPs—safely. *RN, 61*(6), 53–56.

Reinhard, S. C., Young, H. M., Kane, R. A., & Quinn, W. V. (2006). Nurse delegation of medication administration for older adults in assisted living. *Nursing Outlook, 54*(2), 74–80.

Schroeder, S. (2006). Picking up the PACE: A new template for shift report. *Nursing 2006, 36*(10), 22–23.

Spencer, S. A. (2001). Education, training, and use of unlicensed assistive personnel in critical care. *Critical Care Nursing Clinics of North America, 13*(1), 105–118.

Springhouse. (2004). *Nurse's legal handbook* (5th ed.). Philadelphia: Lippincott.

Springhouse. (2009). *Charting made incredibly easy* (4th ed.). Philadelphia: Lippincott.

Thomas, L. (1999). Is delegation the answer? *Elder Care, 11*(4), 1.

Town, J. (1993). Changing to computerized documentation—PLUS. *Nursing Management, 24*(7), 44–46, 48.

Walton, J. C., & Waszkiewicz, M. (1997). Managing unlicensed assistive personnel: Tips for improving quality outcomes. *MEDSURG Nursing, 6*(1), 24–28.

Wilkinson, J., & Treas, L. (2011). *Fundamentals of nursing* (2nd ed.). Philadelphia: F. A. Davis.

Zimmerman, P. G. (1997). Delegating to unlicensed assistive personnel. *Nursing 97, 27*(5), 71.

Chapter 9

Agency for Healthcare Research and Quality. (2007). *Nurse staffing and quality of patient care.* Evidence Report/Technology Assessment Nol. 151; AHRQ Publication No. 07-E005. Retrieved July 16, 2010, from http://www.ahrq.gov/downloads/pub/evidence/pdf/nursestaff/nursestaff.pdf.

American Nurses Association. (1976). *ANA quality assurance workbook.* Kansas City, MO: Author.

American Nurses Association. (1995). *Nursing report card for acute care.* Washington, DC: American Nurses Publishing.

American Nurses Association. (1997). *Implementing nursing's report card. A study of RN staffing, length of stay and patient outcomes.* Washington, DC: Author.

American Nurses Association. (1999). *Nursing quality indicators: Guide for implementation* (2nd ed.). Washington, DC: Author.

American Nurses Association. (2001). *Code of ethics for nurses with interpretive statements.* Washington, DC: Author.

American Nurses Association. (in press). *Nursing: Scope and standards of practice* (2nd ed.). (Public Comment draft, January). Silver Spring, MD: Author. Available at http://nursebooks.org.

Anonymous. (2001). Baldrige criteria spur ongoing change. *QI TQM.11*(8), 89.

Anonymous. (2002). Baldridge National Quality Program. *Health care criteria for performance excellence.* Retrieved January 24, 2008, from http://www.quality.nist.gov.

Anonymous. (2002). ISO 9000: A system-oriented approach to quality management. *QI TQM, 12*i(1), 1–5.

Boucher, K. T. (2004). Home health quality initiative: What it means for nurses. *Nevada RNformation, 13*(2), 19.

Buckley, T., Burns, S., & Bleck, T. (2005). A process improvement project: Achieving quality outcomes. *Journal of Nursing Administration, 35*(2), 94–100.

Carson, V. B. (1989). *Spiritual dimensions of nursing practice.* Philadelphia: W. B. Saunders.

Centers for Medicare and Medicaid Services. (2005). Overview. Retrieved July 27, 2010, from http://www.cms.hhs.gov/OASIS.

Duffy, J. R., Hoskins, L., & Dudley-Brown, S. (2005). Development and testing of a caring-based intervention for older adults with heart failure. *Journal of Cardiovascular Nursing, 20*(5), 325–333.

Duffy, M. E. (2005). The Agency for Healthcare Research and Quality: A valuable resource for evidence-based practice. *Clinical Nurse Specialist, 19*(3), 117–120.

Elliott, K. (2001). Implementing nursing clinical indicators. *Professional Nurse, 16*(6), 1158–1161.

Gibberd, R., Pathmeswaran, A., & Burtenshaw, K. (2000). Using clinical indicators to identify areas for quality improvement. *Journal of Quality in Clinical Practice, 20*(4), 136–144.

Hopkins, D. L. (2002). Evaluating the knowledge deficits of registered nurses responsible for supervising nursing assistants. A learning needs assessment tool. *Journal of Nursing Staff Development, 18*(3), 152–156.

Jacobson, A. F., & Winslow, E. H. (2005). Variables influencing intravenous catheter insertion difficulty and failure: An analysis of 339 intravenous catheter insertions. *Heart Lung, 34*i(5), 345–359.

Johnson, K., Hallsey, D., Meredith, R. L., & Warden, E. (2006). A nurse-driven system for improving patient quality outcomes. *Journal of Nursing Care Quality, 21*(2), 168–175.

Joint Commission for the Accreditation of Healthcare Organizations. (2008). *Hospital accreditation standards: Accreditation policies, standards, elements of performance, scoring.* Oakbrook Terrace, IL: Author.

Lamb, G., Jennings, B., Mitchell, P., & Lang, N. (2004). Quality agenda: Priorities for action recommendations of the American Academy of Nursing Conference on Health Care Quality. *Nursing Outlook, 52*(1), 60–65.

Meyer, G. S., & Massagli, M. P. (2001). The forgotten component of the quality triad: Can we still learn something from "structure"? *Joint Commission Journal on Quality Improvement, 27*(9): 484–493.

Miller, L. J., Corbett, G., Herold, M., Tavares, D., Kirchner, L., & Heath, J. (2005). Journey to the Beacon Award: The Georgetown University Hospital perspective. *Critical Care Nursing Clinics of North America, 17*(2), 155–161.

Moorhead, S., Johnson, M., Maas, M., & Swanson, E. (2008). *Nursing Outcomes Classification (NOC)* (4th ed.). St. Louis: Mosby.

NANDA International. (2009). *Nursing diagnoses definitions and classifications 2009–2011.* Oxford: Wiley-Blackwell.

Oermann, M., & Huber, D. (1999). Patient outcomes: A measure of nursing's value. *American Journal of Nursing, 99*(9), 40–48.

Pelletier, L. R. (2000). Error-free healthcare: Mission possible! *Journal for Healthcare Quality, 22*(2), 2, 9.

Pelletier, L. R., Beaudin, C. L., & van Leeuwen, D. (1999). The use of a prioritization matrix to preserve quality resources. *Journal for Healthcare Quality, 21*(5), 36–38.

Poole, L. (2001). PEPP: Collaborating to improve quality. *Journal of the American Health Information Management Association, 72*(4), 43–47.

Rantz, M. J., Popejoy, L., Petroski, G. F., Madsen, R. W., Mehr, D. R., Zwygart-Stauffacher, M., Hicks, L. L., Grando, V., Wipke-Tevis, D. D., Bostick, J., Porter, R., Conn, V. S., & Maas, M. (2001). Randomized clinical trial of a quality improvement intervention in nursing homes. *Gerontologist, 41*(4), 525.

Watterson, L. (2004). Using indicator development to revise infection control activities in an acute NHS trust. *Journal of Nursing Management, 12*(6), 403–410.

Wilkinson, J. (2009). *Nursing diagnosis handbook* (9th ed.). Upper Saddle River, NJ: Pearson/Prentice Hall.

Wilkinson, J., & Treas, L. (2011). *Fundamentals of nursing* (2nd ed.). Philadelphia: F. A. Davis.

Wilson, L. (2000). "Quality is everyone's business": Why this approach will not work in hospitals. *Journal of Quality in Clinical Practice, 20*(4), 131–135.

Woodring, B. C. (2000). If you have taught – have the child and family learned? *Pediatric Nursing, 26*(5), 505–509.

Zucker, M., & LaDuca, F. (2004). Monitoring in the NICU—The value of point-of-care testing. *Neonatal Intensive Care, 17*(2), 44–46.

Appendix A

Benner, P. (1984) *From novice to expert*. Menlo Park, CA: Addison-Wesley Publishing Co.

Schraeder, B., & Fischer, D. (1987). Using intuitive knowledge in the neonatal intensive care nursery. *Holistic Nursing Practice, 1*(3), 45–51.

Index